Suicide: Phenomenology and Neurobiology

Keri E. Cannon · Thomas J. Hudzik
Editors

Suicide: Phenomenology and Neurobiology

Springer

Editors
Keri E. Cannon
Global Safety Pharmacology
Pfizer, Inc.
Groton, CT
USA

Thomas J. Hudzik
Preclinical Safety
AbbVie
North Chicago, IL
USA

ISBN 978-3-319-37701-8 ISBN 978-3-319-09964-4 (eBook)
DOI 10.1007/978-3-319-09964-4

Springer Cham Heidelberg New York Dordrecht London

Softcover reprint of the hardcover 1st edition 2014

Printed on acid-free paper

Springer is part of Springer Science+Business Media (www.springer.com)

Foreword

We can remember as youngsters watching the television show, Mork and Mindy. We laughed along, while sometimes feeling unable to keep up with the soaring and roaring wit that was Robin Williams. But sometimes we were able to catch on to a suspender and fly along with him for a time, and that was a ride that inspired awe. His dramatic roles were no less inspiring; for example, Awakenings played a role in some of our career choices, Good Morning Vietnam in political perspectives.

We wonder, now, how he could have kept up that quick cognitive pace, and what was required to do so. Did we imagine, later in his life, that when he puffed up the smile on his lips, the light sank from his eyes? Mr. Williams may have exemplified some of the risk factors known to be associated with suicidal behavior. But maybe these were hidden in plain sight, or just plain hidden.

The present volume represents current thought and research on suicidal ideation and behavior, bringing together some of the top thought leaders in the field. All authors have contributed with the hope that application of the methods and theory that is discussed within along with increased momentum in research will assist in understanding this human vulnerability, with the aim of reducing the numbers of tragic outcomes.

Thomas J. Hudzik, Ph.D.
Keri E. Cannon, Ph.D.

Contents

Chapter 1
Introduction

Thomas J. Hudzik and Keri E. Cannon

Abstract Each year, an astonishing number of lives are lost to suicide which highlights an imperative that research efforts and attention be focused upon understanding the causes and contributing factors in suicide. The present volume approaches suicidal behavior and ideation from many different perspectives, which, of course, is necessary because of the complexity associated with these phenomena. In the present chapter, concepts and research efforts that will be discussed in detail in later chapters are introduced and encompass the areas of epidemiology and predictive tools, risk factors, and clinical and preclinical neurobiology.

Nearly 1 million people worldwide die by suicide each year. The World Health Organization (WHO) has estimated that the number of suicides exceeds the number of homicides and deaths due to warfare combined (WHO 2013, p. 4244). The accuracy of these estimates likely is affected by a number of factors, including under-reporting due to social stigma, to accidents with unclear precipitating factors, or even method of legal determination (Sainsbury and Jenkins 1982; O'Donnell and Farmer 1995). In the United States alone, it is the third leading cause of death among teens (12–19) and second leading cause of death for young adults aged 25 to 34 (CDC 2004, 2007; Minino 2010, 2013). In addition, the financial and social consequences of suicide are extensive representing 2.5 % of the global burden of disease, (Murray and Lopez 1996; WHO 2013, p. 4244). The US Centers for Disease Control and Prevention estimated that in 2010, the cost associated with suicide was more than 30 billion dollars in lost earnings, medical expenses, and associated costs (CDC 2010). These statistics and observations in toto highlight an imperative that research efforts and attention be focused upon understanding the causes and contributing factors in

---

T.J. Hudzik (✉)
AbbVie Global Pharmaceutical Research and Development, One N. Waukegan Rd, North Chicago, IL 60064, USA
e-mail: thomas.hudzik@abbvie.com

K.E. Cannon
Global Safety Pharmacology, Pfizer Global Research and Development, Pfizer, Inc., Eastern Point Road MS 8274-1303, Groton, CT 06340, USA
e-mail: Keri.cannon@pfizer.com

K.E. Cannon and T.J. Hudzik (eds.), *Suicide: Phenomenology and Neurobiology*,
DOI 10.1007/978-3-319-09964-4_1

Table 1.1 Some common risk factors in suicidal behavior and ideation

Traumatic brain injury	Genetics	Social isolation
Early life trauma	Serotonergic dysfunction	Mental pain
PTSD	Family history of suicide	chronic physical pain
Acute physical pain	Low serotonergic tone	Life outlook
Chronic disease	Gender	Life goals
Previous attempt	Poor communication skills	Level of cultural acceptance
Psychiatric illness	Unemployment	Ethnicity
Substance use disorders	Economic downturn	Rumination
Access to lethal means	Incarceration	Intrusive thoughts
Current ideation	Vicarious conditioning	Cognitive impairment
Bullying (receiving and conducting)	Employment stress	Physical appearance/self-perception
Religious affiliation	Familial interactions	Age

suicide, continuing to identify high-risk individuals and populations, and developing effective prevention and treatment strategies.

Suicide results from a complex convergence of many possible neurobiological, sociocultural, and genetic factors, the exact composition of which will vary somewhat in each case. Despite the uniqueness of each situation, it is thought that such factors, combining into a 'perfect storm' that can tilt ideation into behavior. Table 1.1 summarizes some of these risk factors in suicidal behavior and ideation. These risk factors can interact with each other, be a product of each other, as well as operate independently, and as such are difficult to categorize, for example, as purely dispositional versus environmental. Among the most important are lack of social support, previous attempt, access to firearms, and other lethal means and concomitant mental illness, including chronic substance abuse. Clinicians and scientists are greatly interested in understanding the complexity of the interaction of these factors in order to increase the ability to predict the risk of suicide in patients. It is important to consider that risk factors may vary by subpopulation identified, and those which may drive ideation in and behavior in Autism Spectrum Disorder, for example, may be quite different from those which affect patients with a history of drug dependence. Only after further understanding of suicidal behavior and ideation is achieved can such predictive tools be applied. The analysis of these various genetic and psychiatric risk factors is providing a blueprint for clinical endophenotypes that may be associated with suicidal behavior and ideation.

Throughout this volume, several terms will be used to describe the spectrum of "suicidality" (hereafter, suicidal ideation and behavior), and as such it is important to establish some clear definitions upfront. Suicidal behavior (Niedzwiedz et al. 2014; Mann and Arango 1992, p. 4361; Mann and Currier 2012) encompasses completed suicide, suicide attempt, and preparatory acts toward imminent suicidal behavior (Meyer et al. 2010). It is important to consider that suicidal behavior does not encompass "death wish", which is often operationally defined as a positive response to the question similar to "do you ever wish to go to sleep and not wake up" or "have you ever felt like life is not worth living?" Death wish is probably necessary but not sufficient for suicidal behavior and ideation to be present. In their draft guidance, the United States Food and Drug Administration (FDA) adopted definitions of the various events encompassed by suicidal behavior and ideation (Services, Administration, and CDER 2012). Self-injurious actions that resulted in fatality and were associated with at least some intent to die as a result of the behavior are considered a completed suicide. Suicide attempts are those potentially self-injurious behaviors that are associated with at least some intent to die as a result of the act. It is important to note, suicide attempts may or may not result in actual injury. Preparatory actions toward imminent suicide suicidal behavior are those actions that an individual takes to injure him- or herself. Suicidal behaviors are classified in this category when the preparatory actions are stopped by self or others from starting the self-injurious act before the potential for harm has begun. Finally, suicidal ideations are thoughts about the desire to die or active thoughts about killing oneself that are not accompanied by preparatory behavior. It would be of obvious great value to be able to distinguish between patients with pure ideation and those with concomitant behavior.

1.1 Epidemiology and Predictive Tools

In the first section, Dr. Oleske begins with analysis of the epidemiologic data obtained on the various areas of suicidal behavior and ideation. One section of the chapter will present information in support of relationships between certain socioeconomic conditions and suicidal behavior and ideation. In addition, one section will report on trends of suicide risk across demographic factors such as geography, ethnicity, and occupation. The role of gender in evaluating suicide risk will be discussed as well as patterns and associations in relation to age and suicidal behavior and ideation explored.

In Chap. 4, Dr. Posner reviews the leading tool used in the clinic to assess suicidal behavior and ideation, its current applications, and thoughts on future application. Finally, in Chap. 3, Dr. Ratcliffe et al. discuss the recent concept of treatment-emergent suicidal ideation and behavior and the impact it has had on public concern, regulatory guidance, and pharmaceutical development. This chapter also reviews current practices that have been implemented in clinical trials to detect treatment-emergent suicidal behavior and ideation and special considerations that must be made when adding these assessments into trials.

1.2 Risk Factors

The second section of this volume addresses some of the risk factors that have been associated with suicidal behavior and ideation. Chap. 5 examines in depth recent developments in relation to the stress-diathesis model—a paradigm that describes the interplay of stressful events and vulnerability traits as a significant contributor to suicidal behavior and ideation (van Heeringen et al. 2012). Although the original stress-diathesis model has greatly assisted in the understanding of suicidal behavior, new research suggests that neurodevelopmental alterations that occur prenatally, postnatally, or in adolescence may contribute to suicidal behavior in later life. This has led to the generation of a neurodevelopmental hypothesis (Jollant et al. 2011) to explain the pathophysiology of suicidal behavior. This hypothesis is expanded upon in Chap. 6, in which Nazem et al. provide an overview of the epidemiology and association with suicidal behavior of PTSD, TBI (mild, moderate, and severe), and co-occurring PTSD and TBI with particular attention paid to military personnel and veterans. This chapter describes the neurocognitive working model of suicidal behavior and suggests its use in understanding the association between PTSD and/or moderate to severe TBI and associated functional neuroanatomy, with suicidal behaviors.

The Stress-Diathesis model for suicide, attributed to Mann and Colleagues, incorporates the notion of genetic predisposition that can manifest as heightened vulnerability to stressors. In Chap. 7, Drs Sarchiapoine and D'Aulerio review the literature on the role of genetics, including polymorphisms in candidate genes that may amplify risk in certain populations. In Chap. 8, Fawcett speculates on the ability to clinically prevent suicide and discusses some of the limited evidence that addresses this concept. He discusses some of the psychiatric risk factors that have been linked to suicidal behavior that clinicians have relied upon to detect suicidal behavior, and makes suggestions for refinements in the clinical interview that may assist in prediction of suicide.

In Chap. 9, Drs. Hudzik and Marek examine suicidal ideation and behavior in neurological disease. Autism spectrum disorder, attention deficit hyperactivity disorder (ADHD), chronic pain and headache, Parkinson's, Tourrette's syndrome, and epilepsy are discussed in relation to comorbidities with psychiatric disease. Dr. Szanto addressed the concept of age as a risk factor for suicidal behavior and focuses on the increasingly important issue of suicide in the elderly in Chap. 10. This chapter reviews accumulating evidence that cognitive decline, deficits in decision making, and impulsivity play a critical role in suicide in the elderly, which links well with the concepts presented in the chapter by Nazem et al. Finally, Chap. 11 discusses early life trauma (ELT) as a risk factor for suicidal ideation and behavior. An overview of the origins of ELT is presented as well as its interaction with other risk factors associated with suicide.

1.3 Treatment Approaches

The third section of this volume reviews the current state of treatment approaches for suicidal behavior and ideation. One major gap in suicide prevention is that, currently, there is only a single drug, clozapine, which has a reduction in suicidal behavior as an indication. Arguably, lithium is effective in this regard as well, but has not received approval for the indication. Chapter 12 discusses the experimental pharmacological approaches in the prevention of suicidal behavior and ideation with a particular focus on experimental therapeutics that have demonstrated rapid, robust, and sustained reductions in suicidal thoughts. Ballard et al. also review novel putative targets, including the purinergic system, for intervention and prevention of suicidal behavior and ideation. But no drug, no matter how effective, can truly operate upon processes as complex as those that contribute to suicide without psychotherapeutic support. In Chap. 13, Chesin et al. provides a review of psychotherapeutic treatments to prevent suicidal behavior and ideation in high-risk groups. In addition, Chesin et al. speculate on future directions that could lead to the refinement of psychotherapeutic treatments and the development of additional interventions. Finally, Thase provides a comprehensive review of cognitive therapy as a means for suicide prevention in Chap. 14 and summarizes the results obtained thus far using this type of approach.

1.4 Clinical and Preclinical Neurobiology

The final section of this volume focuses on current clinical and nonclinical research efforts. Chapter 15 reviews clinical neuroimaging studies of suicidal behavior and its major risk factors, and discusses the relevance of the findings in relation to the understanding, prediction, and prevention of suicide. Furthermore, van Heeringen et al. describes a picture that emerges from neuroimaging studies that reflects the involvement of a fronto-cingulo-striatal network in the development of suicidal behavior. In Chap. 16, Ferris attempts to probe neuroanatomical pathways of suicidal behavior and ideation in the rat via non-invasive, ultra-high field, functional magnetic resonance imaging (fMRI) studies. Utilizing fMRI in awake animals, Ferris examined the neural imaging finger prints a few marketed compound that contain black box warning labels for suicidal behavior and ideation. The results from Ferris's preliminary work provide an early foundation for future work that could identify similarities in the patterns of neural activity among therapeutics that have been associated with suicidal behavior and ideation. Chapter 17 introduces the role of microRNAs (miRNAs) in neural plasticity, stress responses, major depression, and suicide pathogenesis. Dwivedi also provides support for the use of miRNAs as a biomarker for depression and suicidal behavior and ideation. Finally, in Chap. 18, animal models of risk factors associated with suicide are reviewed by Stuart et al. This chapter provides an overview of traditional and novel models of several risk factors, including depression, behavioral despair, anhedonia, impulsivity, and aggression. In addition, this chapter reviews more novel cognitive neuropsychological models of depression.

1.5 Summary

The present volume approaches suicidal behavior and ideation from many different perspectives, which, of course, is necessary because of the complexity associated with these phenomena. The purpose of such a multitiered approach is to help to further advance identification of risk, prediction of outcome, and tailoring of treatment to achieve the best possible quality of life for patients, and their families. Considering the question raised in the title of Chap. 9, "Is Suicide Clinically Preventable?," as clinicians and scientists we believe that research can and will continue to bring us toward a positive answer to the question.

References

(CDC) Centers for Disease, Control, and Prevention (2004) Methods of suicide among persons aged 10–19 years–United States, 1992–2001. MMWR Morb Mortal Wkly Rep 53.22:471–474

CDC (2007) Suicide trends among youths and young adults aged 10–24 Years–United States, 1990–2004. MMWR Morb Mortal Wkly Rep 56.35:905–908

CDC (2010) Web-based injury statistics query and reporting system (Wisqars). National Center for Injury Prevention and Control, CDC. http://www.cdc.gov/injury/wisqars/index.html. Accessed 13 March 13

CDC (2013) Suicide among adults Aged 35–64 years–United States, 1999–2010. MMWR Morb Mortal Wkly Rep 62.17:321–325

(CDER) (2012) Guidance for industry: suicidal ideation and behavior: prospective assessment of occurrence in clinical trials. Published Online: http://www.fda.gov/downloads/Drugs/GuidanceComplianceRegulatoryInformation/Guidances/UCM225130.pdf

Jollant F et al (2011) The suicidal mind and brain: a review of neuropsychological and neuroimaging studies. World J Biol Psychiatry 12.5:319–339

Mann JJ, Arango V (1992) Integration of neurobiology and psychopathology in a unified model of suicidal behavior. J Clin Psychopharmacol 12.2 Suppl:2S–7S

Mann JJ, Currier D (2012) Medication in suicide prevention insights from neurobiology of suicidal behavior. In: Dwivedi Y (ed) The neurobiological basis of suicide Frontiers in Neuroscience, Boca Raton

Meyer A et al (2010) Mood disorders hospitalizations, suicide attempts, and suicide mortality among agricultural workers and residents in an area with intensive use of pesticides in Brazil. J Toxicol Environ Health A 73.13–14:866–877

Minino A (2010) Mortality among teenagers Aged 12–19 years: United States, 1999–2006. NCHS Data Brief 37:18

Minino AM (2013) Death in the United States, 2011. NCHS Data Brief 115:1–8

Murray CJ, Lopez AD (1996) Evidence-based health policy–lessons from the global burden of disease study. Science 274.5288:740–743

Niedzwiedz C et al (2014) The definition and epidemiology of clusters of suicidal behavior: a systematic review. Suicide Life Threat Behav. doi:10.1111/sltb.12091. Published online April, 2017

O'Donnell I, Farmer R (1995) The limitations of official suicide statistics. Br J Psychiatry 166.4:458–461

Posner K et al (2007) Columbia classification algorithm of suicide assessment (C-Casa): classification of suicidal events in the Fda's pediatric suicidal risk analysis of antidepressants. Am J Psychiatry 164.7:1035–1043

Sainsbury P, Jenkins JS (1982) The accuracy of officially reported suicide statistics for purposes of epidemiological research. J Epidemiol Community Health 36.1:43–48

van Heeringen K (2012) Stress-diathesis model of suicidal behavior. In: Dwivedi Y (ed) The neurobiological basis of suicide. Frontiers in Neuroscience. CRC Press, Boca Raton

World Health Organization (2013) Investing in mental health: evidence for action. WHO Library Cataloguing-in-Publication Data. ISBN 978 92 4 156461 8

Part I
Epidemiology and Predictive Tools

Chapter 2
Epidemiology

Denise M. Oleske

Abstract Suicide is a complex global health problem with consequences extending far beyond the estimated annual 800,000 fatalities. According to World Mental Health Surveys, the lifetime prevalences of suicidal ideation, plans, or attempts are 9.2, 3.1, and 2.7 %, respectively. There are somewhat different patterns among nations regarding who are at risk and factors contributing to this risk. An understanding of the epidemiology of suicide and suicidal thoughts and other suicidal behaviors, namely the pattern of their distribution in populations and the factors which could be attributed to their occurrence, provide an insight into those at risk for whom preventive efforts may be targeted. Concepts, sources of epidemiological data, and key findings are presented in this chapter.

2.1 Introduction

Self-directed violence encompasses a range of violent behaviors, including acts of fatal and nonfatal suicidal behavior, and nonsuicidal intentional self-harm (i.e., behaviors where the intention is not to kill oneself, as in self-mutilation). Suicidal behavior is a complex health problem with fatal and nonfatal components. Suicide, the fatal behavior, is according to the proverbial epidemiological paradigm is only the "tip of the iceberg" of self-directed violence. Suicide, nonfatal suicidal behaviors and suicidal ideations lead to considerable utilization of health care resources, specifically emergency department visits and hospitalizations, with variable outcomes from these encounters (Fig. 2.1). An understanding of the epidemiology of suicide and suicidal thoughts and behaviors, namely the pattern of their distribution in populations and the factors which could be attributed to their occurrence, provide an insight into those at risk for whom preventive efforts may be targeted. Concepts, sources of epidemiological data, and key findings are presented in this chapter.

D.M. Oleske (✉)
Global Surveillance and Pharmacoepidemiology, AbbVie, North Chicago, IL 60064, USA
e-mail: denise.oleske@abbvie.com

K.E. Cannon and T.J. Hudzik (eds.), *Suicide: Phenomenology and Neurobiology*,
DOI 10.1007/978-3-319-09964-4_2

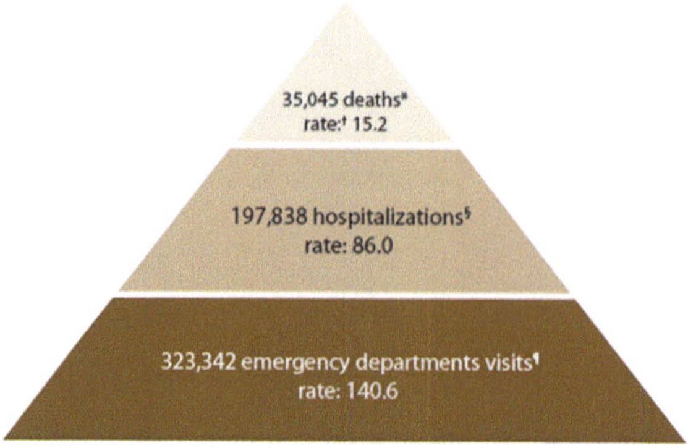

Fig. 2.1 Public health burden of suicidal behavior among adults aged ≥18 years—United States, 2008 (*Source* Crosby et al. 2011). **Source* CDC's National Vital Statistics System. All rates per 100,000 population. § Agency for Healthcare Research and Quality's Healthcare Cost and Utilization Project–Nationwide Inpatient Sample. ¶ CDC's National Electronic Injury Surveillance System–All Injury Program

2.2 Suicide

Suicide is defined as the fatal event of self-directed violence. The death certificate is the source document for the identification of cases of suicide in epidemiologic studies and in vital statistics. Suicide, including accidental poisonings, on the death certificate in the "cause of death" field can be identified through the ICD-10 codes displayed in Table 2.1. In the UK, the definition of suicide includes deaths given an underlying cause of intentional self-harm or an injury/poisoning of undetermined intent. However, it cannot be applied to children due to the possibility that these deaths could have been attributed to neglect, abuse, or unverifiable accidents. The risk suicide is defined as the number of events of death from suicide in a defined population occurring at the same time the population was enumerated and multiplied by a factor of 10. Risk of suicide is represented as a rate measure when referring to the frequency of its occurrence in a general population, where:

Rate = Number of events in a specified time interval/Average population during the same time interval × 10^k

In 2010, the population of the U.S. was 308,746,000 and there were 38,364 deaths from suicide. Using the above formula and applying a power of 10 multiplier (10^k) to convert the fraction into a rate (usually 100,000 for vital statistics), the suicide rate was 12.4 per 100,000 population. This means that for every 100,000 persons, there were about 12–13 suicides in this one year in the U.S.

Table 2.1 International classification of disease codes (ICD-10) for suicide—including accidental poisonings

General code groupings	
X60–X84	Intentional self-harm
Y10–Y34	Injury/poisoning of undetermined intent
Y87.0–Y87.2	Sequelae of intentional self-harm /injury/poisoning of undetermined intent
Y87.0–Y87.2	Sequelae of intentional self-harm /injury /poisoning of undetermined intent
Specific intent codes	
Accidental poisoning: ICD-9 codes E850-E854, E858, E862, E868; ICD-10 codes X40-X42, X46, X47	
Poisoning with undetermined intent: ICD-10 codes Y10-Y12, Y16, Y17	
Self-inflicted poisoning: ICD-9 codes E950-E952, ICD-10 codes X60-X69	
Self-inflicted injury by hanging, strangulation, and suffocation: ICD-9 code E953, ICD-10 code X70	
Self-inflicted injury by drowning: ICD-9 code E954, ICD-10 code X71	
Self-inflicted injury by firearms and explosives: ICD-9 code E955, ICD-10 codes X72-X75	
Self-inflicted injury by smoke, fire, flames, steam, hot vapors, and hot objects: ICD-9 codes E958.1, E958.2; ICD-10 codes X76, X77	
Self-inflicted injury by cutting and piecing instruments: ICD-9 code E956; ICD-10 codes X78, X79	
Self-inflicted injury by jumping from high places: ICD-9 code E957, ICD-10 code X80	
Self-inflicted injury by jumping or lying before a moving object: ICD-9 code E958.0, ICD-10 code X81	
Self-inflicted injury by crashing of motor vehicle: ICD-9 code E958.5, ICD-10-CA code X82	
Self-inflicted injury by other and unspecified means: ICD-9 codes E958.3, E958.4, E958.6-E958.9; ICD-10 codes X83, X84	
Late effects of self-inflicted injury: ICD-9 code E959	

2.2.1 Data Sources for Suicide Statistics

National vital statistics systems are the primary sources of country-specific suicide mortality statistics. These statistics are derived from a death certificate, the format and procedures for completing differ by regional laws and practices. The listing of a cause of death on a death certificate is influenced by many factors, including cultural factors, availability of an informant, provisions regarding confidentiality of the cause of death, and local laws governing forensic investigation. Death rates may also be affected by the age structure of a population and any temporal trends within age subgroups. In general, any suicide rate may be underestimated. For example, suicide rates generally exclude those aged <10 years (aged <15 years in the UK) because intent for self-harm is typically not attributed to young children. Thus, when interpreting suicide rates, it is important to keep in mind how these factors could influence the rate and use caution in interpreting rates across countries.

The World Health Organization (WHO) compiles suicide statistics by country. Data, search tools, and reports can be obtained through the Global Health

Observation (GHO) at http://ww.who.int/GHO/. Data from the WHO reveal that suicide is a worldwide health problem with more than 800,000 people worldwide dying every year from suicide.

In the U.S., **WISQARS™** (Web-based Injury Statistics Query and Reporting System) is an interactive database system that provides customized reports of suicide and other injury-related data. Suicide was the 10th leading cause of death among all ages and the leading cause of injury death in 2012. In Canada, CANSIM is a data base updated daily which provides the latest statistics for Canada, including health conditions. Suicide mortality data by age, gender, and year are available as downloadable tables.

In addition to recording death information in a vital records system, some countries and organizations have specialized surveillance systems or registries for obtaining more detailed information about a suicide event and its causes. In the U.S., surveillance data is obtained through the National Violent Death Reporting System (NVDRS). This system links information from death certificates, medical examiners, law enforcement, and forensic laboratories. Circumstances surrounding the suicide by age group, such as depressed mood, declining health, and disclosure of suicidal intent are compiled. The U.S. Department of Defense has a similar system and employs a more standardized and detailed collection of medical, military, and personal history information as a potential model for other organizations (Gahm et al. 2012). The National Suicide Registry in Malaysia also engages psychiatrics and staff members of psychiatric and mental health departments for the collection of the information on the demographics of the decedent, characteristics of the suicidal act, and risk factors (Hayati et al. 2008). The National Poison Data System is a near real-time surveillance database tracking poisonings and their sources in the U.S. Information is collected from calls by the public and health professionals to poison centers nationwide, consolidated, and evaluated. Suspected suicides, fatal (and non-fatal) cases are among the human exposure cases analyzed. The system is maintained by the American Association of Poison Control Centers (www.aapcc.org) with annual reports published in the journal Clinical Toxicology.

2.2.2 Age, Sex, Race/Ethnicity, Geographical Region, and Other Population Subgroups

There is marked variation in suicide rates by age, sex, race/ethnicity, and geographic region.

By age group, among the highest suicide rates are noted to occur in midlife in Canada, the U.K., and the U.S. Suicide rates by age reveal a peak in adolescence in the U.S. (ONS 2014; Navaneelan 2012) (Fig. 2.2). In the U.S., the rates of suicide exceed homicide rates for all age groups except for the age groups of 18–24, where the homicide rate exceeds the suicide rate and for under age 10, where suicide rates are not reported (Fig. 2.2). In contrast, the highest suicides rates across European nations, the highest suicide rates are reported among people aged 65+ (21.9 per

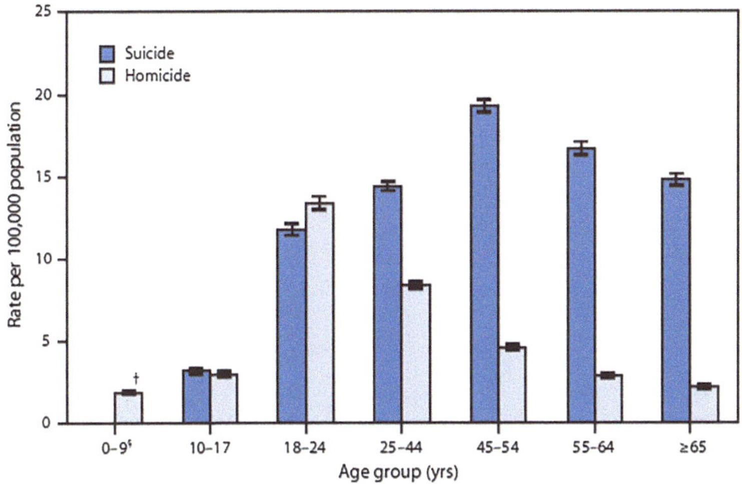

Fig. 2.2 Suicide and Homicide Rates,* by Age Group—United States, 2009. MMWR:July 20, 2012:61(28);543. * Per 100,000 population in age group. Suicides are coded as *U03, X60–X84, and Y87.0, and homicides are coded as *U01–*U02, X85–Y09, and Y87.1 according to the *International Classification of Diseases, 10th Revision*. † 95 % confidence interval. § Suicide data for persons aged 0–9 years are suppressed based on a child's inability to form and understand suicidal intent and consequences

100,000 population and those aged 45–59 (21.5 per 100,000 population) (WHO 2014). Higher rates have been reported among those aged 85 years and older in China ranging from 68.41 per 100,000 in large cities to 191.74 per 100,000 in rural areas (Simon et al. 2013).

The male predominance of suicide (as much as three times higher than females) is noted for all age groups across all nations with the exception in China, where overall it is higher among females (Table 2.2).

Suicide rates are two-times higher among whites than nonwhites. Between 1999 and 2010, the suicide rates among whites increased 20.4 % from 11.3 deaths per 100,000 population to 13.6 per 100,000 (Fig. 2.3) (CDC 2013, April 5, 2013/62 (13);257**)**. Ethnicity contributes to suicide risk when those groups are immigrants. Suicide occurs at a disproportionately higher rate among persons in higher income countries than among those in low- and middle-income countries with the exception of low- and middle-income countries of Europe and Southeast Asia (Table 2.2) (Norton and Kobusingye 2013).

Other population subgroups at risk for suicide include military personnel and veterans, young parents, and those with various chronic medical conditions (e.g., schizophrenia, certain dementias, bipolar disorder, chronic pain, post traumatic stressdisorder, and traumatic brain injury) (Trofimovich et al. 2012; Fawcett 2014; Fazel et al. 2014; Hooley et al. 2014; Niederkrotenthaler et al. 2012).

Table 2.2 Suicide rates per 100,000 by country, year and sex, for most recent year available as of 2011

Country	Year	Males	Females
Albania	03	4.7	3.3
Antigua and Barbuda	95	0	0
Argentina	08	12.6	3
Armenia	08	2.8	1.1
Australia	06	12.8	3.6
Austria	09	23.8	7.1
Azerbaijan	07	1	0.3
Bahamas	05	1.9	0.6
Bahrain	06	4	3.5
Barbados	06	7.3	0
Belarus	07	48.7	8.8
Belgium	05	28.8	10.3
Belize	08	6.6	0.7
Bosnia and Herzegovina	91	20.3	3.3
Brazil	08	7.7	2
Bulgaria	08	18.8	6.2
Canada	04	17.3	5.4
Chile	07	18.2	4.2
China (selected rural and urban areas)	99	13	14.8
China (Hong Kong Sar)	09	19	10.7
Colombia	07	7.9	2
Costa rica	09	10.2	1.9
Croatia	09	28.9	7.5
Cuba	08	19	5.5
Cyprus	08	7.4	1.7
Czech Republic	09	23.9	4.4
Denmark	06	17.5	6.4
Dominican Republic	05	3.9	0.7
Ecuador	09	10.5	3.6
Egypt	09	0.1	0
El salvador	08	12.9	3.6
Estonia	08	30.6	7.3
Finland	09	29	10
France	07	24.7	8.5
Georgia	09	7.1	1.7
Germany	06	17.9	6
Greece	09	6	1
Grenada	08	0	0
Guatemala	08	5.6	1.7
Guyana	06	39	13.4

(continued)

Table 2.2 (continued)

Country	Year	Males	Females
Haiti	03	0	0
Honduras	78	0	0
Hungary	09	40	10.6
Iceland	08	16.5	7
India	09	13	7.8
Iran	91	0.3	0.1
Ireland	09	19	4.7
Israel	07	7	1.5
Italy	07	10	2.8
Jamaica	90	0.3	0
Japan	09	36.2	13.2
Jordan	08	0.2	0
Kazakhstan	08	43	9.4
Kuwait	09	1.9	1.7
Kyrgyzstan	09	14.1	3.6
Latvia	09	40	8.2
Lithuania	09	61.3	10.4
Luxembourg	08	16.1	3.2
Maldives	05	0.7	0
Malta	08	5.9	1
Mauritius	08	11.8	1.9
Mexico	08	7	1.5
Netherlands	09	13.1	5.5
New Zealand	07	18.1	5.5
Nicaragua	06	9	2.6
Norway	09	17.3	6.5
Panama	08	9	1.9
Paraguay	08	5.1	2
Peru	07	1.9	1
Philippines	93	2.5	1.7
Poland	08	26.4	4.1
Portugal	09	15.6	4
Puerto Rico	05	13.2	2
Republic of Korea	09	39.9	22.1
Republic of Moldova	08	30.1	5.6
Romania	09	21	3.5
Russian Federation	06	53.9	9.5
Saint Kitts and Nevis	95	0	0
Saint Lucia	05	4.9	0
Saint vincent and the Grenadines	08	5.4	1.9
Sao Tome and principe	87	0	1.8

(continued)

Table 2.2 (continued)

Country	Year	Males	Females
Serbia	09	28.1	10
Seychelles	08	8.9	0
Singapore	06	12.9	7.7
Slovakia	05	22.3	3.4
Slovenia	09	34.6	9.4
South Africa	07	1.4	0.4
Spain	08	11.9	3.4
Sri lanka	91	44.6	16.8
Suriname	05	23.9	4.8
Sweden	08	18.7	6.8
Switzerland	07	24.8	11.4
Syrian Arab Republic	85	0.2	0
Tajikistan	01	2.9	2.3
Thailand	02	12	3.8
Tfyr Macedonia	03	9.5	4
Trinidad and Tobago	06	17.9	3.8
Turkmenistan	98	13.8	3.5
Ukraine	09	37.8	7
United Kingdom	09	10.9	3
United States of America	05	17.7	4.5
Uruguay	04	26	6.3
Uzbekistan	05	7	2.3
Venezuela	07	5.3	1.2
Zimbabwe	90	10.6	5.2

2.2.3 *Agents of Suicide*

Agents of suicide exhibit variation by characteristics of the population and their environmental circumstances. In the U.S., firearm suicides comprised 51 % (6.3 per 100,000 population) of the 38,364 suicide deaths in 2010. Of the drug-induced deaths, 13.1 % were suicidal drug poisoning. Although access to lethal agents are thought to be major risk factors, in nations where firearms are greatly restricted, elevated structures, substances, or other means may prevail. For example, suffocation has become the predominant method for committing suicide among adolescents in Canada, hanging, strangulation and suffocation among men in the U.K., and access to toxic substances, such as pesticides in rural China (Li et al. 2012; ONS 2014; Skinner and McFaull 2012).

Globally, European nations have among the highest suicide rates. The average suicide rate in Europe is 13.9 per 100,000, with the highest rates in the Commonwealth of Independent States (CIS) (21.4 per 100,000), followed by the new

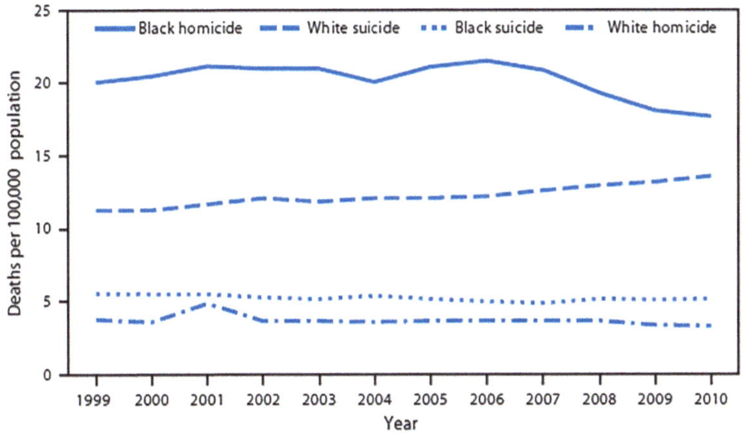

Fig. 2.3 Annual Age-Adjusted Death Rates*† for Suicide and Homicide, by Black or White Race —United States,§ 1999–2010. April 5, 2013/62(13);257. * Deaths are coded as *U03, X60–X84, and Y87.0 for suicide, and *U01–*U02, X85–Y09, and Y87.1 for homicide, as underlying causes of death, according to the *International Classification of Diseases 10th Revision*. Rates include deaths related to the events of September 11, 2001. † Rates have been revised by using populations enumerated as of April 1, for 2000 and 2010, and intercensal estimates as of July 1 for all other years. Therefore, the rates might differ from those published previously. § U.S. residents only

EU countries (13.8 per 100,000). Even within the European Union, where the overall average rate is 10.1 per 100,000 population, it rises as high as 30.7 per 100,000 population in Lithuania, 21.5 per 100,000 in Hungary, and 18.5 per 100,000 in Finland, and 18.4 per 100,000 in Slovenia (WHO 2014).

2.2.4 Risk Factors for Suicide

There are a number of risk factors identified for suicide. The most common ones cited in the literature are displayed in Table 2.3. There is no single risk factor on its own known to be causative, although depression is the most commonly identified from forensic autopsies and other studies of those who have committed suicide. Suicide typically results from a combination and interaction of a number of personal factors, including mental illness, marital difficulties, specifically divorce, financial hardship, deteriorating physical health, fearlessness about death, a major loss, as well as environmental factors such as lack of social support, economic downturns (Europe, Americas) and residence in rural areas (China) (Chang et al. 2013; Fassberg et al. 2012; Hooley et al. 2014; Hor and Taylor 2010; Li et al. 2012; Tang and Crane 2006). More recently, the social environment such as bullying and social internet media providing advice on aspects of suicide methods are playing a more prominent role as potential risk factors.

Table 2.3 Risk factors for completed suicide

Risk factor
Schizophrenia
Downward economic cycle/unemployment
Easy access to lethal methods (e.g., access to firearms)
Family history of suicide
Family history of violence, including physical or sexual abuse
Previous suicide attempt(s)
History of or current mental disorders, particularly clinical depression
History of or current alcohol and substance abuse
Feelings of hopelessness
Impulsive or aggressive tendencies
Cultural and religious beliefs (e.g., belief that suicide is noble resolution of a personal dilemma)
Exposure to suicidal behavior of others, including from media
Isolation, a feeling of being cut off from other people
Barriers to accessing mental health treatment
Loss (relational, social, work, or financial)
Chronic medical conditions (e.g., chronic pain)
Unwillingness to seek help because of the stigma attached to mental health and substance abuse disorders or to suicidal thoughts

2.3 Suicidal Thoughts and Nonfatal Suicidal Behaviors

When obtaining information about suicidal thoughts, plans, or attempts, it is important to take note of the time interval in which the event occurred. Common time periods ascertained are lifetime, recent history (<6 months), baseline (within 30 days), or some prospective measurement (since baseline, since last visit, within one year). Historical measures are subject to recall bias. This means that respondents tend to recall events in the recent past better than those occurring more distantly. This could reflect why certain groups would have a lower prevalence of these behaviors if their event was 12 months or more prior to the survey compared with others, whose event was only one month prior to the survey. Persons in the former group might not report their event because of recall bias, and so the finding might not mean that their rates were actually lower. Prospective measurements are subject to survivorship bias meaning individuals who died from suicide or other means may not have lived and thus might be different from persons available for subsequent interviews.

2.3.1 Data Sources for Nonfatal Suicidal Events

Population based data on nonfatal suicidal events provide important background context for evaluating the impact of any programmatic or therapeutic intervention or change in public policy.

The World Mental Health (WMH) Survey Initiative is a source of information about suicidal behavior and various mental disorders, risk factors, and their treatment in the general. The WMH surveys were conducted 17 countries in Africa, the Americas, Asia, and the Pacific, Europe, and the Middle East (Nock et al. 2008).

The National Comorbidity Survey Replication (NCS-R) is a probability sample of the United States carried out a decade after the original 1992 NCS (NCS-1) was conducted. The NCS-R repeats many of the questions from the NCS-1 and also expands the questioning to include assessments based on the diagnostic criteria of the American Psychiatric Association as reported in the Diagnostic and Statistical Manual-IV (DSM-IV), 1994. The two major aims of the NCS-R were first, to investigate time trends and their correlates over the decade of the 1990s, and second, to expand the assessment in the baseline NCS-1 in order to address a number of important substantive and methodological issues that were raised by the NCS-1. The NCS-R is part of the Collaborative Psychiatric Epidemiology Surveys (CPES) data collection. Data and documentation for NCS-R can be accessed through the CPES Web site. The NCSR conducted the first national survey of US adolescents (NCS-Adolescent Suppl3ment) assessing a wide range of DSM-IV suicidal behaviors using structured diagnostic interviews (Nock et al. 2013).

The National Survey on Drug Use and Health (NSDUH) is an annual nationwide survey of a representative sample of the civilian, noninstitutionalized U.S. population aged ≥12 years. NSDUH collects data on adverse health consequences related to the use of illicit drugs, alcohol, and tobacco; initiation of substance use; substance use disorders and treatment; health care; and mental health. The suicide-related questions from NSDUH may be correlated with population demographics and the presence of a risk factor (e.g., major depressive episode), its duration and severity.

2.3.2 Age, Sex, Race, and Geographical Region Variations in Suicidal Thoughts and Nonfatal Suicidal Behaviors

There is marked variation in the prevalence of suicidal thoughts, plans, and attempts by age, sex, gender, and other demographic characteristics across nations and within nations (Casey et al. 2006; Crosby et al. 2011; Nock et al. 2008; Simon et al. 2013). Demographic, social, and access to health care could explain most of the cross-country variation, although there are some similarities in patterns. Results from the World Mental Health Surveys display the prevalences of these behaviors for individuals 18+ years are displayed in Table 2.4. Across all countries studied, the lifetime prevalence (standard error) of suicidal ideation, plans, and attempts is 9.2 % (0.1), 3.1 % (0.1), and 2.7 % (0.1). The prevalence of each of these varied widely by country. Although these prevalences appear small, when translated on a population basis, the extent of the impact becomes profound. For example, in the U.S., during 2008–2009, 0.5 % of the adult population reported having made a suicide attempt or an estimated 1 million (annual average) persons. Sixty percent of transitions from ideation to plan and attempt were estimated to occur within the first year after ideation onset in both adults and children (Nock et al. 2008, 2013). Further details on the prevalences of these according to more detailed population characteristics for the U.S. adults are listed in Table 2.5. By comparison, among adolescents in the U.S., the lifetime prevalences of suicide ideation, plans, and attempts were 12.1, 4.0, and 4.1 %, respectively, rates higher than in the overall adult population (Nock et al. 2013). Noteworthy in these statistics combined are that suicidal thoughts (or ideas) are not uncommon in the population ranging from 15.9 % in New Zealand to 3.0 % in Italy. Accordingly, plans are less frequently reported, ranging from 5.6 % in New Zealand to 0.9 % in China. The prevalence of attempts is of similar magnitude to prevalence of those making suicidal plans, ranging from 0.5 % in Italy to 5.0 % in the U.S. (Table 2.4).

2.3.3 Risk and Protective Factors for Suicidal Thoughts and Behavior

There are a number of risk factors for nonfatal suicidal thoughts and behavior many of which are also associated with a fatal suicide (Table 2.6). Similarly, these also vary by age, gender, race, and ethnic group. Consistently among countries, the strongest association with suicidal thoughts and behaviors is depression, particularly severe depression, despite variability in the prevalence of this factor across nations (Casey et al. 2006; Nock et al.2008). Other populations at risk for self-harm include those with dementia or psychiatric disorders, particularly schizophrenia. In these populations, the risk is further increased with the presence of comorbidites such as depression (Haw et al. 2009; Radomsky et al. 1999). An increased risk of suicide attempts after benzodiazepine and/or antidepressant use has been reported (Neutel and Patten 1997). Caution should be used in attributing prescription drug use and suicidal thoughts and behavior among persons with psychiatric behaviors as the association may be from a confounding by indication. Protective factors should also be considered as these are associated with a lower risk of suicidal behaviors. Both are listed in Table 2.6.

Table 2.4 Lifetime prevalence of suicide-related outcomes in the world mental health surveys (Knock et al. 2008)

	Total sample											
	Ideation				Plan				Attempt			
	(%)	(se)	(sd)	(n)	(%)	(se)	(sd)	(n)	%	(se)	(sd)	(n)
The Americas												
Colombia	12.4[b]	(0.7)	(46.6)	(587)	4.1[b]	(0.4)	(26.6)	(204)	4.7[b]	(0.4)	(26.6)	(224)
Mexico	8.1[a]	(0.5)	(38)	(488)	3.2	(0.3)	(22.8)	(192)	2.7	(0.3)	(22.8)	(166)
USA	15.6[b]	(0.5)	(48.2)	(1462)	5.4[b]	(0.3)	(28.9)	(507)	5.0[b]	(0.2)	(19.3)	(469)
Europe												
Belgium	8.4	(0.9)	(44.3)	(209)	2.7	(0.4)	(19.7)	(77)	2.5	(0.4)	(19.7)	(66)
France	12.4[b]	(0.7)	(37.7)	(391)	4.4[b]	(0.4)	(21.5)	(143)	3.4	(0.4)	(21.5)	(115)
Germany	9.7	(0.7)	(41.7)	(347)	2.2[a]	(0.3)	(17.9)	(78)	1.7[a]	(0.3)	(17.9)	(64)
Italy	3.0[a]	(0.3)	(20.6)	(144)	0.7[a]	(0.1)	(6.9)	(33)	0.5[a]	(0.1)	(6.9)	(26)
Netherlands	8.2	(0.6)	(29.2)	(223)	2.7	(0.5)	(24.4)	(78)	2.3	(0.3)	(14.6)	(64)
Spain	4.4[a]	(0.3)	(22.2)	(272)	1.4[a]	(0.2)	(14.8)	(84)	1.5[a]	(0.2)	(14.8)	(80)
Ukraine	8.2[a]	(0.5)	(34.4)	(389)	2.7	(0.3)	(20.6)	(126)	1.8[a]	(0.2)	(13.7)	(80)
Africa and the Middle East												
Israel	5.5[a]	(0.3)	(20.9)	(268)	1.9[a]	(0.2)	(13.9)	(93)	1.4[a]	(0.2)	(13.9)	(66)
Lebanon	4.3[a]	(0.6)	(32.1)	(117)	1.7[a]	(0.4)	(21.4)	(39)	2.0[a]	(0.3)	(16)	(54)
Nigeria	3.2[a]	(0.2)	(16.4)	(237)	1.0[a]	(0.1)	(8.2)	(70)	0.7[a]	(0.1)	(8.2)	(46)
South Africa	9.1	(0.7)	(46)	(394)	3.8	(0.4)	(26.3)	(171)	2.9	(0.3)	19.7)	(140)

(continued)

Table 2.4 (continued)

	Total sample											
	Ideation				Plan				Attempt			
	(%)	(se)	(sd)	(n)	(%)	(se)	(sd)	(n)	%	(se)	(sd)	(n)
Asia and the Pacific												
China	3.1[a]	(0.2)	(14.4)	(160)	0.9[a]	(0.2)	(14.4)	(42)	1.0[a]	(0.2)	(14.4)	(49)
Japan	10.9[b]	(0.5)	(24.7)	(264)	2.1[a]	(0.3)	(14.8)	50)	1.9[a]	(0.3)	(14.8)	(48)
New Zealand	15.9[b]	(0.5)	(56.5)	(2212)	5.6[b]	(0.3)	(33.9)	(814)	4.6[b]	(0.3)	(33.9)	(688)
Total	9.2	(0.1)	(29.1)	(8164)	3.1	(0.1)	(29.1)	(2801)	2.7	(0.1)	(29.1)	(2445)

[1] n = 84,850

[a] The upper end of the 95 % confidence interval of the estimate is below the prevalence estimate for the total sample

[b] The lower end of the 95 % confidence interval of the estimate is above the prevalence estimate for the total sample

Source (Nock et al. 2008)

Table 2.5 Annual average estimated number* and percentage of adults aged ≥18 years who had suicidal thoughts or engaged in suicidal behaviors during the previous year, by selected demographic characteristics—National Survey on Drug Use and Health, United States, 2008–2009†

Characteristic	Thought			Plan			Attempt		
	No.	(%)	(95 % CI)	No.	(%)	(95 % CI)	No.	(%)	(95 % CI)
Sex									
Male	3,789	3.5	(3.2–3.8)	1,045	1.0	(0.8–1.1)	442	0.4	(0.3–0.5)
Female	4,571	3.9	(3.7–4.2)	1,218	1.0	(0.9–1.2)	616	0.5	(0.4–0.6)
Age group (yrs)									
18–29	2,865	5.7	(5.4–6.0)	821	1.6	(1.5–1.8)	477	1.0	(0.8–1.1)
≥30	5,494	3.1	(2.9–3.4)	1,442	0.8	(0.7–0.9)	581	0.3	(0.3–0.4)
Race/ethnicity									
White, nonhispanic	6,044	3.9	(3.7–4.1)	1,616	1.0	(0.9–1.2)	663	0.4	(0.4–0.5)
Black, nonhispanic	911	3.5	(3.1–4.0)	262	1.0	(0.8–1.3)	182	0.7	(0.5–0.9)
Hispanic§	933	3.0	(2.6–3.6)	267	0.9	(0.6–1.2)	144	0.5	(0.3–0.6)
Asian, nonhispanic	208	2.1	(1.6–2.8)	37	0.4	(0.2–0.6)	23	0.2	(0.1–0.6)
Education									
Less than high school	1,373	4.0	(3.5–4.4)	429	1.2	(1.0-1.5)	247	0.7	(0.6–0.9)
High school graduate¶	2,823	4.0	(3.7–4.4)	730	1.0	(0.9–1.2)	393	0.6	(0.5–0.7)
Some college	2,359	4.1	(3.8–4.5)	672	1.2	(1.0–1.4)	304	0.5	(0.4–0.7)
College graduate or higher	1,805	2.8	(2.5–3.2)	433	0.7	(0.5–0.9)	113	0.2	(0.1–0.3)
Current employment									
Full-time	3,679	3.1	(2.9–3.3)	844	0.7	(0.6–0.8)	351	0.3	(0.2–0.4)
Part-time	1,380	4.5	(4.0–5.0)	405	1.3	(1.1–1.6)	200	0.6	(0.5–0.9)
Unemployed	768	6.5	(5.6–7.5)	244	2.1	(1.6–2.7)	118	1.0	(0.8–1.3)
Other**	2,532	3.9	(3.6–4.3)	770	1.2	(1.0–1.4)	389	0.6	(0.5–0.8)

(continued)

Table 2.5 (continued)

Characteristic	Thought			Plan			Attempt		
	No.	(%)	(95 % CI)	No.	(%)	(95 % CI)	No.	(%)	(95 % CI)
County type									
Large metropolitan area††	4,353	3.6	(3.4–3.9)	1,148	1.0	(0.8-1.1)	559	0.5	(0.4–0.6)
Small metropolitan area§§	2,692	3.9	(3.6–4.3)	777	1.1	(1.0–1.3)	351	0.5	(0.4–0.6)
Nonmetropolitan area¶¶	1,315	3.5	(3.2–4.0)	338	0.9	(0.8–1.1)	148	0.4	(0.3–0.5)
*Total***	8,359	3.7	(3.5–3.9)	2,263	1.0	(0.9–1.1)	1,058	0.5	(0.4–0.5)

Abbreviations CI = confidence interval; thought = had serious thoughts of suicide; plan = made any suicide plan; attempt = attempted suicide

* In thousands

† Estimates are based only on responses to suicide items in the Mental Health module. Respondents with unknown suicide information were excluded

§ Persons of hispanic origin can be of any race

¶ Includes persons with a general education diploma

** Includes retired persons, disabled persons, homemakers, students, or other persons not in the labor force

†† Area with a population of ≥1 million persons

§§ Area with a population of <1 million persons

¶¶ Area that is outside of a metropolitan statistical area; includes urbanized counties with a population of ≥20,000 persons in urbanized areas, less urbanized counties with a population of ≥2,500 persons but <20,000 persons in urbanized areas, and completely rural counties with a population of <2,500 persons in urbanized areas

** Totals exclude persons with missing or unknown race and ethnicity. Totals might vary due to rounding

Source (Crosby et al. 2011)

Table 2.6 Risk and protective factors for suicidal thoughts and nonfatal suicidal behaviors

Risk factor (See also Risk Factors in Table 2.3)
Low birth weight
Young maternal age at birth
Young paternal age at birth
Life events without help (women)
Severity of depressed mood (Beck's depression inventory score $\geq$13)
Schizophrenia
Post traumatic stress disorder
Major depressive disorder
Disruptive behavior disorders
Certain forms of dementia
Protective factors
Effective clinical care for mental, physical, and substance abuse disorders
Easy access to a variety of clinical interventions and support for help seeking
Family and community support (connectedness)
Support from ongoing medical and mental health care relationships
Skills in problem solving, conflict resolution, and nonviolent ways of handling disputes
Cultural and religious beliefs that discourage suicide and support instincts for self-preservation

2.4 Conclusion

There are a number of challenges in assessing suicide risk and suicidal behavior in populations. Among these are changing environmental factors and their differential distribution among population subgroups. But uniform in concern is that suicide rates are trending upwards in many countries and population subgroups despite a recognition that suicide data may be under reported due to the difficult nature of classifying suicide and the time lag in determining this as a cause of death. The epidemiological concepts underlying suicide and suicidal behavior illustrate a complex pathway to either fatal or nonfatal self-harm and present a challenge in developing preventive strategies. The factors that give rise to these events are highly subject to personal and environmental characteristics, whose influences are changed over time because of social, cultural, and economic conditions. Thus, the interpretations of any measures of such must consider to what degree biases enter into how their measurement and reporting could affect the underlying true rates.

References

Bossarte RM, Knox KL, Piegari R, Altieri J, Kemp J, Katz IR (2012) Prevalence and characteristics of suicide ideation and attempts among active military and veteran participants in a national health survey. Am J Pub Health 102:S38–S40

Casey PR, Dunn G, Kelly BD, Birkbeck G, Dalgard OS, Lehtinen V, Britta S, Ayuso-Mateos JL, Dowrick C (2006) Factors associated with suicidal ideation in the general population: five-centre analysis from the ODIN study. Br J Psychiatry 189:410–415

Chang S-S, Stuckler D, Yip P, Gunnell D (2013) Impact of 2008 global economic crisis on suicide: time trend study in 54 countries. BMJ 17(347):f5239

Crosby AE, Han B, Ortega LAG, Parks SE, Gfroerer J (2011) Suicidal thoughts and behaviors among adults aged ≥18 years—United States, 2008–2009. MMWR 60(SS-13):1–22

Fassberg MM, van Orden KA, Duberstein P, Erlangsen A, Lapierre S, Bodner E, Canetto SS, DeLeo D, Szanto K, Waern M (2012) A systematic review of social factors and suicidal behavior in older adulthood. Int J Environ Res Pub Health 9:722–745

Fazel S, Wolf A, Pillas D, Lichtenstein P, Langstrom N (2014) Suicide, fatal injuries, and other causes of premature mortality in patients with traumatic brain injury: a 41-year Swedish population study. JAMA Psychiatry 71:326–333

Gahm GA, Reger MA, Kinn JT, Luxton DD, Skopp NA, Bush NE (2012) Addressing the surveillance goal in the national strategy for suicide prevention: the Department of Defense suicide event report. Am J Pub Health 102:S24–S28

Haw C, Harwood D, Hawton K (2009) Dementia and suicidal behavior: a review of the literature. Int Psychogeriatr 21:440–453

Hayati AN, Abdullah AA, Shah MM (eds) (2008) National suicide registry Malaysia: preliminary report July–Dec 2007. Kuala Lumpur

Hooley JM, Franklin JC, Nock MK (2014) Chronic pain and suicide: understanding the association. Curr Pain Headache Rep 18:435

Hor K, Taylor M (2010) Suicide and schizophrenia: a systematic review of rates and risk factors. J Psychopharmacology 24(Suppl 4):81–90

Knock MK et al (2008) Cross-national prevalence and risk factors for suicidal ideation, plans, and attempts. Br J Psychiatry 192:98−105

Li Y, Li Y, Cao J (2012) Factors associated with suicidal behaviors in mainland China: a meta-analysis. BMC Publ Health 12:524

Navaneelan T (2012) Suicide rates: an overview. Statistics Canada Catalogue no. 82-624-X

Neutel CI, Patten SB (1997) Risk of suicide attempts after benzodiazepine and/or antidepressant use. Ann Epidemiol 7:568–574

Niederkrotenthaler T, Rasmussen F, Mittendorfer-Rutz E (2012) Perinatal conditions and parental age at birth as risk markers for subsequent suicide attempt and suicide: a population based case-control study. Eur J Epidemiol 27:729–738

Nock MK, Borges G, Bromet EJ, Alonso J, Angermeyer M, Beautrais A, Bruffaerts R, Chiu WT, de Girolamo G, Gluzman S, de Graaf R, Gureje O, Haro JM, Huang Y, Karam E, Ronald C (2008) Cross-national prevalence and risk factors for suicidal ideation, plans, and attempts. Br J Psychiatry 192:98–105

Nock MK, Green JG, Hwang I, McLaughlin KA, Sampson NA, Zaslavsky AM, Kessler RC (2013) Prevalence, correlates, and treatment of lifetime suicidal behavior among adolescents. JAMA Psychiatry 70:300–310

Norton R, Kobusingye O (2013) Injuries. New Engl J Med 368:1723–1730

Office for National Statistics (ONS) (2014) Suicides in the United Kingdom, 2012 Registrations. ONS: United Kingdom

Radomsky ED, Haas GL, Mann JJ, Sweeney JA (1999) Suicidal behavior in patients with schizophrenia and other psychotic disorders. Am J Psychiatry 156:1590–1595

Simon M, Chang E-S, Zeng P, Dong X (2013) Prevalence of suicidal ideation, attempts, and completed suicide rate in Chinese aging populations: a systematic review. Arch Gerontol Geriatr 57:250–256

Skinner R, McFaull S (2012) Suicide among children and adolescents in Canada: trends and sex differences, 1980-2008. CMAJ 184:1029–1034

Tang NKY, Crane C (2006) Suicidality in chronic pain: a review of the prevalence, risk factors and psychological links. Psychol Med 36:575–586

Trofimovich L, Skopp NA, Luxton DD, Reger MA (2012) Health care experiences prior to suicide and self-inflicted injury, active component, U.S. Armed Forces, 2001–2010. MSMR 19:2–6

WHO (2014) Data and statistics: fact sheet mental health. http://www.euro.who.int/en/health-topics/noncommunicable-diseases/mental-health/data-and-statistics/fact-sheet-mental-health. Accessed 20 May 2014

Chapter 3
Treatment Emergent Suicidal Ideation and Behavior

Sian L. Ratcliffe, Phillip B. Chappell, Janel Boyce-Rustay, Svetlana Gloukhova and Denise M. Oleske

Abstract The concept of treatment emergent suicidality during clinical trials has been a subject of regulatory and research interest, especially since the early 1990s. A key series of analyses have shaped the regulatory environment for expectations of prospective assessment of suicidal ideation and behavior (SIB) in clinical trials. The development of a scale for prospective assessment of these events has been a key priority in order to detect emergent signs during the course of a clinical trial and to assist in patient selection criteria of suicide risk. The maturing regulatory environment and increasing evolution in thinking on definitions of SIB have underpinned significant changes in the main assessment scale, the Columbia Suicide Severity Rating Scale (C-SSRS), as well as in the standard adopted by the FDA for coding, summarizing, and analyzing SIB data, the Columbia Classification Algorithm for Suicide Assessment (C-CASA). For new drugs undergoing clinical development, assessment of SIB is incorporated into benefit/risk decision-making and continuing risk management approaches throughout the pharmaceutical industry and academia. A number of companies have developed internal guidances, which may include quantitative decision-criteria (i.e., based on binding data at CNS targets) or qualitative clinical judgment (i.e., based on mechanistic understanding

S.L. Ratcliffe (✉) · P.B. Chappell
Pfizer Inc, Groton, CT, USA
e-mail: sian.ratcliffe@pfizer.com

P.B. Chappell
e-mail: philip.chappell@pfizer.com

J. Boyce-Rustay · S. Gloukhova · D.M. Oleske
AbbVie, North Chicago, IL, USA
e-mail: boyceruj@gene.com

S. Gloukhova
e-mail: lana.gloukhova@abbvie.com

D.M. Oleske
e-mail: denise.oleske@abbvie.com

Present Address:
J. Boyce-Rustay
Genentech Inc., South San Francisco, CA, USA

K.E. Cannon and T.J. Hudzik (eds.), *Suicide: Phenomenology and Neurobiology*,
DOI 10.1007/978-3-319-09964-4_3

and emerging safety profiles) of drug candidates that may require the inclusion of prospective SIB tools. In this chapter, we will provide an overview of the regulatory history surrounding treatment emergent SIB and will outline a number of structured qualitative steps for prospective SIB assessment.

3.1 Introduction

The detection of treatment emergent suicidal ideation and behavior (SIB) during clinical trials has been a subject of interest for researchers and regulators alike since the early 1990s with the controversial possibility that antidepressants might paradoxically contribute to the risk of suicide ideation (i.e., suicidal thinking) and suicidal behavior (i.e., suicide attempts, preparatory behaviors or suicide completions).

Research into suicide is fraught with methodological problems, including lack of definition and clarity. The problem of definition has been complicated by the use of the term "suicidality", which lumps together suicidal ideation, self-injurious behavior, suicide attempts, and completed suicide despite their very different consequences to the patient. The general term suicidality is not considered to be adequately specific or as clinically useful as more precise terminology (ideation, behavior, attempts, and suicide). In addition, epidemiological findings suggest that suicidal ideation is not a strong predictor of a suicide attempt, although approximately one-third of those who think about suicide at some point in their lives later make a suicide attempt (Nock et al. 2009a, b). Furthermore, psychological autopsy studies have found frequent expression of suicidal thoughts before completed suicide, with one meta-analysis showing 50–66 % of people who complete suicide have disclosed their ideation or intent to those around them (Cavanagh et al. 2003).

The use of more precise terms to describe SIB has now emerged following expert working groups, systematic historical clinical trial analyses, clinical trial methodology workshops and discussion with regulatory authorities. SIB refers to suicidal behavior (completed suicide, suicide attempts, interrupted attempts, aborted attempts, and preparatory acts toward imminent suicide) and suicidal ideation (active and passive). Suicidal behavior must be distinguished from self-injurious acts or behaviors without suicidal intent that may actually be a mechanism to gain attention and/or attempts to manipulate the environment.

The development of a scale for prospective assessment of these events has been a key priority in order to detect emergent signs during the course of a clinical trial and to assist in patient selection criteria of suicide risk. While it is important for prospective risk assessment to include specific focused questions on suicidal ideation, narrowing the time period for this has been the subject of methodological discussion. The expression of suicidal ideation and threats is relatively common. Therefore, it is difficult to identify the small percentage of a large number of ideators who will progress to a suicide attempt. Narrowing down the timeframe to the past 12 months is one way to ensure better identification of those ideators who may subsequently be at greater risk of suicide attempt (Nock et al. 2009a).

In addition to considering the specific manifestations of SIB, it is important to recognize that there are other risk factors that influence the risk of suicide. There is no clearly defined combination of risk factors that has sufficient sensitivity and specificity to predict who among a group at risk will make an attempt or completion, or the circumstances or timing of this (Goodwin and Jamison 2007), as there are a number of general, chronic, and short-term risk factors for suicide. Interestingly, and somewhat surprisingly, subjects with depression and suicidal ideation, although a risk group, are not the leading group at risk for progression to a suicide attempt. Ideators with anxiety or impulse control disorders (i.e., conduct disorder and post-traumatic stress disorder, PTSD) showed a higher likelihood, or predictive power, for making a suicide attempt as reported in the National Comorbidity Survey Replication in US adults (Nock et al. 2009a, b). An anxiety disorder is an independent risk factor for suicidal ideation and suicide attempts. Comorbid anxiety and mood disorders have been shown to further increase the risk compared with a mood disorder alone (Sareen et al. 2005).

There have been a key series of analyses of drug classes that have shaped the development of scales, in particular, the Columbia scale and algorithm and the regulatory expectation of its broad application across many clinical trials. The most prominent of these are the meta-analyses of antidepressant clinical trial data that underpinned the FDA's conclusions that: (1) the risk of SIB was greatest among children and adolescents taking antidepressants versus placebo OR = 2.2 (95 % CI 1.4 − 3.6), followed by young adults aged 18–24 OR = 1.55 (95 % CI 0.91 − 2.7), and the risk appears to go down with age (e.g., ages 25–30, OR = 1.00; ages 31–64, OR = 0.77; ages 65+, OR = 0.39); and (2) the risk of suicidality was stronger for non-depressed psychiatric patients as compared with depressed ones. (Institute of Medicine 2010; Hammad et al. 2006; Stone et al. 2009). This latter finding led to ramifications for antidepressant and other centrally acting medicines, especially in indications other than depression. Other post hoc analyses have indicated that antiepileptic drugs (AEDs) might also increase suicide risk (FDA analysis 2008; Pompili and Tatarelli 2010; Pompili et al. 2010). Several recent studies, however, have yielded inconsistent findings in relation to risks with specific AEDs, nevertheless levetiracetam, lamotrigine, and topiramate were among the top three anticonvulsants associated with the highest observed risk of suicidal behaviors in at least two of the six reported analyses (FDA analysis 2008; Gibbons et al. 2009; Andersohn et al. 2010; Van Cott et al. 2010; Patorno et al. 2010; Olesen et al. 2010). Most of the studies as well as epidemiological studies identify psychiatric comorbidities in epilepsy as important factors that increase the propensity toward suicide and suicidal behaviors (Arana et al. 2010; Pompili and Baldessarini 2010).

In addition to the regulatory and clinical focus on identifying suicidal ideation associated with antidepressant use, research has been ongoing into potential genetic markers of susceptibility to treatment emergent suicidal ideation (TESI). Although family and twin studies have been conducted and have estimated the heritability of suicidal behavior to be 30–55 % (Brent and Mann 2005; Statham et al. 1998), no such formal evidence has been established for TESI, probably due to the rareness and transience of the event that cannot be assessed by the usual genetic epidemiological methods. A genetic influence on this trait could be likely, based on a number of reports about the association of TESI with genetic markers (Brent et al. 2010; Perroud 2011). Two genome wide association studies (GWAS) have identified association between genetic variants and emergent or worsening suicidal ideation upon antidepressant treatment. In the Sequenced Treatment Alternatives to Relieve Depression (STAR*D) trial, variants in the genetic loci encoding papilin and the IL-28 α-receptor were identified (Laje et al. 2009). In the Genome-Based Therapeutic Drugs for Depression (GENDEP) study, a genetic marker in the vicinity of the *guanine deaminase* (*GDA*) gene has been associated with emergent or worsening of suicidal ideation (Perroud et al. 2012). In a recent GWAS study that investigated associations between TESI and single nucleotide polymorphisms (SNPs) in a naturalistic pharmacogenetic study of patients with depressive disorder, a subset of 14 SNPs were associated with TESI and had supportive genetic evidence (Menke et al. 2012). Of these, nine variants were located in or nearby genes previously linked to bipolar disorder (*RHEB*, *TMEM138* and *CYBASC3*) and one variant in a gene also associated with schizophrenia and neurodegeneration (*PIK3C3*). Despite the limited sample size, the results from this GWAS study suggest that genetic markers may be used as tools to identify patients at risk of TESI in the future.

3.2 Historical Perspectives and Regulatory History

Assessment of SIB in clinical trials continues to be an area of active regulatory concern. Reviewing the US regulatory history is important to put into context the current guidance for prospective assessment of SIB in clinical trials. The maturing regulatory environment and increasing evolution in thinking on definitions of SIB have underpinned significant changes in the main assessment scale, the C-SSRS, as well as in the standard adopted by the FDA for coding, summarizing and analyzing SIB data, the C-CASA.

While a number of global regulatory authorities have expressed interest in the prospective assessment of SIB in clinical trials, few other than the FDA have provided specific guidance on assessment tools and expectations for industry. The FDA issued a number of communications pertaining to the risk of SIB with individual drugs or classes of drugs via post-marketing safety updates. Thus, the regulatory history provides a useful background to the current global landscape and recommendations in the FDA Guidance document, as discussed below (see Fig. 3.1).

European Regulators were the first to post restrictions on the use of antidepressants. In 2003, the UK Medicines and Healthcare Products Regulatory Agency (MHRA) initiated urgent safety restrictions to contraindicate the use of selective serotonin reuptake inhibitor (SSRI) antidepressants, with the exception of

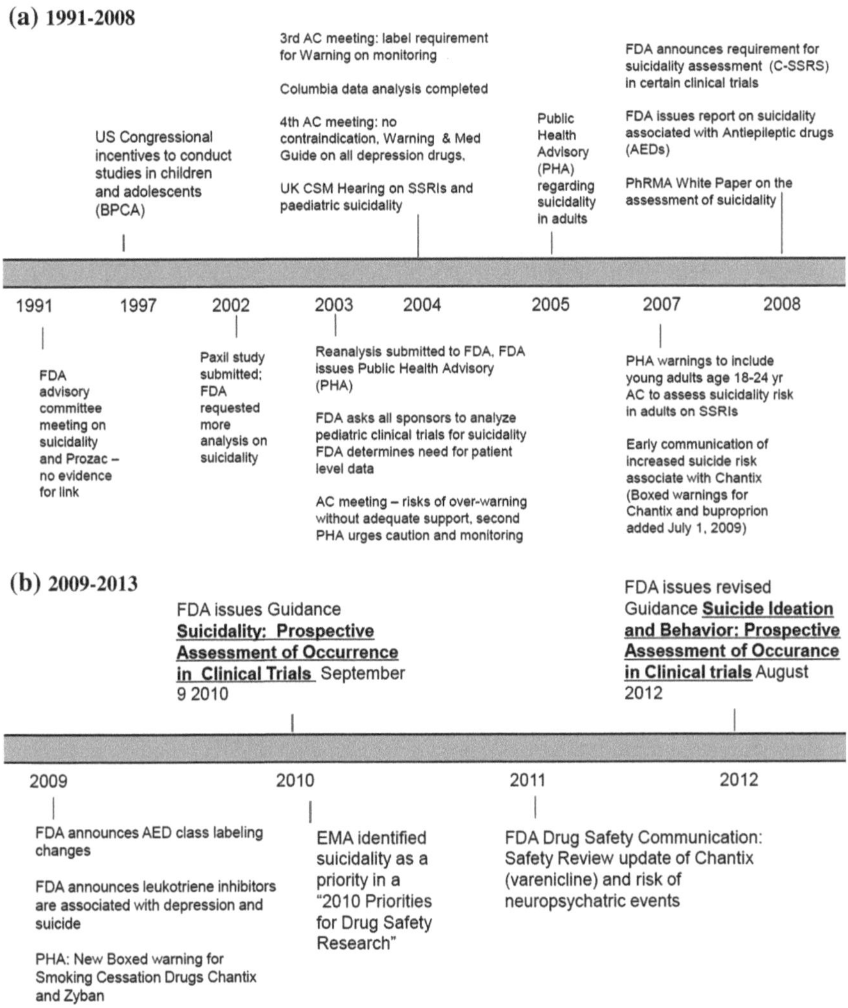

Fig. 3.1 Regulatory history and perspectives on SIB assessment. **a** 1991–2008 **b** 2009–2013

fluoxetine, in children and adolescents. This had followed comprehensive reviews of pediatric depression clinical trial data by the Committee on Safety of Medicines (CSM). The MHRA stated that "on the basis of this review of the available clinical trial data, CSM has advised that the balance of risks and benefits for the treatment of major depressive disorder (MDD) in under 18s is judged to be unfavorable for sertraline, citalopram, and escitalopram, and is unassessable for fluvoxamine. Only fluoxetine (Prozac) has been shown in clinical trials to have a favorable balance of risks and benefits for the treatment of MDD in the under 18s" (MHRA 2003).

Subsequently in 2004, after lengthy analysis and review of clinical trial data, FDA required that labeling of specific antidepressants carry black box warnings, intended to alert healthcare providers and patients to increase monitoring of troubling symptoms. At the time of these regulatory actions, many public health and mental health professionals (MHPs) were concerned that deterring the prescription of antidepressants might lead to undertreatment of depression and in turn to an increase in suicide rates for untreated MDD. Two published studies highlighted this concern, indicating that between 2003 and 2005 in the US there was a 20 % reduction in prescription of antidepressants and, at the same time from 2003 to 2004, an increase in youth suicide rate by 14 % (Gibbons et al. 2007) and new diagnoses of depression in pediatric populations dropped by 44 % (Libby et al. 2009). In addition, previous pharmacoepidemiologic studies had reported that adolescent suicide rates had declined in the early 1990s, related to increasing use of antidepressant drugs in this population (Fergusson et al. 2000, 2005; Gibbons et al. 2006; Olfson et al. 2003; Sondergard et al. 2006; Simon 2006; Valuck et al. 2007).

Subsequent to the regulatory reviews of antidepressant medication, TESI was the focus of further analyses for other classes of centrally acting drugs, particularly anticonvulsants, antipsychotics, and anxiolytics. These analyses resulted in a number of regulatory labeling changes and/or risk management actions as a result (see Table 3.1 for further details). Risk management actions typically focus on ensuring appropriate warnings and wording are reflected in patient materials, such as medication guides, as well as the physician prescribing information. Not all warning language in the product information includes both SIB. For example, product information for Strattera (atomoxetine) described suicidal ideation risks. While a number of the regulatory analyses and reviews were conducted as class reviews (e.g., antidepressants, antiepileptic drugs), not all assessments of SIB relied on data from across compounds (e.g., Strattera is the only ADHD medication with specific warning language for suicidal ideation). A consistent feature across the product labeling for compounds (Table 3.1) is the inclusion of other psychiatric symptoms that may be associated with increased risk of SIB, including mood disturbances, anxiety and/or disturbing thoughts. In addition, recent labeling inclusions for antidepressants have referenced a lowering of suicidal risk in the >65-year age group, based on reviews showing lowered relative risk of events in this age group.

3.3 US Regulatory Guidance on SIB

The result of the regulatory focus on SIB is the need to implement prospective assessment for treatment emergent SIB in clinical trials for CNS-active medicines. In addition, the same assessment tools can be used to measure prior history of suicidal ideation or behavior, and the implementation of other psychiatric screening tools are helpful to elucidate current or history of psychiatric comorbidities.

The FDA's first draft guidance document, entitled "Suicidality: Prospective Assessment of Occurrence in Clinical Trials" was issued in September 2010. The main rationale for this document was to "Ensure patients who are experiencing suicidality are properly recognized and adequately treated." In addition, the

Table 3.1 Summary of labeling changes for FDA reviews of different medication classes for suicidal ideation and behavior (as of March 2011)

Drug class	Drugs	Class labeling	Black box	Warnings	REMS	Med guide	Comments
Antidepressants		√	√	√		√	Black box—suicidality and antidepressants
							Children, adolescents, young adults
							Reduction in risk in 65+ years
Antiepileptics		√		√		√[a]	Warnings and precautions—suicidal behavior or ideation; antiepileptic drugs increase the risk of suicidal thoughts
ADHD							
	Strattera		√	√		√	Black box—suicidal ideation: children or adolescents
							Wording also in patient counseling info
	other stimulants					√	No focused language for suicidality
Antipsychotics (depression)							
	Abilify, Seroquel		√	√		√	Black box—suicidal thinking and behavior: children, adolescents, young adults
Smoking cessation							
	Chantix, Zyban		√	√	√	√	Black box—suicide ideation, suicide attempt and completed suicide reported in patients
Leukotriene inhibitors							
	Singulair			√			Suicidal thinking and behavior (including suicide)
	Accolate, Zyflo						Warnings for neuropsychiatric events *not* suicide

(continued)

Table 3.1 (continued)

Drug class	Drugs	Class labeling	Black box	Warnings	REMS	Med guide	Comments
Sedative/hypnotics							
	Lunesta	√		√		√	Suicidal thoughts and actions (including completed suicides)
							Also in dosing section
	Ambien	√		√		√	Suicidal thoughts and actions (including completed suicides)
							Warning in special populations (depressed patients)
	Ativan	√					Precaution and AE section
Acne							
	Accutane			√			Suicidal ideation, suicide attempts, suicide
							Patient informed consent for suicidal thoughts, suicide attempts, suicide
Other indications							
GERD	Reglan			√		√	Based on post-marketing events
							Warnings/CNS effects: suicidal ideation and suicide
Huntington's disease	Xenazine		√		√	√	Clinical trial events including completed suicide
Multiple sclerosis	Interferons	√		√			Suicidality based on post-marketing events

[a] *Note* in 2009 communication, all AEDs should have MedGuide, as of 1 Apr 2011, this has not occurred

guidance was intended to "Ensure collection of more timely and more complete data on suicidality to better detect increased suicidality in individual studies and in pooled analyses. This is important whether or not a particular drug is known to be associated with treatment-emergent SIB." Subsequently, in August 2012, the FDA issued a revised draft guidance document, entitled "SIB: Prospective Assessment of Occurrence in Clinical Trials". The revised FDA guidance reflects the FDA's current thinking on the importance of assessment of SIB in psychiatric and non-psychiatric drug trials conducted under Investigational New Drugs (INDs) and general principles for how best to accomplish SIB assessment in drug development.

The major revisions in the FDA's revised draft guidance of August 2012 include the following:

- The term *suicidality* is replaced with the phrase *suicidal ideation and behavior.*
- An expanded set of the C-CASA categories is provided, along with definitions and explanations.
- The advice on particular trials and patients that would need assessments of SIB and the timing of such assessments is revised.
- Concerns about the time burden of assessments are addressed.
- Questions about the possible value of the assessments providing protection for patients in the trials themselves are discussed.
- It is made clear that use of an assessment instrument that directly classifies relevant thoughts and behaviors into C-CASA categories eliminates the need for any additional coding.
- Additional advice on evaluation of alternative instruments is provided.

The scope of the revised FDA draft guidance encompasses both psychiatric and neurologic drugs as well as drugs for nonpsychiatric indications (e.g., isotretinoins, other tretinoins, beta blockers, reserpine, smoking cessation drugs, and drugs for weight loss). The revised FDA draft guidance was adopted by the Division of Psychiatry Products, and the Division of Neurologic Products. It is anticipated that the draft guidance will become the standard approach for other FDA divisions as well [such as the Division of Pulmonary, Allergy and Rheumatology Products (with regard, especially, to leukotriene-modifying drugs)]. It is unclear when the 2012 draft guidance will be finalized.

3.4 The Columbia Suicide Severity Rating Scale

The 2010 draft FDA guidance recommended the use of a particular SIB assessment, the C-SSRS. This instrument was designed to be used prospectively in clinical trials and was intended to systematically ascertain and document the occurrence of suicidal events. These events were defined as indicative of SIB based on the use of the retrospective tool, the C-CASA (Posner 2009; see Table 3.2). The C-CASA was developed by Kelly Posner and her team at Columbia University. C-CASA

Table 3.2 C-CASA classification scheme from 2010 FDA guidance

Events	2010 C-CASA classification
Suicidal	1 Completed suicide
	2 Suicide attempt
	3 Preparatory actions toward imminent suicidal behavior (including interrupted attempt or aborted attempt)
	4 Suicidal ideation
Indeterminate	5 Self-injurious behavior with unknown intent: (suicidal or non-suicidal self-injurious behavior)
	6/9 Not enough information: (suicidal or "other") 6 Death 9 Non-death
Non-suicidal	7 Self-injurious behavior without suicidal intent
	8 Other: accidental, psychiatric, medical

Note Light gray boxes were FDA "primary analysis" (includes events deemed suicidal): *light and dark boxes* were FDA "sensitivity analysis" (includes any event that could possibly be suicidal)

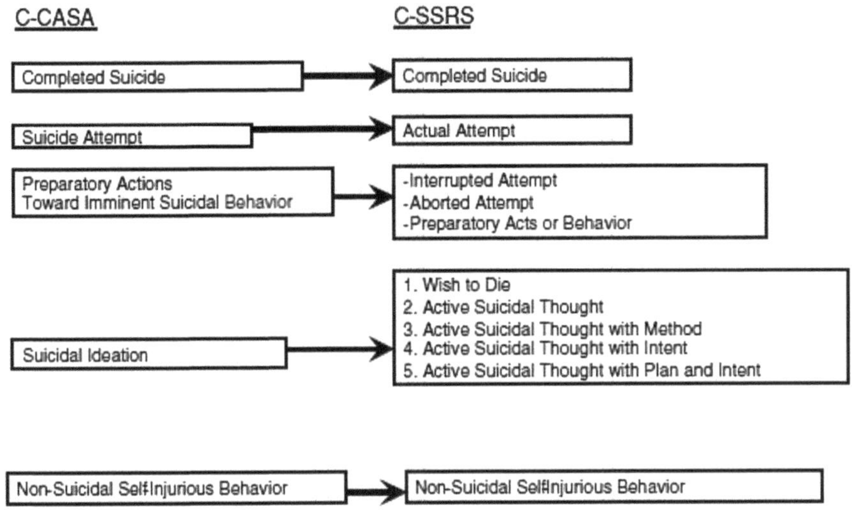

Fig. 3.2 C-SSRS and C-CASA mapping per Posner (2009)

provided a common language to classify SIB data derived from retrospective examination of clinical trial submitted to FDA.

C-CASA is the retrospective counterpart of the more detailed prospective classification instrument, the C-SSRS. It contains a 1–5 numerical rating scale for suicidal ideation of increasing severity (from a "wish list to die" to an "active thought of killing oneself with plan and intent"). By contrast, the C-CASA in the 2010 FDA guidance only had one ideation item (classification 4). How the C-CASA and C-SSRS mapping is done is shown in Fig. 3.2.

The 2012 revision continues to emphasize the use of the C-SSRS and highlights that it classifies SIB events directly to the 11 expanded C-CASA categories without the need for additional narratives or coding. This direct classification of events is viewed by the FDA as one of the C-SSRS's strengths.

The standard adopted by the FDA for coding, summarizing and analyzing SIB data in the 2012 revision of the draft guidance is an expanded version of the C-CASA. This version has 11 categories in total: 5 for suicidal ideation, 5 for suicidal behavior, and 1 for self-injurious behavior with no suicidal intent. Data collected for assessment (whether retrospectively or prospectively) must be classified into these 11 categories as defined by the FDA (see Table 3.3 for a listing of the categories).

The revised draft FDA guidance does state that other appropriate prospective SIB assessments can be used and instructs sponsors to discuss proposed alternatives with the relevant review division prior to implementing them. For example, the FDA's view of the Sheehan Suicide Tracking Scale (S-STS) and in particular its ability to classify SIB events into the 11 expanded C-CASA categories, is not clear at this time.

Table 3.3 Revised guideline (2012) suicidal ideation and behavior events and categories[a]

Category	Event
Suicidal ideation	
1	Passive
2	Active: nonspecific (no method, intent, or plan)
3	Active: method, but no intent or plan
4	Active: method and intent, but no plan
5	Active: method, intent, and plan
Suicidal behavior	
1	Completed suicide
2	Suicide attempt
3	Interrupted attempt
4	Aborted attempt
5	Preparatory actions toward imminent suicidal behaviors
Self-injurious behavior, no suicidal intent	Self-injurious behavior, no suicidal intent

[a] From the revised FDA Guidance (August 2012): "according to the C-SSRS, the definition of plan includes intent (i.e., intent to complete suicide is implicit with the concept of plan). Thus, there is no need for the category *method and plan, but no intent.*"

3.5 European Regulatory Guidance

Unlike the FDA, the European Medicines Agency (EMA) has not yet produced a guidance document specific to assessing SIB in clinical trials. However, in 2010, the EMA identified SIB as a priority in a "2010 Priorities for Drug Safety Research" paper calling for increased research into suicide research methodologies (Issued 4 August 2009). Of particular interest in this paper, are methods to separate suicide associated with certain diseases from treatment for those diseases. In addition, SIB was incorporated into disease specific guidances as part of underlying disease as well as the risk assessment thereof. Disease-specific guidances that encompass suicidal ideation and behaviour include those for: Alcohol dependence, Attention Deficit Hyperactivity Disorder, Depression, Epileptic Disorders, Multiple Sclerosis, Obsessive Compulsive Disorder, Panic Disorder, Post Traumatic Stress Disorder, and Treatment of Smoking. The most recently issued guidances include a statement that C-CASA is an available tool that can be used in these assessments, although there is no explicit expectation to use this tool. Many European clinical trial investigators are familiar with use of the MINI neuropsychiatric interview for assessment of suicide risk at baseline, and have used depression scale suicide-specific items/questions for detection of suicidal symptoms. There is growing familiarity with the use of C-SSRS in global clinical trials, although the construct of the scale is still thought to be very US-centric. Product labels in Europe incorporate similar warning language in the *Special Precautions and Warnings for Use* section of the Summary of Product Characteristics for all of the products with suicidality warning in the US Product Information.

3.6 Impact of FDA Guidance on Clinical Trials

For new drugs undergoing clinical development, assessment of SIB is incorporated into benefit/risk decision-making and continuing risk management approaches throughout the pharmaceutical industry and academia. A number of companies have developed internal guidances, which may include quantitative decision-criteria (i.e., based on binding data at CNS targets) or qualitative clinical judgment (i.e., based on mechanistic understanding and emerging safety profiles) of drug candidates that may require the inclusion of prospective SIB tools. In this section, we will outline a number of structured qualitative steps that are common throughout most large pharmaceutical companies.

Based on the 2012 revision of the FDA guidance, trials conducted under an IND in the following specific categories should address plans for SIB monitoring:

- *CNS Drug Candidates*:
  Prospective SIB assessments should be carried out in all inpatient and outpatient clinical trials involving any drug being developed for a psychiatric indication (i.e., those indications managed in the Division of Psychiatry Products), as well as for all antiepileptic drugs and other neurologic drugs with CNS activity. These trials include multiple-dose Phase 1 trials involving healthy volunteers. Questions on what constitutes CNS activity can be directed to the Division of Neurology Products, although some companies make this decision based on CNS clinical signs in preclinical studies, evidence of or expected brain penetration, as well as functional pharmacological data on typical CNS target receptors, ion channels, or transporters (typically through in vitro profiling).
- *Non-CNS drug Candidates*:
  Although prospective SIB assessments are not required for compounds/drugs that do not have overt CNS effects, there are some types of trials in this category for which the draft FDA guidance recommends that prospective SIB assessments be performed. This includes all clinical trials for drugs that are pharmacologically similar to drugs where possible signals of risk for SIB have been identified, including isotretinoin and other tretinoins, beta blockers (especially those entering the brain), reserpine, drugs for smoking cessation, and drugs for weight loss.

Leukotriene-modifying drugs are not explicitly discussed in the August 2012 Guidance; however, emerging regulatory intelligence for similar agents suggests that there is an expectation by the Division of Pulmonary, Allergy, and Rheumatology Products for inclusion of SIB assessment with agents acting in the leukotriene pathway.

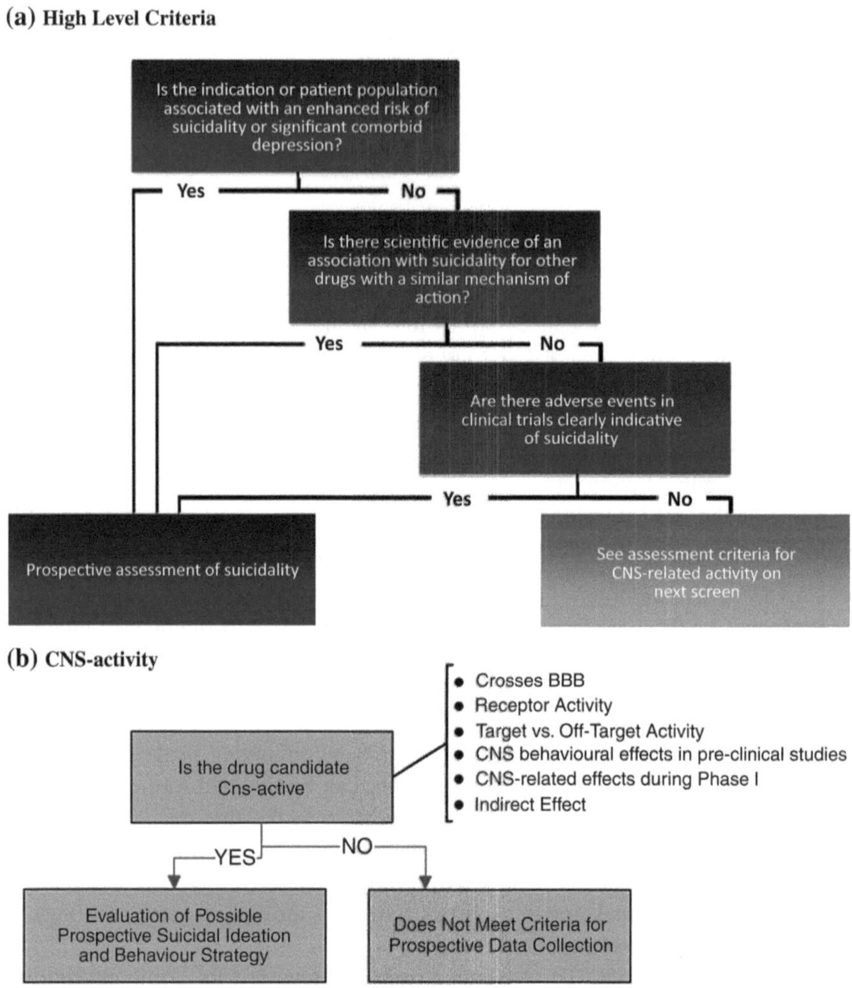

Fig. 3.3 Structured criteria for inclusion of SIB assessment in clinical trials **a** High level criteria. **b** CNS-activity

In addition to mechanistic assessment of new treatments under development, the underlying disease under study and patient population specific considerations need to be taken into account when evaluating prospective SIB assessment. In particular, if the intended indication is one in which the background rate of SIB is considered to be elevated compared with the general population, or if patients have overlapping comorbidity with mood and/or anxiety disorders, then prospective assessment of SIB is recommended. Figure 3.3 outlines a high level structured decision tree for evaluation of SIB in clinical trials.

Besides the C-SSRS or alternative structured SIB assessment tool, collection of narratives can also add valuable information, especially if there are additional notes from MHP referral in response to the C-SSRS questions. A pre-planned Safety Narrative Plan for a trial should describe what events will require a narrative for the clinical study report and consideration should be made for events associated with SIB. Information for the narrative should be obtained from screening and baseline evaluations, data collected during the subject's participation in the trial and any MHP assessments. For drug candidates for which a medically significant SIB concern has not been identified, treatment emergent SIB adverse events that are spontaneously reported should have additional information collected at the time the event is reported to facilitate retrospective coding to C-CASA, if required. The following information is useful to obtain in a Narrative Guide to facilitate supplementary data collection and to help understand full details of a patient's risk for SIB.

Adverse events that may trigger a SIB narrative:

- Suicidal ideation
- Suicidal behaviors and gestures, including preparatory acts for suicide and actual attempts
- Self-injurious behavior or injury
- Completed suicides
- Adverse events that might initially appear accidental or unrelated to SIB, but could potentially have suicidal/self-injurious intent (Overdose, Poisoning, Intoxication, Motor vehicle accidents, Cuts/lacerations, Burns, Gunshot injuries)
- Other Deaths (drowning, asphyxiation/suffocation, etc.)
- Potential SIB-related adverse events or other clinical observations may, based on the judgment of the investigator, trigger a narrative. Suicidal Ideation

Supplemental data to collect for a SIB narrative:

- Suicidal Ideation
  - *Passive* ideation ("wish to be dead"; thoughts of wanting to be dead without plan or intent)
  - *Nonspecific* suicidal thoughts (general thoughts of killing oneself without actual intent or plan)
  - *Active* suicidal ideation (thoughts of killing oneself with actual plan and intent)
- Suicidal Behavior
  - Were there any *preparatory* acts? (Steps toward suicide such as buying a gun, hoarding medications)
  - Was there an *actual attempt*? (Including attempts stopped by the subject or interrupted by someone else)
  - Was there evidence that the patient *intended* to die by his/her behaviors? (Putting affairs in order, giving away personal possessions, writing a note)
- Was there *self-injurious* behavior without suicidal intent? (e.g., manipulative gesture)
- Was the event or behavior due to an underlying psychiatric condition?

- Was the event or behavior due to an accident or underlying medical condition?
- If a Completed Suicide
  - How and where did the patient kill himself/herself?
  - How was the patient discovered and by whom?
  - Did the patient leave a note?
  - Did the patient make or relay active plans or preparations? Were there any warning signs?
  - Was a triggering event identified?
  - Did the patient overdose on study drug?
- Did the event occur in the context of any of the following: Symptoms of depression, mania, psychosis, Drug or alcohol abuse

Useful information to determine relevant risk factors:

- Social*/family stressors
- School/academic stressors (e.g., failing classes, lack of peer acceptance)
- Drug/alcohol use by subject
- Physical or sexual abuse
- Traumatic personal event—specify
- Depressed mood/despair/hopelessness
- Severe psychotic symptoms (e.g., command voices, guilt delusions)
- Comorbidity (physical or mental)
- (*Social stressors might include separation, bereavement, moving house, financial, legal, medical, unemployment, housing, dependents, workplace stress)
- Is there a history of *previous* suicidal ideation/plans or attempts?
- Previous suicidal ideation or plans
- Previous suicidal attempts or behaviors
- Is there a history of *previous* deliberate self-injurious behaviors
- Is there a family history of suicide ideation/plans/behaviors or completed suicide?
- Is there a family history of psychiatric illness, substance or alcohol abuse/ dependence?

Is there any previous psychiatric history in the subject and/or family not documented above?

3.6.1 Phase 1 Studies

The FDA Guidance (August 2012) specifies that in multiple dose inpatient Phase 1 studies, the SIB assessment should be completed at any visit where a symptom assessment (scheduled or unscheduled) is conducted, but is not necessary when non symptom assessments are performed (e.g., vital signs). For multiple dose studies with dosing periods longer than 1-week in duration, it is helpful to extend the SIB assessment to be administered at least weekly while the subject is being dosed. The SIB assessment can also be administered at the discretion of the investigator, based on any reasonable concern, at any time during the study.

According to the revised FDA Guidance (August 2012), it is no longer necessary to perform prospective SIB assessments in Phase 1 single dose trials in healthy volunteers or in microdose trials (i.e., using doses that are not expected to have a measurable pharmacological effect). However, SIB adverse events that are spontaneously reported in this category of trials should have additional information collected at the time the event is reported (see above narrative guide insets).

If a positive finding suggestive of SIB is detected in a Phase 1 study, an SIB risk assessment (by a qualified mental health professional) should be completed within a clinically reasonable timeframe as determined by the study principle investigator, taking into account the severity of the finding and subject history.

3.6.2 SIB Assessment in Phase 2/3 Blinded, Controlled Trials

This section will focus on the use of screening instruments to exclude or assess the baseline risk of subjects entering in psychiatric and neurologic clinical trials, and the detection of potential treatment emergent SIB. A number of scales in addition to the required C-SSRS assessment are often implemented by many companies conducting clinical studies. As the C-SSRS is a clinician-administered scale, it is often helpful to balance this with self-rated instruments or other instruments that assess psychiatric comorbidity also.

3.6.3 Selection and Screening Instruments: Psychiatric Trials

Studies of adult subjects with psychiatric indications are now expected to include the C-SSRS, and many companies also include a self-rated instrument such as the Suicidal Behaviors Questionnaire-Revised (SBQ-R; Osman et al. 2001) at the screening visit to detect possible SIB. In typical practice, a risk assessment is required by a qualified MHP to assess whether it is safe for the subject to participate in the trial if the subject's responses on any of the screening instruments indicate: (1) the subject may have had suicidal ideation associated with actual intent and a method or plan in the past year, (2) any history of suicidal behavior in the past 5 years, (3) any lifetime history of serious or recurrent SIB, (4) the subject meets criteria on the SBQ-R (i.e., total score ≥ 8), or (5) in the investigator's judgment a risk assessment is required. (The recommended look-back period for suicidal behavior is 5 years; however, a longer look-back period may need to be used dependent on the patient population or indication.)

A qualified MHP is a clinically-qualified MHP with appropriate training in the assessment of suicide risk, according to local clinical practice standards and regulations, who would normally evaluate the risk for SIB in a patient. In the United States, in addition to psychiatrists (board certified or board eligible), clinically qualified MHPs include the following: (1) Psy. D. or Ph.D. level Clinical Psychologists, (2) licensed Master's level Clinical Social Workers (LCSW), or (3) licensed Psychiatric Nurse Practitioners (PNP), who have specific training and experience in the assessment and management of acutely suicidal patients. The qualification of MHPs has been the subject of previous regulatory scrutiny of clinical trial conduct, and therefore these details are critically important to the quality of data obtained in such clinical trials.

3.7 Selection and Screening Assessments for Adult Patients (Neurologic Indications)

Studies in adult subjects with neurologic indications (epilepsy, neuropathy, stroke, etc.) are expected to include the C-SSRS, and other instruments such as the Suicidal Behaviors Questionnaire Revised (SBQ-R), and the Patient Health Questionnaire-8 (PHQ-8; Kroenke and Spitzer 2002) are helpful at the screening visit to detect possible SIB and depression. Subjects may either be excluded or have a risk assessment done by a qualified MHP to assess whether it is safe for them to participate in the trial if the subject's responses on any of the screening instruments or other screening information indicate:

- Suicidal ideation associated with actual intent and a method or plan in the past year: "Yes" answers on items 4 or 5 of the C-SSRS.
- Previous history of suicidal behaviors in the past 5 years: "Yes" answer (for events that occurred in the past 5 years) to any of the suicidal behavior items of the C-SSRS.
- Any lifetime history of serious or recurrent suicidal behavior. [Non-suicidal self-injurious behavior is not a trigger for a risk assessment unless in the investigator's judgement it is indicated.]
- SBQ-R total score ≥ 8.
- Clinically significant depression: PHQ-8 when the total score ≥ 15.
- The presence of any current major psychiatric disorder that is not explicitly permitted in the inclusion/exclusion criteria.
- In the investigator's judgment a risk assessment or exclusion is required.

3.8 Detection of Emergent SIB During the Course of Clinical Trials (Psychiatric and Neurologic Indications)

Studies of adult subjects in psychiatric and neurologic indications typically include the C-SSRS at every visit to detect possible SIB. At the baseline (randomization) visit, if there are "yes" answers on items 4, 5, or on any behavioral question of the C-SSRS, a risk assessment should be done prior to randomization by a qualified MHP to determine whether it is safe for the subject to continue to participate in the trial. At post-baseline visits, if there are "yes" answers on items 4, 5, or on any behavioral question of the C-SSRS, a risk assessment by a qualified MHP should be done to determine whether it is safe for the subject to continue to participate in the trial.

Subjects who answer "yes" on items 4, 5, or on any behavioral question of the C-SSRS *on more than one occasion* during a trial should either have their SIB managed appropriately by the Principal Investigator (PI) together with a qualified MHP (or the PI alone if the PI is a qualified MHP), or be discontinued from the trial, depending on the specifics of the subject and the trial. Studies that allow for the possibility of subjects with recurrent SIB of this severity to continue to participate in the trial must provide guidance on how to manage SIB of this severity in the study protocol. One example of how to operationalize the National Institute of Mental Health (NIMH) guidance on managing suicidal subjects in clinical trials has been published (Nierenberg et al. 2004). When there is a positive response to any question on the C-SSRS, the PI should determine whether an adverse event has occurred. Data collected from SIB assessments such as the C-SSRS directly map to the 11 categories the FDA has adopted in the August 2012 guidance for classifying SIB events.

3.9 Special Population Considerations

Populations that require special consideration include children and adolescents, the elderly, cognitively impaired subjects, and subjects with illnesses associated with significant mortality (e.g., oncology trials shortly after first diagnosis or following relapse). For cognitively impaired subjects and children, involvement of a third party (e.g., proxy) to assist with completion of SIB assessments can often be useful and may be necessary.

3.9.1 SIB Assessment in the Elderly (>65 Years)

Elderly subjects and subjects with illnesses associated with significant mortality may think about death or dying in an adaptive way (Bartels et al. 2002; Szanto et al.

2003). This is often termed "death ideation" and is different from suicidal ideation. As such, evaluation of SIB in the elderly requires the clinician to distinguish bereavement and end of life ruminations from suicidal ideation. In addition, research clinical trials enrolling the elderly should have clearly articulated inclusion/exclusion criteria with respect to SIB and psychopathology, which may increase suicide risk.

As with other studies in adults for psychiatric (non-dementia) indications, studies of elderly subjects in psychiatric indications should include at the screening visit the C-SSRS and include a self-administered scale such as the SBQ-R. In neurologic indications, the PHQ-8 is helpful to detect possible depression. A risk assessment should be done by a MHP skilled in the evaluation of SIB in the elderly by virtue of training or experience (e.g., psychiatrist, geriatric psychiatrist/licensed clinical psychologist, geriatrician or neurologist, social worker or psychiatric nurse practitioner) to determine whether it is safe for the subject to participate in the trial in the same way as for other adult patient. Treatment emergent SIB should be assessed using the C-SSRS at every visit throughout the study.

3.9.2 Patients with Alzheimer's Disease or Mild Cognitive Impairment

In the FDA's revised draft guidance, August 2012, the inclusion of prospective SIB assessments in studies of patients with Mild Cognitive Impairment and in studies of patients with mild to moderate Alzheimer's Disease (or other dementia) are recommended. In subjects with a diagnosis of Mild Cognitive Impairment, involvement of a third party (e.g., proxy) to assist with completion of SIB assessments may be required, depending on the severity of cognitive impairment. In subjects with a diagnosis of Alzheimer's disease, the assessments should not depend solely upon patient self-report, but should systematically utilize information provided by third parties such as spouses, caregivers, or the patient's medical providers.

The 2012 version of the FDA guidance indicates that prospective SIB assessments in studies of patients with advance cognitive impairment such as severe Alzheimer's Disease may be omitted under some circumstances, although FDA needs to be consulted prior to the finalization of the study protocol.

In addition to the C-SSRS, studies of subjects with MCI or mild to moderate Alzheimer's Disease should include additional tools at the screening visit such as the SBQ-R and the Cornell Scale for Depression in Dementias (CSDD; Alexopoulos et al. 1988) or the Neuropsychiatric Inventory (NPI; Cummings et al. 1994; Cummings 1997) Depression/dysphoria domain to detect possible SIB and depression, respectively (Kaufer et al. 1998; Wood et al. 1999). Selected additional questions from the NPI may be added to assist in identifying the behavioral aspects of dementia. (It should be noted that the NPI Depression/dysphoria domain is not an adequate substitute for the CSDD as a screen for DSM-IV Major Depressive Disorder in AD.)

Special considerations for risk assessment, above and beyond those mentioned above, include the endorsement of clinically significant depression as determined by the scores on the CSDD or the NPI Depression/dysphoria domain with additional optional information provided by other items of the NPI (e.g., Agitation/Aggression, Apathy/Indifference, Irritability/Lability).

Although the C-SSRS is widely used in studies of patients with MCI, Alzheimer's Disease, and other dementias, it has not been specifically validated for the prospective assessment of SIB in elderly or cognitively impaired patients nor does it have scope for caregiver input. Integration of information from third parties (spouses, caregivers, medical providers) essential in this patient group, but there have been no systematic studies on:

- The best method of obtaining third party input to SIB assessments,
- Who is qualified to provide third party input
- At what level of cognitive impairment third party input is necessary
- How discrepancies between patient and caregiver input should be reconciled

Additional challenges in assessing SIB in patients with dementia include:

- the tendency of elderly to minimize symptoms of depression,
- the reluctance of many elderly to speak directly about thoughts of suicide
- the risk of confounding age appropriate "death ideations" with passive suicidal ideation
- interview burden in patients with physical limitations (visual and hearing problems, motor impairments)
- complicated by progressive cognitive and functional decline associated with dementia.

3.9.3 Children and Adolescent Patients

Studies of adolescent subjects (age 12–17) in psychiatric indications that do not involve cognitive impairment (as in the case of mental retardation or autism) should include the adult version of C-SSRS at the screening visit. Additional validated scales such as the SBQ-R or the Suicidal Ideation Questionnaire (SIQ; Reynolds 1987) or SIQ-junior (SIQ-JR; Reynolds and Mazza 1999) should also be considered to enhance the screening for subjects at risk. The use of alternative instruments to the C-SSRS would have to be discussed and agreed upon with the FDA *prior* to study start. If the SIQ/SIQ-JR is chosen, the SIQ should be used for subjects aged 15–17, while the SIQ-JR should be used for subjects aged 12–14. The risk assessment for participation in the study needs to take into account not only the C-SSRS answers, but also scores on the SBQ-R and/or suicide specific items on the SIQ/SIQ-JR. For non-psychiatric indications, the Quick Inventory of Depressive Symptomatology—Self-report (QIDS-SR; Rush et al. 2003) should also be administered to screen for depression at the screening visit.

The risk assessment must be done by a clinically qualified child and adolescent mental health provider (MHP). In the United States, in addition to Child and Adolescent Psychiatrists (board certified or board eligible), clinically qualified MHPs include the following: (1) general psychiatrists, (2) Psy. D. or Ph.D. level Clinical Psychologists, (3) LCSW, or (4) PNP who have training and experience in the diagnosis and treatment of children and adolescents with psychiatric disorders. In other countries, the risk assessment should be done by a clinically-qualified MHP who would normally evaluate the risk of suicide in children and adolescents, according to local clinical practice standards and regulations.

Studies of adolescents (age 12–17) in psychiatric and neurologic indications should use the adult version of the C-SSRS at every post-screening visit to detect possible SIB as described above for adult psychiatric and neurologic indications.

There are challenges in using the C-SSRS in this population, given the limited psychometric data available. While the C-SSRS has been validated in adolescents aged 12–17, no psychometric data is available for any version of the instrument in children <12 years of age. In addition, there have been no studies of the validity and reliability of the pediatric version of the C-SSRS. The pediatric version for children 6–11 years of age has age appropriate probes (see the children's baseline screening assessment on the C-SSRS website at http://www.cssrs.columbia.edu/documents/C-SSRS6-23-10-ChildrenBaselineScreening.pdf). There is general guidance on how best to conduct joint interviews of the child and parent, but only limited specific guidance on how to do this in children of different ages and developmental stages, which can be a complication in clinical trials in this patient group. The instrument has been simplified for use in this age group, with the intensity subscale (with the exception of frequency) omitted in this age group. The lethality section needs to be addressed by a parent if the subject is younger than 13 years old.

The revised draft FDA guidance (August 2012) acknowledges that assessment of suicidal thoughts and behavior in young children is challenging since they are not at a point of cognitive development that allows for an understanding of the concept of death. In such cases, it is recommended to discuss potential options, including a waiver, directly with the FDA. In studies of children age ≤11 years and in children and/or adolescents with disorders involving cognitive impairment (e.g., mental retardation or autism), the use of specific scales needs to be customized appropriately.

3.10 Special Considerations for Use of the C-SSRS: Look-Back Period

The revised 2012 FDA Draft Guidance (2012) states that the C-SSRS "is conducted at baseline (this would be a lifetime SIB assessment) and at each patient visit." Use of a lifetime assessment for the purpose of determining treatment emergence or between group differences could be very problematic in certain patient populations (e.g., lifetime assessments in elderly subjects might artificially inflate the baseline).

Table 3.4 Recommended look-back periods for SIB assessments

Visit	Look-back period	Purpose
Screen	Lifetime[a]	Provides lifetime SIB history; meets FDA recommendations and, per this guidance, for determination if a risk assessment should be obtained in children and adolescents before subject can be randomized
Screen	1 year active suicidal ideation; 5 years suicidal behaviors	Per this guidance, for determination if a risk assessment should be obtained before subject can be randomized
Baseline	Since last visit (screen)	Detect emergence of SIB since screen visit
Baseline	1 month active suicidal ideation; 3 months suicidal behaviors	Provides recent history of SIB to be used in determining treatment emergence

[a] In children and adolescents, the lifetime look-back should be used to determine if a risk assessment is required prior to enrolment of the subject

There is ongoing debate over what is the most relevant look-back period for measuring baseline SIB status (Table 3.4).

The definition of the baseline look-back period can significantly impact ability to detect both treatment emergent SIB adverse events (worsening) and beneficial effects of treatment (improvement). Longer look-back periods (as in lifetime assessments) may inflate baseline rates of suicidal ideation or suicidal behavior, particularly in the elderly or in conditions with high background rates of SIB. In addition, a longer look-back period may capture SIB events that are remote from the time of the study and not relevant for determination of current status and are sensitive to recall bias or selective recall. In addition, look-back periods used in study exclusion criteria need to be selected with care to avoid overlapping of the exclusion look-back period with the baseline look-back period, which could lower baseline rates.

Currently, clinical trials methodologists (Gassman-Meyer et al. 2011) recommend the approach of obtaining a more recent SIB history for the purpose of determining treatment emergence (i.e., 1 month look-back from the Baseline Visit for active suicidal ideation and a 3 months look-back for suicidal behaviors). A summary of the recommended look-back periods for SIB assessments at the Screening Visit and at the Baseline Visit is provided in the following table. Different baseline look-back periods may have greater pertinence depending on the patient population and indication under study.

Post-baseline SIB can be displayed without regard to recent history, or as treatment emergent, new onset, or worsening relative to recent history. In general, the recommended look-back period for recent history is 1 month for suicidal ideation and 3 months for suicidal behavior. Any incident of reported post-baseline SIB is typically defined as a new onset if the subject reported no ideation and no behavior during the recent history period. Treatment emergent SIB includes both new onset and worsening. Worsening of existing SIB is defined as movement to a higher numbered C-CASA ideation category than was reported during the recent history period. A subject who reports on-study behavior is considered to have worsened provided no behavior was reported during recent history, regardless of reported ideation during recent history. On-study movement to a lower number behavior category is considered worsening.

3.11 Special Considerations for Use of the C-SSRS: Analysis

One of the critical unresolved questions and issue with the 2012 revised FDA Draft Guidance (2012) on SIB remains the lack of detailed guidance on statistical analysis of SIB clinical trial data. In particular, how analysis might be impacted by the use of "expanded" C-CASA, which increases the multiplicity of categories.

There are no formal analysis recommendations for C-SSRS and C-CASA data, however, there are precedented formats for data presentation. No formal statistical hypothesis testing is recommended for individual studies as only few events are typically observed, and a listing of the events or descriptive summary statistics will often suffice. Exceptions may occur with large trials or trials in which an "enriched" population is under investigation. If statistical analyses are to be performed, then exact estimation (and testing) methods should be considered.

Subject listings of both expanded C-CASA categories as well as the underlying scale data are helpful. In addition, a summary table of C-CASA categories for life-time, recent history, and post-baseline should be considered. Alternately, C-CASA summaries may be displayed by visit. Tabulation of new onset, worsening, and/or treatment emergent SIB relative to recent history is also helpful to assess treatment emergent SIB risk in selected populations, such as schizophrenia or depression, where there could be a sufficient number of events for meaningful interpretation.

It is important to exercise caution when pooling data across studies and to account for variability associated with methods of data collection (retrospective vs. prospective, different prospective SIB scales, etc.), as well as varying patient populations, extent of exposure, and cultural norms.

There is not one standard analysis as yet and the most appropriate analyses for any given program will depend on the population and compound under study. Sufficient analyses need to be conducted to characterize the level of SIB present in the clinical trial database.

The primary focus of analyses of program level data is to accurately estimate the rates of SIB in the treated and the placebo groups. There are several analysis methods available for the evaluation of SIB at the program level, including the examples highlighted below:

- Odds Ratio (OR)
- Incidence Rate
- Exposure Adjusted Incidence Rate
- Time-to-Event Analyses
- Sensitivity Analysis Methods to corroborate findings or assumptions

3.12 Conclusion

Despite the absence of specific analysis guidance by regulatory agencies, the prospective assessment of SIB in industry sponsored trials is now standard practice. With the growing use of the prospective tools, there are a number of emerging issues that have been encountered, including the specific challenges mentioned above. In addition, there are emerging data on the psychometric qualities of SIB assessments currently being used in clinical trials that warrant further study and the growth of trials in challenging and vulnerable patient groups (i.e., dementia, young children, and children and adolescents with autism) now means that valid assessment methods are of increasing priority. SIB assessment in these patient populations may require a range of different tools and approaches, which can be adapted to their changing cognitive and functional status. An additional challenge is the need for guidance on the best method to obtain and integration of third party input for such patient populations also. There also continue to be questions about the selection and training of raters, and this can become not only a regulatory quality issue, but also one of importance to clinical quality when conducting large, global clinical trials.

Acknowledgements The authors would like to acknowledge additional members of the Suicidal Ideation and Behavior Working Group [Michelle Stewart, Sarah Dubrava, Donna Palumbo, Susan Anway, Nathan Chen, Brendon Binneman, Keri Cannon, Deborah Light and Douglas Kalunian (now at Group Health Permanente), Douglas Feltner (now at AbbVie)] for their contributions to internal and cross-industry guidance on SIB assessment in clinical trials.

References

Alexopoulos GA, Abrams RC, Young RC, Shamoian CA (1988) Cornell Scale for depression in Dementia. Biol Psychiatry 23:271–284

Andersohn F, Schade R, Willich SN, Garge E (2010) Use of antiepileptic drugs in epilepsy and the risk of self-harm or suicidal behavior. Neurology 75:335–340

Arana A, Wentworth CE, Ayuso-Mateos JL, Arellano FM (2010) Suicide-related events in patients treated with antiepileptic drugs. N Engl J Med 363:542–551

Bartels SJ, Coakley E, Oxman TE, Constantino G, Oslin D, Chen H, Zubritsky C, Cheal K, Durai UN, Gallo JJ, Llorente M, Sanchez H (2002) Suicidal and death ideation in older primary care patients with depression, anxiety and at-risk alcohol use. Am J Geriatric Psychiatry 10:417–427

Brent DA, Mann JJ (2005) Family genetic studies, suicide, and suicidal behavior. Am J Med Genet C 133:13–24

Brent D, Melhem N, Turecki G (2010) Pharmacogenomics of suicidal events. Pharmacogenomics 11:793–807

Cavanagh JT, Carson AJ, Sharpe M, Lawrie SM (2003) Psychological autopsy studies of suicide: a systematic review. Psychol Med 33(3):395–405

Cummings JL, Mega M, Gray K, Rosenberg-Thompson S, Carusi DA, Gornbein J (1994) The Neuropsychiatric Inventory: comprehensive assessment of psychopathology in dementia. Neurology 44(12):2308–2314

Cummings JL (1997) The Neuropsychiatric Inventory: assessing psychopathology in dementia patients. Neurology 48(5 Suppl 6):S10–S16

FDA (2008) Statistical review and evaluation: anti-epileptic drugs and suicidality. http://www.fda.gov/ohrms/dockets/ac/08/briefing/2008-4372b1-01-FDA.pdf

Fergusson D, Doucette S, Glass KC, Shapiro S, Healy D, Hebert P, Hutton B (2005) Association between suicide attempts and selective serotonin reuptake inhibitors; systematic review of randomised controlled trials. BMJ 330(7488):396

Fergusson DM, Woodward IJ, Horwood IJ (2000) Risk factors and life processes associated with the onset of suicidal behavior during adolescence and early adulthood. Psychol Med 30 (1):23–29

Gassman-Meyer C, Jiang K, McSorley P, Arani R, DuBrava S, Suryawanshi S, Webb DM, Nilsson M (2011) Clinical and statistical assessment of suicidal ideation and behavior in pharmaceutical trials. Clin Pharmacol Therapeutics 90(4):554–560

Gibbons RD, Brown CH, Hur K, Marcus SM, Bhaumik DK, Erkens JA, Herings RM, Mann JJ (2007) Early evidence of the effects of regulators' suicidality warnings on SSRI prescriptions and suicide in children and adolescents. Am J Psychiatry 164(9):1356–1363

Gibbons RD, Hur K, Brown CH, Mann JJ (2009) Relationship between antiepileptic drugs and suicide attempts in patients with bipolar disorder. Arch Gen Psychiatry 66:1354–1360

Gibbons RD, Hur K, Bhaumik DK, Mann JJ (2006) The relationship between antidepressant prescription rates and rate of early adolescent suicide. Am J Psychiatry 163(11):1898–1904

Goodwin F, Jamison K (2007) Manic–depressive illness: Bipolar disorders and recurrent depression. 2nd edn. Oxford University Press, Oxford, England

Hammad TA, Laughren T, Racoosin J (2006) Suicidality in pediatric patients treated with antidepressant drugs. Arch Gen Psychiatry 63(3):332–339

Institute of Medicine (IOM) (2010) CNS clinical trials: suicidality and data collection. In: Workshop summary. The National Academies Press, Washington DC

Kaufer DI, Cummings JL, Christine D, Bray T, Castellon S, Masterman D, MacMillan A, Ketchel P, Dekosky ST (1998) Assessing the impact of neuropsychiatric symptoms in Alzheimer's Disease: the neuropsychiatric inventory caregiver distress scale. J Am Geriatric Soc 46:210–215

Kroenke K, Spitzer RL (2002) The PHQ-9: a new depression diagnostic and severity measure. Psychiatric Ann 32:509–515

Laje G, Allen AS, Akula N, Manji H, John Rush A, McMahon FJ (2009) Genome-wide association study of suicidal ideation emerging during citalopram treatment of depressed outpatients. Pharmacogenet Genomics 19:666–674

Libby AM, Orton HD, Valuck RJ (2009) Persisting decline in depression treatment after FDA warnings. Arch Gen Psychiatry 66:633–639

Medicines and Healthcare Products Regulatory Agency (2003) Selective serotonin reuptake inhibitor—use in children and adolescents with major depressive disorder. http://www.mhra.gov.uk/home/groups/pl-p/documents/websiteresources/con019492.pdf

Menke A, Domschke K, Czamara D, Klengel T, Hennings J, Lucae S, Baune BT, Arolt V, Muller-Myschok B, Holsboer F, Binder EB (2012) Genome-wide association study of antidepressant treatment-emergent suicidal ideation. Neuropsychopharmacology 37:797–807

Nierenberg AA, Trivedi MH, Ritz L, Burroughs D, Greist J, Sackeim H, Kornstein S, Schwartz T, Stegman D, Fava M, Wisniewski SR (2004) Suicide risk management for the sequenced treatment alternatives to relieve depression study: applied NIMH guidelines. J Psychiatric Res 38(6):583–589

Nock MK, Hwang I, Sampson N, Kessler RC, Angermeyer M, Beautrais A, Borges G, Bromet E, Bruffaerts R, de Girolamo G, de Graaf R, Florescu S, Gureje O, Haro JM, Hu C, Huang Y, Karam EG, Kawakami N, Kovess V, Levinson D, Posada-Villa J, Sagar R, Tomov T, Viana MC, Williams DR (2009a) Cross-national analysis of the associations among mental disorders and suicidal behavior: Findings from the WHO world mental health surveys. PLoS Med 6(8): e1000123

Nock MK, Hwang I, Sampson NA, Kessler RC. (2009b). Mental disorders, comorbidity and suicidal behavior: Results from the National Comorbidity Survey Replication. *Mol Psychiatry* (31 March 2009)

Olesen JB, Hansen PR, Erdal J, Abildstrøm SZ, Weeke P, Fosbøl EL, Poulsen HE, Gilason GH (2010) Antiepileptic drugs and risk of suicide: a nationwide study. Pharmacoepidemiol. Drug Safety 19:518–524

Olfson M, Shaffer D, Marcus SC, Greenberg T (2003) Relationship between antidepressant medication treatment and suicide in adolescents. Arch Gen Psychiatry 60(10):978–982

Osman A, Bagge CL, Gutierrez PM, Konick LC, Kopper BA et al (2001) The suicidal behaviors questionnaire-revised (SBQ-R): validation with clinical and nonclinical samples. Assessment 8 (4):443–454

Patorno E, Bohn RL, Wahl PM, Avorn J, Patrick AR, Liu J, Schneeweiss S (2010) Anticonvulsant medications and the risk of suicide, attempted suicide or violent death. JAMA 303:1401–1409

Perroud N (2011) Suicidal ideation during antidepressant treatment: do genetic predictors exist? CNS Drugs 25:459–471

Perroud N, Uher R, Ng MY, Guipponi M, Hauser J, Henigsberg N et al (2012) Genome–wide association study of increasing suicidal ideation during antidepressant treatment in the GENDEP project. Pharmacogenomics 12(1):68–77

Pompili M, Baldessarini RJ (2010) Risk of suicidal behavior with antiepileptic drugs. Nature Rev Neurol 6:651–653

Pompili M, Tatarelli R (eds) (2010) Evidence-based practice in suicidology: a sourcebook. Hogrefe, Gottingen

Pompili M, Tatarelli R, Girardi P, Tondo L, Baldessarini RJ (2010) Suicide risk during anticonvulsant treatment. Pharmacoepidemiol Drug Safety 19:525–528

Posner K (2009) C-CASA and C-SSRS in CNS clinical trials: development and implementation. In: Presentation at the IOM workshop on CNS clinical trials: suicidality and data collection, Washington DC, June 16

Reynolds WM (1987) Suicidal ideation questionnaire (SIQ): professional manual. Psychological Assessment Resources, Odessa

Reynolds WM, Mazza JJ (1999) Assessment of suicidal ideation in inner-city children and young adolescents: reliability and validity of the suicidal ideation questionnaire-Jr. Sch Psychol Rev 28:17–30

Rush AJ, Trivedi MH, Ibrahim HM, Carmody TJ, Arnow B, Klein DN, Markowitz JC, Ninan PT, Kornstein S, Manber R, Thase ME, Kocsis JH, Keller MB (2003) The 16-item quick inventory of depressive symptomatology (QIDS), clinician rating (QIDS-C), and self-report (QIDS-SR): a psychometric evaluation in patients with chronic major depression. Biol Psychiatry 54:573–583

Sareen J, Cox BJ, Afifi TO, de Graaf R, Asmundson GJ, ten Have M, Stein MB (2005) Anxiety disorders and risk for suicidal ideation and suicide attempts: a population based longitudinal study of adults. Arch Gen Psychiatry 62(11):1249–1257

Simon GE (2006) How can we know whether antidepressants increase suicide risk? Am J Psychiatry 163(11):1861–1863

Sondergard I, Kvist K, Andersen PK, Kessing LV (2006) Do antidepressants precipitate youth suicide?: a nationwide pharmacoepidemiological study. Eur Child Adolesc Psychiatry 15 (4):232–240

Statham DJ, Heath AC, Madden PA, Buchholz KK, Bierut L, Dinwiddie SH, Martin NG (1998) Suicidal behaviour: an epidemiological and genetic study. Psychol Med 28:839–855

Stone M, Laughren T, Jones L, Levenson M, Holland PC, Hughes A, Hammad TA, Temple R, Rochester G (2009) Risk of suicidality in clinical trials of antidepressants in adults: analysis of proprietary data submitted to US food and drug administration. BMJ 339:b2880

Szanto K, Mulsant BH, Houck P, Drew MA, Reynolds CF 3rd (2003) Occurrence and course of suicidality during short-term Treatment of late-life depression. Arch Gen Psychiatry 60 (6):610–617

Valuck RJ, Libby AM, Orton HD, Morrato EH, Allen R, Baldessarini RJ (2007) Spillover effects on treatment of adult depression in primary care after FDA advisory on risk of pediatric suicidality with SSRI's. Am J Psychiatry 164(8):1198–1205

Van Cott AC, Cramer JA, Copeland LA, Zeber JE, Steinman MA, Dersh JJ, Glickman ME, Mortensen EM, Amuan ME, Pugh MJ (2010) Suicide-related behaviors in older patients with new anti-epileptic drug use: data from the VA hospital system. BMC Med 8:4–11

Wood S, Cummings JL, Hsu M-A, Barclay T, Wheatley MV, Yarema KT, Schnelle JE (1999) The use of the neuropsychiatric inventory in nursing home residents: characterization and measurement. Am J Geriatric Psychiatry 8:75–83

Chapter 4
From Uniform Definitions to Prediction of Risk: The Columbia Suicide Severity Rating Scale Approach to Suicide Risk Assessment

Kelly Posner, Randy Subramany, Leora Amira and J. John Mann

Abstract Suicide prevention is of high national and international importance as suicide remains one of the world's greatest public health crises. Identification is the key to prevention, and therefore the ideal suicide risk assessment instrument enables identification of high risk individuals, monitors for suicide risk factors, and predicts future suicidal behavior in both research and practice. However, research and clinical practice have been challenged by nomenclature and methodological limitations regarding assessment of suicidal ideation and behavior. Systematic assessment for suicidal risk is feasible and provides more reliable outcomes, establishes operationalized criteria, and specifies parameters for triggering referrals, thereby decreasing unnecessary referral and burden. Therefore, assessment of suicidal ideation and behavior should be routinely integrated across public health settings. Knowledge of the full range of suicidal ideation and behaviors and key criteria for differentiating suicidal and non-suicidal events is paramount to the advancement of suicide risk assessment. The Columbia Suicide Severity Rating Scale (C-SSRS), a brief, standardized research-supported risk assessment tool, identifies individuals at increased risk for suicide to lower the overall disease burden and potentially the numbers of unnecessary deaths.

K. Posner (✉)
Center for Suicide Risk Assessment, New York State Psychiatric Institute,
Columbia University College of Physicians and Surgeons, New York, USA
e-mail: posnerk@nyspi.columbia.edu

R. Subramany · L. Amira
Child and Adolescent Psychiatry, New York State Psychiatric Institute,
Columbia University, New York, NY, USA
e-mail: subrama@nyspi.columbia.edu

L. Amira
e-mail: amirale@nyspi.columbia.edu

J. John Mann
Department of Psychiatry, New York State Psychiatric Institute,
Columbia University, New York, NY, USA

K.E. Cannon and T.J. Hudzik (eds.), *Suicide: Phenomenology and Neurobiology*,
DOI 10.1007/978-3-319-09964-4_4

4.1 Introduction

Suicide is a global public health crisis and the magnitude of its global disease burden is under-recognized. In the US alone, an adult dies by suicide every 13 min (WISQARS 2011), yet, the public health impact and disease burden of suicide are under-recognized (Insel 2010). Nearly 10 % of high school students report having attempted suicide in the past year (Eaton et al. 2012). $141 billion in annual medical costs lost are incurred and millions of years of life globally, while in the US alone nonfatal suicide attempts cost $6 billion a year (WISQARS 2011). Identification of individuals at high risk is crucial for any prevention effort. However, identification and detection are hampered by failure to screen adequately or at all by critical gatekeepers (See Fawcett, this volume).

A report by the U.S. Institute of Medicine concluded that "research on suicide is plagued by many methodological problems…definitions lack uniformity…[and] reporting of suicide is inaccurate" (Goldsmith 2002). Diverse terminology for identical suicidal phenomena (O'Carroll et al. 1996; Posner et al. 2007) negatively impacts instrument validity and reliability and the utility of epidemiological statistics. Across all age groups, as many as 45 % of those who died by suicide have had contact with their primary care providers within one month prior to their death; 90 % of adolescents and 77 % across all age groups visit their primary care provider within one year of their death (Luoma et al. 2002; McCarty et al. 2011). Yet, fewer than 3 % of these visit records contain a comment about suicide risk (Appleby et al. 1996). Moreover, a large number of adolescent suicide attempters present to emergency departments for nonpsychiatric reasons and can be easily missed (King et al. 2009). An even lower percentage of those who die by suicide have contact with mental health professionals (e.g., 20–25 % of adolescents within a year of suicide (Gould et al. 2003). Predictably, only 19 % of primary care providers compared with 59 % of psychiatric practitioners knew about the suicidal intentions of their patients who died by suicide (Suominen et al. 2004).

The consistent use of a standardized instrument with clinically appropriate, specific, and comprehensive terminology can greatly enhance detection, monitoring, and prediction in the suicidal patient. The ideal suicide risk assessment instrument enables identification of high-risk individuals, ongoing monitoring of risk factors for suicide (i.e., suicidal ideation and behavior) and prediction of future suicidal behavior both in research and practice.

4.2 Suicide Risk Assessment

Importantly, traditional of assessing suicide risk, which include relying on open-ended questions, have been problematic. When instructed to ask two open-ended questions about suicide, clinicians tended to over-detect suicidal ideation and under-detect suicidal behavior in adolescent patients (Holi et al. 2008). Structured or semi-structured tools, on the other hand, improve detection in routine clinical assessments (Bongiovi-Garcia et al. 2009). In one study, the use of a structured questionnaire detected 29.7 % of patients with suicidal ideation and 18.7 % of patients with a history of a suicide attempt that were undetected by an open-ended clinician interview (Bongiovi-Garcia et al. 2009). Overall, evidence has shown that performing routine intakes identifies only 25 % of patients with a history of suicide attempt when compared to 100 % of patients identified through structured risk assessment instruments (Hawton 1987).

In a national emergency department study, a structured telephone follow-up using the Columbia-Suicide Severity Rating Scale (C-SSRS) improved detection (59 %) of suicide attempts by more than 40 % when compared to hospital chart reviews detection (18 %) (Arias et al. 2014). Furthermore, utilizing evidence-supported instruments facilitates clinical decision-making and fosters confidence in the determination of next steps for individuals identified with various levels of suicide risk. A scale with thresholds for clinical management streamlines interpretation of assessment results and when matched with triage protocols should result in more efficient use of mental health services and patient management during trials (Peñta and Caine 2006).

Therefore, a comprehensive and successful implementation of structured suicide risk assessment programs should include policies and protocols that allow for assessment, intervention, and monitoring (AIM). Evidence of such implementation is apparent in the policies of various institutions and settings. The New York State Office of Mental Health has developed a comprehensive systems approach to suicide prevention for all adult and youth behavioral health care organizations in which all patients are screened using the C-SSRS. Furthermore, C-SSRS and Safety Planning online learning modules are used in training all NYSOMH staff. Additionally, the National Action Alliance, in its commitment to a vision of zero suicide, now provides a suicide toolkit that contains training in the C-SSRS and safety planning intervention. Also, Georgia has begun a state-wide dissemination and linking of systems with the C-SSRS, in which providers are implementing the C-SSRS in all services, between services, and in systems of care.

4.3 Assessment of Suicidal Ideation and Behavior

The stress-diathesis model of suicidal behavior proposes that suicidal behavior may manifest through individual traits (e.g., impulsivity) that can be influenced by genetic and epigenetic effects on stress responses, mood regulation and decision-making. This array of traits is determined by genetic and early life experience resulting in a preexisting susceptibility or diathesis. The diathesis interacts with current stressors (e.g., psychosocial crisis or exacerbation of psychiatric illness) to create the risk of suicidal behavior (Mann et al. 2005; Oquendo et al. 2003; Mann 2003) (Nazem, this volume, Lopez-Castroman et al., this volume). Approximately 90 % of people who die by suicide have a diagnosable and treatable mental disorder

Suicidal Ideation

Passive suicidal ideation: wish to be dead

Patient has thoughts about a wish to be dead or not alive anymore, or wish to fall asleep and not wake up.

Active suicidal ideation: nonspecific (no method, intent, or plan)

General nonspecific thoughts of wanting to end one's life or commit suicide (e.g., "I've thought about killing myself") without general thoughts of ways to kill oneself/associated methods, intent, or plan during the assessment period.

Active suicidal ideation: method, but no intent or plan

Patient has thoughts of suicide and has thought of at least one method during the assessment period. This situation is different than a specific plan with time, place, or method details worked out (e.g., thought of method to kill self but not a specific plan). Includes person who would say, "I thought about taking an overdose but I never made a specific plan as to when, where, or how I would actually do it . . . and I would never go through with it."

Active suicidal ideation: method and intent, but no plan

Active suicidal thoughts of killing oneself, and patient reports having some intent to act on such thoughts, as opposed to "I have the thoughts but I definitely will not do anything about them."

Active suicidal ideation: method, intent, and plan

Thoughts of killing oneself with details of plan fully or partially worked out and patient has some intent to carry it out (i.e., some degree of intent is implicit in the concept of plan).

Suicidal Behavior

Suicide

A self-injurious behavior that resulted in fatality and was associated with at least some intent to die as a result of the act. Evidence that the individual intended to kill him- or herself, at least to some degree, can be explicit or inferred from the behavior or circumstance

Fig. 4.1 Suicidal ideation and behavior categories and definitions (FDA 2012)

at the time of death (Hjelmeland and Knizek 1999). Specifically, mood, substance use, impulse control, and personality disorders and schizophrenia spectrum disorders confer the highest risk (Turecki et al. 2012; Mann and Currier 2010; Jiménez et al. 2013; Dwivedi and Mann 2012; Baca-Garcia et al. 2010; Bennett 2013) (Fig. 4.1).

Suicidal ideation and a history of suicidal behavior are among the most salient short- and long-term risk factors for suicide (Beck et al. 1999; Brown et al. 2000; Kuo et al. 2001; Nordström et al. 1995). Many individuals die from their first suicide attempt (Isometsa 1998), which underscores the importance of assessing

Suicide attempt

A potentially self-injurious behavior, associated with at least some intent to die as a result of the act. Evidence that the individual intended to kill him - or herself, at least to some degree, can be explicit or inferred from the behavior or circumstance. A suicide attempt may or may not resultin actual injury.

Interrupted suicide attempt

When the person is interrupted (by an outside circumstance) from starting a potentially self-injurious act (if not for that, actual attempt would have occurred).

Aborted suicide attempt

When person begins to take steps toward making a suicide attempt, but stops before actually engaging in any self-destructive behavior. Examples are similar to interrupted attempts, except that the individual stops before being stopped by something else.

Preparatory acts

This category can include anything beyond a verbalization or thought, but it stops short of a suicide attempt, an interrupted suicide attempt, or an aborted suicide attempt. This might include behaviors related to assembling a specific method (e.g., buying pills, purchasing a gun) or preparing for one's death by suicide (e.g., giving things away, writing a suicide note).

Self-Injurious Behavior Without Suicidal Intent

Self-injurious behavior associated with no intent to die. The behavior is intended purely for other reasons, either to relieve distress (often referred to as *self-mutilation* (e.g. superficial cuts or scratches, hitting or banging, or burns)) or to effect change in others or the environment.

Fig. 4.1 (continued)

risk for this before people make that first suicide attempt. The terminology of suicidal outcomes has historically been diverse, inconsistent and ambiguous (O'Carroll et al. 1996; Posner et al. 2007). Terms that carry value judgments such as "failed attempt," "suicide gesture," "manipulative act", "parasuicide", "deliberate self-harm" and "suicide threat" (Crosby et al. 2011) obscure appropriate identification, and ambiguity and diversity in definitions may result in both over- and under-identification of high-risk individuals. In an effort to establish a meaningful common language for suicidal behavior, the United States Centers for Disease Control (CDC) has adopted terminology developed by a group of Columbia University suicidologists and recommends a standardized scale, the C-SSRS, to elicit the required information from respondents. The C-SSRS distinguishes between the following suicidal behaviors: (a) suicide, (b) suicide attempt, (c) interrupted attempt,

Uniform Definitions

Definitions

Self-directed violence (analogous to self-injurious behavior)

Behavior that is self-directed and deliberately results in injury or the potential for injury to oneself.

This does not include behaviors such as parachuting, gambling, substance abuse, tobacco use or other risk taking activities, such as excessive speeding in motor vehicles. These are complex behaviors some of which are risk factors for SDV but are defined as behavior that while likely to be life-threatening is not recognized by the individual as behavior intended to destroy or injure the self. (Farberow, N. L. (Ed) (1980). The Many Faces of Suicide. New York: McGraw-Hill Book Company). These behaviors may have a high probability of injury or death as an outcome but the injury or death is usually considered unintentional. Hanzlick R, Hunsaker JC, Davis GJ. *Guide for Manner of Death Classification*. National Association of Medical Examiners. Available at: http://www.charlydmiller.com/LIB03/2002NAMEmannerofdeath.pdf. Accessed 1 Sept 2009.

Self-directed violence is categorized into the following

Non-suicidal (as defined below)

Suicidal (as defined below).

Non-suicidal self-directed violence

Behavior that is self-directed and deliberately results in injury or the potential for injury to oneself.

There is no evidence, whether implicit or explicit, of suicidal intent. Please see appendix for definition of implicit and explicit.

Suicidal self-directed violence

Behavior that is self-directed and deliberately results in injury or the potential for injury to oneself.

There is evidence, whether implicit or explicit, of suicidal intent.

Undetermined self-directed violence

Behavior that is self-directed and deliberately results in injury or the potential for injury to oneself.

Suicidal intent is unclear based on the available evidence.

Suicide attempt

A non-fatal self-directed potentially injurious behavior with any intent to die as a result of the behavior.

A suicide attempt may or may not result in injury.

Interrupted self-directed violence – by self or by other

By other - A person takes steps to injure self but is stopped by another person prior to fatal injury. The interruption can occur at any point during the act such as after the initial thought or after onset of behavior.

By self (in other documents may be termed "aborted" suicidal behavior) - A person takes steps to injure self but is stopped by self prior to fatal injury.

Source: Posner K, Oquendo MA, Gould M, Stanley B, Davies M. Columbia Classification Algorithm of Suicide Assessment (C-CASA): Classification of Suicidal Events in the FDA's Pediatric Suicidal Risk Analysis of Antidepressants. Am J Psychiatry 2007; 164:1035-1043. http://cssrs.columbia.edu/

SELF-DIRECTED VIOLENCE SURVEILLANCE: UNIFORM DEFINITIONS AND RECOMMENDED DATA ELEMENTS 21

Fig. 4.2 CDC and Columbia uniform definitions

(d) self-interrupted/aborted attempt, and (e) preparatory acts or behavior (Crosby et al. 2011) (Fig. 4.2). The U.S. Food and Drug Administration (FDA) adopted the C-SSRS categories of both behavior and the five subtypes of suicidal ideation, for the systematic, prospective monitoring of suicidal occurrences in clinical trials (See http://www.cssrs.columbia.edu). Self-injurious behavior without suicidal intent was also included in the list of outcomes in order to help distinguish suicide attempts from non-suicidal self-injurious behavior. These 11 categories are the FDA standard used for the detection of pre-existing risk and treatment-emergent suicidal ideation and behavior in all clinical trials involving drugs with central nervous system (CNS) activity (Food and Drug Administration 2012) (Fig. 4.1). Once one is assessing patients for treatment-emergent suicidal ideation and behavior, then it is also possible to detect beneficial effects of medications on ideation and behavior.

Suicide risk assessment instruments should aim to delineate suicidal ideation and behavior categories and their severity for more accurate determination of suicide risk. The following elements in a suicide risk assessment instrument are critical for the identification of high-risk individuals: a full range of suicidal behaviors and suicidal ideation.

4.3.1 The Full Range of Suicidal Behaviors

Historically a suicide risk assessments or screening queried solely about lifetime or recent suicide attempts, which resulted in the omission of other types of significant suicidal behaviors. Behaviors in which steps are taken imminently before a suicide attempt or suicide would have otherwise occurred (e.g., putting a noose around one's neck and changing one's mind, being rescued by another before running in front of traffic) and behaviors in preparation of suicide (e.g., buying a knife, collecting pills, writing a suicide note) are important subtypes of suicidal behavior that often go undetected by clinicians and gate keepers. This was confirmed in a 3,776 patient sample, in which attempts comprised only 13 % of reported suicidal behaviors, while the remaining 87 % consisted of the other three types (Mundt et al. 2011). While these events were rare (approximately one percent of 35,000 assessments), it is critical to more appropriately identify high-risk individuals. This is evidenced by the fact that, over a short-term follow-up, these other lifetime behaviors significantly predicted subsequent suicidal behavior, with all behaviors being similarly predictive. Furthermore, the total number of different suicidal behaviors increased risk (Posner 2012).

While a history of a suicide attempt is the most consistent predictor of future suicide attempts or death by suicide (Brown et al. 2000; Fawcett et al. 1990; Harris and Barraclough 1997; Malone 1995; Steer et al. 1988). Other categories of suicidal behavior also predict the risk of future suicide attempts including interrupted and aborted attempts and preparatory activities (Mundt et al. 2013). Finally, the most severe lifetime suicidal ideation predicts the risk for suicide.

Importantly, interrupted attempt, self-interrupted/aborted attempt, or preparatory acts or behavior constitute the majority of suicidal behaviors engaged in by high-risk individuals (Mundt et al. 2011) and are salient risk factors for suicide or suicide attempt, with similar risk ratios (Steer et al. 1988; Barber et al. 1998; Marzuk et al. 1997; Beck et al. 1999). Lastly, ideation is also a significant risk factor: the most severe lifetime suicidal ideation is a significant predictor for future suicide. Thus, it is critical that the full range of suicidal behaviors and ideation is assessed.

4.3.2 Intent to Die

With a history of a suicide attempt being the number one risk factor for future attempts or death by suicide, improved identification of past behavior is essential. Identification, in turn, critically hinges on the clear and accurate distinction between suicidal and non-suicidal behavior. Suicidal behavior is any type of self-injurious behavior (Crosby 2010), carried out with some intent to die. A critical criterion of suicidal behavior for its distinction from nonsuicidal self-injurious behavior is the presence of intent to die. Intent to die requires the desire to bring about one's own death and is distinct from the motivations for desiring such an outcome (Hjelmeland and Knizek 1999). Such behavior is considered suicidal irrespective of the motivations surrounding the behavior, which are often affective in nature, such as ending emotional pain. A self-injurious behavior is suicidal if it is a result of any intent to die, and is strictly non-suicidal if it is not a result of any intent to die. Thus, the same behavior across individuals may be classified as suicidal or nonsuicidal depending solely on the presence or absence of intent to die. Intent to die need not be stated directly by the individual but may be inferred from additional facts such as high potential lethality of behavior (De Leo et al. 2004; Posner et al. 2011), the individuals' perception of a behavior's high potential lethality (Beck and Greenberg 1971), or additional data from informants (O'Carrol 1989) or medical records (Posner et al. 2007).

4.3.3 Distinction of Suicidal Ideation and Behavior

The prognosis and outcome of suicidal ideation and behavior are different. Suicide attempts are both less common and more closely related to suicide as an outcome. A widely used term "suicidality", conflates ideation and behavior and FDA has recommended to discontinue its use. Distinct, non-overlapping definitions of suicidal ideation and suicidal behavior are critical for accurate assessment of prior ideation and behavior as predictors of future risk and for prospective detection of suicidal phenomena in the context of treatment. In a large multi-trial study lifetime severe suicidal ideation with at least some intent to die was associated with a five-fold increase in the risk of suicidal behavior on trial and a lifetime history of suicidal behavior without severe ideation was associated with a four-fold increase in risk of on trial behavior. Importantly, patients with a history of severe ideation and behavior were nine times more likely to have behavior during trial (Mundt et al. 2013). In an adolescent emergency department follow-up study, ideation was predictive of subsequent suicidal behavior even when a history of attempts was not predictive, reinforcing the need to identify suicidal ideation.

In general, the extant literature suggests separation of ideation and behavior because: (1) suicidal ideation and behavior do not always co-occur (Fawcett 1992), (2) gene variants associated with treatment-emergent suicidal ideation in clinical treatment trials of SSRIs appear to be unrelated to genes primarily associated with suicidal behavior (Laje et al. 2007; Meyer et al. 2010; Perlis et al. 2007; Perroud et al. 2009), (3) suicidal ideation is predictive of or a precursor to suicidal behavior (Posner et al. 2011; Kessler et al. 1999), and (4) ideation and behavior might be more predictive of suicide depending on other factors such as age (Brent et al. 1993; Fergusson et al. 2005; Lewinsohn et al. 1994; Pfeffer et al. 1993; Wichstrom 2000; Brown et al. 2000; Conwell and Thompson 2008; Vannoy et al. 2007; King et al. 2012). Moreover, suicidal ideation may add incremental validity to the prediction of future suicide attempts relative to a history of past suicide attempts alone (Horwitz et al. 2014). Treatment may affect risk of ideation without affecting risk of nonfatal suicide attempts or suicide. These findings confirm the importance of assessing suicidal ideation independently of suicidal behavior.

4.3.4 Suicidal Ideation

Suicidal ideation is a heterogeneous construct. The National Institute of Mental Health (NIMH) Developing Centers for Intervention and Prevention of Suicide specified that wish to die, thoughts of killing oneself, and intent to kill oneself constitute types of suicidal ideation (Brown et al. 2008). Suicidal ideation may be passive (i.e., having a wish to die as opposed to thoughts of killing one self) or active, which can range from range from non-specific thoughts of killing oneself to thoughts with a specific method or plan for killing (Brown et al. 2008). The distinction of passive and active suicidal ideation was first described by Beck et al. (1979) to separate thoughts of desiring one's own death from thoughts of actively killing oneself (Beck et al. 1979). Intent to act demarcates the difference between thoughts of a suicide attempt where the person feels sure they would never act and where they believe they could act on those thoughts of killing themselves. A more severe stage is when the thoughts have a compulsive, or hard to resist quality, and the person may describe a struggle to resist the thoughts of suicide. The evidence base examining predictive properties of these ideation subtypes is growing (Mundt et al. 2013; Posner et al. 2011; Arias 2014; Hesdorffer et al. 2013; Katzan et al. 2013; Posner 2013) which was likely a result of the C-SSRS delineating ideation types more clearly.

4.3.5 Wish to Die

Thus, the PHQ-9 combines a large range of severity of suicidal ideation, blurring and eliminating the distinction between higher and lower risk ideation indicators, making the predictive value of this item poor.

Passive suicidal ideation includes any internal experience that indicates a wish or desire to die ("wish to die") and excludes thoughts of being better off dead, thoughts of one's own death, or that life is not worth living. This definition represents the consensus of the National Institute of Mental Health (NIMH) Developing Centers for Intervention and Prevention of Suicide conference (Brown et al. 2008). Evidence has shown that people with a high wish-to-die/wish-to-live index are six times more likely to die by suicide than those with lower indices (Brown et al. 2005). In turn, these research findings played a pivotal role in the development of the C-SSRS. Prior to this, assessment of suicidal ideation failed to distinguish true passive suicidal ideation (i.e., the wish to die) from other thoughts of death or dying that are not passive suicidal ideation and not predictive of future suicidal behavior. This historical muddling of definitions is evident in the Patient Health Questionnaire (PHQ-9), which spuriously equates thoughts of being "better off dead" with passive suicidal ideation, effectively eliminating the distinction between higher and lower risk indicators. Unsurprisingly, the predictive value of this item is poor. The observed point prevalence of suicidal ideation, behavior, or both was 6.2 % on the C-SSRS compared to 23.8 % on item 9 (the "suicide" item) on the PHQ-9 a nearly four-fold increase in false positive screens (Katzan el al. 2013). The Cleveland Clinic similarly compared the PHQ-9 suicide item to the electronic screening version of the C-SSRS, and found that the PHQ-9 yielded more than three times as many false positives as true positives (Katzan el al. 2013).

4.3.6 *Intent to Act*

Intent to act depends on the extent to which one is ready to act on thoughts of killing oneself. Suicidal thoughts without intent to act are characterized by having thoughts of killing oneself but not feeling that one might do anything about them. The distinction is clinically important because the presence of intent to act confers higher risk for subsequent suicidal behavior, as shown in a study of adolescent suicide attempters, where a lifetime history of severe ideation with at least some intent to die was associated with a 50 % increase in the risk of on-trial suicidal behavior (Posner et al. 2011; Currier et al. 2009).

4.3.7 *Intensity and Worst-Point Ideation*

In addition to types of suicidal thoughts, assessing their intensity and time frame is also very important. Although researchers and clinicians have assumed that one needs to query about current levels of ideation to identify risk, worst point lifetime ideation has been shown to be a better predictor of death by suicide (Beck et al. 1999). Unlike severity, ideation intensity is best seen as a continuous characteristic consisting of five dimensions: duration of thoughts, frequency of thoughts, controllability of thoughts, deterrents from acting on thoughts, and reasons for ideation. Duration of the most severe ideation predicts subsequent suicidal behavior among adolescents (King et al. 2012). In an adolescent emergency department follow-up study, it was demonstrated that duration of thoughts was predictive of subsequent suicidal behavior, while suicide attempts and lifetime attempts were not predictive, thus reinforcing the importance of ideation assessment (King et al. 2012). Significantly, all items on the C-SSRS intensity of ideation subscale (i.e., frequency, duration, controllability, deterrents, and reasons for ideation) were shown to be significantly predictive of suicide on Beck's SSI. Large trial data across multiple indications show that total score on ideation intensity incrementally is associated with a greater risk of suicidal behavior during trial, while minimal intensity of ideation was associated with a six-fold increase in the odds of suicidal behavior on-trial, very severe intensity was associated with a thirty-fold increase in risk (OR=34.39; 95 % CI: 9.23-128.09) (Posner 2014).

4.4 Instruments: Utility and Feasibility

Utilizing an evidence-based and research-supported instrument, such as the C-SSRS, for risk assessment can minimize false negatives and false positives, enable the redirection of scarce resources, and efficiently guide appropriate care to at-risk individuals. To determine whether a particular instrument is optimal and ideal for assessment, monitoring, or screening, consideration should be given to the following administration parameters: administration time, administration methods and delivery, the type of raters, and the level of training required for administration.

4.4.1 Administration: Time

The optimal administration time for any risk assessment instrument should be brief (minutes), which may be facilitated by the instrument's structure. In particular, guided interpretation of patient responses during risk assessment in the form of a decision tree allows for briefer administration time and quicker and more reliable decision-making.

4.4.2 Administration: Methods and Delivery

The most common methods for suicide risk assessment by gate-keepers and clinicians involve a general interview and no systematic questions about ideation, behavior or family history of suicidal behavior. A much better approach involves systematic questioning guided by a checklist or rating scale (Malone 1995).

Self-report instruments have the advantage of making self-disclosure of sensitive issues easier. These types of instruments may facilitate the admission of suicidal ideation and behavior, or any suicide-related phenomena, which may be denied in an in-person, face-to-face interview. As mentioned previously, a telephone follow-up assessment, which used the C-SSRS, improved detection (58 %) of suicide attempts by more than 40 % when compared to hospital chart reviews (18 %) (Arias 2014).

Risk assessment instruments for suicide are available in a variety of paper and electronic formats. Importantly, innovative delivery formats enable a greater number of individuals to be screened, facilitating broader implementation. Timing of assessment is crucial after an at-risk patient is discharged from a hospital, particularly from a psychiatric inpatient unit, as there is an increased risk for suicide in the first week after discharge (Roy 1982).

4.4.3 Administration: Gatekeepers

Suicide risk assessment is not limited to medical settings, even though primary care physicians often see individuals shortly before they attempt suicide, but should include educational, religious, workplace, legal, and forensic settings. As such, settings may include diverse populations, it is crucial that nonmental health professions be able to ask appropriate screening questions. Training in the administration of a risk assessment tool enhances implementation efforts in these settings. In a juvenile justice setting nonclinician raters (gatekeepers) showed good inter-rater reliability when administering a structured risk assessment questionnaire to adolescent girls (Kerr et al. 2014). In the U.S. Marines, all support workers, such as chaplains, family advocacy workers and attorneys, are trained to be aware of suicide risk and warning signs and to administer and utilize the C-SSRS. In rural communities, where access to a mental health professional or practitioner may be limited, the ability of nonmental health professional gatekeepers to screen is essential.

4.4.4 Multiple Sources of Information

In many risk assessment contexts, situational factors render obtaining information directly from a patient impossible. Examples of clinical populations that are challenging span dementias, cognitive impairment, and autism. In all of these cases, collecting information from other reporters and its integration into an overall clinical picture is crucial. The ability of a risk assessment tool to obtain and integrate information from a variety of sources of information provides the necessary flexibility and accuracy.

4.4.5 Risk Management

Assessment scales should have operationalized thresholds that differentiate levels of risk and aid in determining patient disposition. A patient management protocol that specifies next steps after the risk assessment may include referrals to mental health professionals for low-to-moderate risk patients or hospitalization and suicide watch, for high-risk patients. Without a systematic assessment to determine suicide risk level that drives the next steps, providers are less able to properly triage patients. This can lead to overestimation of risk, or a tendency to err on the safe side, resulting in increased burden for mental health professionals, hospitals, and other healthcare facilities and diminished resources to offer the right quality of patient care for those who are most in need.

4.4.6 Generalizability

Suicide risk assessment instruments require parallel forms developed for specific populations. Modifications may include developmentally appropriate questions or addition of population-specific risk factors (e.g., the military) (Peñta and Caine 2006).

4.4.7 Triage

Operationalized thresholds that distinguish higher levels of risk are an essential component of assessment scales, so that appropriate triage steps can be taken. In cases of low-to-moderate risk, such steps may involve referral to mental health professionals for further evaluation, while high-risk cases may require hospitalization or suicide watch. In the absence of built-in thresholds that link to specific triage protocols, providers are forced to worry about every person screened. This could lead to problematic situations such as clinicians believing more patients require one-to-one observation than there is staff available to provide it. In other words, over-estimation of risk leads to misallocation of resources and poorer quality of care. Whether at a hospital or a correctional facility, it is essential for assessment administrators to have access to a screener with research-based next-step protocol, which will in turn impact care delivery and service utilization.

4.5 Risk Factors: Suicidal Behavior and Ideation-Specific Mediators and Moderators and Corresponding Instruments

A thorough evaluation of the benefits and risks of therapeutic interventions and suicide-related outcomes should include a consideration of known risk factors as well as mediating and moderating variables. Mediators are intervening variables that help clarify the nature of and represent potential mechanisms that underlie the relationship between independent and dependent variables. Moderators are characteristics that affect the direction and/or strength of the relationship between the independent and dependent variables. Suicidal behavior and ideation-specific mediators and moderators to be considered include: biological factors (genetic, stress responsivity, developmental anomalies, altered neural circuitry), psychological factors (aggressive and impulsive traits, negative inferential styles, cognitive rigidity, hopelessness, decision-making, problem-solving, mood regulation), psychiatric illness (e.g., major depressive episode), and social support systems (see Hudzik and Cannon, this volume). Knowing mediating and moderating relationships affecting the risk of suicide enhances the understanding of factors that play a role in mitigating or increasing that risk and creates a context for evaluating the effects of treatment. Table 4.1 lists examples of instruments assessing some of these risk factors.

4.6 How Should Instruments Measure Suicide Risk: Characteristics Important for Detection and Prediction

Suicidal behavior occurs in many psychiatric disorders (e.g., depression, schizophrenia) and in many medical conditions (e.g., strokes, epilepsy, head injury and AIDS) (Harris et al. 1994). Thus, monitoring of suicidal ideation and behavior should be part of clinical practice for nonpsychiatrists including neurologists, internists and primary care physicians. In the evaluation of new medications that affect the brain and other systems such as endocrine, measuring the impact of new drugs on suicidal ideation and behavior has been made a requirement by the FDA for all clinical trials. For accurately assessing the comparable importance of risk and protective factors from a clinical and public health perspective.

Prior to FDA mandating prospective monitoring of suicide-related events in drug trials, all previous antidepressant, anticonvulsant, and other non-psychiatric trials were not set-up to adequately assess these events. Suicide risk analyses were based on spontaneously generated adverse events and the higher risk estimates from these analyses may have been a product of ascertainment bias rather than a reflection of a true association.

The choice of a suicide risk assessment instrument and interpretation of the results obtained from the assessment depend on the degree to which the instrument is able to capture concepts of interest (Fig. 4.1). From this point of view, an

Table 4.1 Select risk factors and associated instruments

Risk factor	Assessment instrument	References
Aggression and impulsivity	• Barratt impulsiveness scale • Buss–Durkee hostility inventory • Brown–Goodwin aggression history (AGGHx)	Stanford et al. (2009), Buss and Durkee (1957), Kelip et al. (2006)
Substance abuse	• Mental health screening form-III (MHSF-III) • Simple screening instrument for substance abuse (SSI-SA) • CAGE questionnaire (alcohol) • Drug abuse screening test (DAST) • Michigan Alcoholism Screening test (MAST), • Psychiatric research interview for substance and mental disorders (PRISM)	Sacks et al. (2005), Ewing (1984), Skinner et al. (1982), Selzer et al. (1971), Samet et al. (1996)
Hopelessness	• Beck hopelessness scale (BHS)	Beck et al. (1990)
Distress/mental pain	• Mental pain scale • Self-defeating personality questionnaire (SDPQ) • Self-critical cognition scale • Self-derogation scale • The guilt inventory	Orbach et al. 2003, Shneidman et al. (1993), Schill (1990), Kugler and Jones (1992), Kaplan et al. (1969), Orbach et al. (1991)
Neurocognitive factors	• Iowa gambling task (decision-making) • Stroop task (interference scores; attention) (adapted) • Buschke selective reminding task (SRT) test (memory and learning)	Bowman et al. 2005), Keilp et al. (2014)

instrument which incorporates clear definitions and examples of behaviors that reflect those concepts minimizes variability in clinical judgment.

Science demands uniformity in measurement: moving away from a single instrument inherently degrades the precision of the signal, compounding existing imprecision across research sites and raters (Gibbons, 2010). The impact of imprecision grows when incidence rates are low, such as with death by suicide. At the same time, imprecision with low frequency events is incredibly problematic, as misclassification of one or two cases can have a profound impact on risk estimates and substantially alter conclusions. Even if you assume two measures are equally valid, more measurement variability still equals more noise. This has a particularly large impact when trying to combine studies. The 2012 FDA Guidance echoes this sentiment, stating that "the use of different instruments is likely to increase measurement variability… decreasing the opportunity to identify potential signals" that would inform future analyses and clinical trials. Uniform measurement with a validated instrument like the C-SSRS is crucial for prevention, research, and clinical practice.

Research has shown that systematic monitoring and consistent application of well-operationalized suicidal ideation and behavior criteria result in lower and more precise risk estimates. In a classic example of controversy surrounding safety of antidepressants, analyses commissioned by the FDA showed that consistent application of the C-SSRS' empirically supported definitions of ideation and behavior led to significantly better estimates of risk, with 50 % fewer ascertained suicide attempts (Posner et al. 2007). Similarly, in a large nonpsychiatric trial with 14,000 subjects, systematic monitoring sourcing the C-SSRS revealed 12 suicidal adverse events (AEs) compared to 452 reported spontaneously (Posner January 2009). Reducing false positives is as important as identifying risk in the effort to improve detection and better allocate limited or scarce resources. An initiative organized by the CDC, Department of Defense, National Institute of Mental Health, and the Department of Veterans Affairs is recommending the C-SSRS as one of the consensus measures to be incorporated into large-scale biomedical studies involving human subjects to facilitate data sharing and comparison (http://www.phenxtoolkit.org).

Accuracy and validity of clinical judgment about suicidal ideation and behavior, whether in research or practice, improve when validated measures are used in assessment, which in turn increase their treatment utility. The critical parameters of a valid clinical suicide risk assessment in addition to construct/conceptual validity include sensitivity to clinical change and predictive validity. Scales that take classification in consideration for the measurement of ideation and behavior and incorporate definitions of ideation and behavior subtypes have shown robust sensitivity to change in symptoms as well as predictive validity (Posner et al. 2011). The Beck Scale for Suicide Ideation, a continuous scale, has shown predictive validity for death by suicide in adults in long-term follow-up studies (Brown et al. 2000) but has not performed as well in predicting near-term nonfatal suicidal behavior, whereas the C-SSRS has demonstrated such predictive qualities (Posner et al. 2011). Identifying specific types of suicidal ideation and including the full range of behaviors (including preparatory acts or behavior and self and other interrupted attempts) instead of aggregating characteristics along a continuum may be more useful for risk stratification. In support, research on the SSI has shown that empirically derived factors such as "plans" and "desire" have different predictive patterns using past attempts and suicide as outcomes (Beck et al. 1997; Joiner et al. 2003). Lifetime history of a specific *type* of ideation—with intent to act—has been shown to be a stronger predictor of subsequent suicidal behavior than ideation without intent to act (Mundt et al. 2013; Posner et al. 2011).

4.7 Inclusion/Exclusion of Suicidal Individuals in Clinical Trials

Cross-national studies suggest that suicidal ideation and suicide attempts are relatively common (Nock et al. 2008). In fact, suicidal ideation and behavior are prevalent across all medical disorders; in those with one or more general illnesses, 25.2 % have suicidal ideation and 8.9 % make a suicide attempt (Druss and Pincus 2000). Consequently, there exists the expectation that increased suicide risk may be present in psychiatric and nonpsychiatric clinical trials and that such risk should be assessed and managed. The various approaches to any suicidal phenomena in clinical trials have included: (a) exclusion of those at risk for suicidal behavior from participation, (b) removal from trial if suicidal ideation or behavior emerge during the trial, (c) management of suicidal issues in the context of the trial, or (d) any combination of these approaches (Pearson et al. 2001). Possible exclusion of those at risk for suicidal behavior from participation may have been the result of active and/or significant past suicidal ideation, a recent suicide attempt, or a history of suicidal behavior. Seventy-seven antidepressant (SSRI) clinical trials of fluoxetine, citalopram, paroxetine, and sertraline (Prozac, Celexa, Paxil, and Zoloft, respectively) between 1984 and 2001 were reviewed for inclusion and exclusion criteria for suicidal phenomena (Stanley 2009). Approximately 10 % (8 out of 77) of these trials allowed some level of suicidal ideation, history of behavior but excluded those with recent suicidal behavior in their research subjects; thus, these trials told very little about how antidepressants would affect suicidal patients (Stanley 2009).

The issue of exclusion of suicidal patients from clinical trials arises in relation to the balancing of scientific and safety concerns. Understandibly, exclusion of suicidal individuals offers the advantages of minimizing risk to participants and investigators, lowering costs for monitoring, and maintaining homogeneity of the sample. However, exclusion is potentially unfair to a segment of the population that is in need of treatment. It leads to the false assumption that treatments found effective for nonsuicidal persons with certain mental disorders can be effective in reducing suicidal behavior among persons with that disorder as well. Exclusion hampers generalizability, as the desired applicability for a study is usually an entire diagnostic group and not just a specific segment of the group (Stanley 2009). Protection by exclusion has a cost and may not be protective; expert consensus has consistently indicated that suicidal patients should not be excluded from clinical trials (Meyer et al. 2010). Suicidal individuals have been deprived of access to effective treatments tailored to their needs, similar to the effects of the historical exclusion of women of childbearing age, children and adolescents, and ethnic minorities. Thus, the optimal approach would include the active management of suicidal ideation, behavior, and attempts through the addition of risk-mitigating procedures (Pearson et al. 2001). Such procedures would include additions to the study planning process, alteration in the consent process, increased staff training, and managing increased suicidal risk via increased monitoring and crisis intervention procedures. Managing suicidal ideation and behavior in the context of clinical trials will allow for increased generalizability as both suicidal and nonsuicidal individuals will be included.

Studies have demonstrated the ethical and clinical feasibility of including individuals with suicidal ideation and/or recent suicidal behavior as participants in clinical trials (Liu 2009; Safer and Zito 2007). Therefore, it is difficult to argue for the exclusion of individuals considered at risk for suicide from clinical trials as many individuals with these symptoms will be receiving these medications, after FDA approval, in the absence of systematic premarketing data on the associated risks and benefits related to suicidal ideation and suicidal behavior (Meyer et al.

2010). Clinical trials in which suicide is the primary outcome measure will need to be so much larger and longer than the usual 8-week study (Meyer et al. 2010) that such studies are not practical. Nonfatal suicide attempts are a higher base rate outcome that is more realistic in terms of sample size and study duration. Informed consent forms for such a study must explain that suicidal ideation and behavior are outcome variables and the limits of confidentiality should an individual become suicidal, and describe the assessment and treatment individuals will receive if they withdraw from the study (Meyer et al. 2010). A balance between research assessment and clinical care can be established to preserve patient safety and the validity of the clinical trial results.

4.8 The Columbia-Suicide Severity Rating Scale (C-SSRS)

The Columbia-Suicide Severity Rating Scale (C-SSRS) maximizes feasibility of suicide risk assessment. It is a semi-structured, rater-based interview that prospectively assesses the severity and frequency of suicidal ideation and behaviors. The C-SSRS was developed by leading experts and researchers at the University of Pennsylvania and Columbia University, in collaboration with Aaron Beck's research group, over 10 years ago in the context of a National Institute of Mental Health (NIMH) research effort, in response to the need for a measure to assess outcome, change, and severity. The C-SSRS identifies the full range of suicidal ideation and behavior, monitors change from visit to visit, and predicts safety referral criteria derived from studies.

The C-SSRS was designed to (1) provide definitions of suicidal ideation and behavior and corresponding probes; (2) quantify the full spectrum of suicidal ideation and suicidal behavior and gage their severity over specified periods; (3) distinguish suicidal behavior and nonsuicidal self-injurious behavior; and (4) employ a user-friendly format that allows integration of information from multiple sources (e.g., direct patient interview, family and other interviews, and medical records). As reviewed by Meyer et al. (2010), these criteria are considered essential for judging the utility of scales assessing suicide-related phenomena. The C-SSRS is unique among rating instruments in meeting all of these criteria. The C-SSRS has received wide acceptance in the US and worldwide. It has been translated into 116 languages and is also used in clinical trials to screen for suicide and prevention efforts across the US. The C-SSRS is used in many county and state screening and prevention programs, in the military, and by many large private medical centers and health care networks. The C-SSRS provides reliable outcomes, establishes operationalized criteria, specifies parameters for triggering referrals, which decreases unnecessary burden, and impacts care delivery and triage.

As a result, the C-SSRS has been endorsed and adopted into policies across a variety of national and international settings and institutions. In particular, the Substance Abuse and Mental Health Services Administration (SAMHSA) and Health Resources Service Administration's jointly funded Center for Integrated

Health Solutions has endorsed the C-SSRS as one of three screening tools that should be utilized to assess suicide risk; the other two are the Suicide Assessment Five-Step Evaluation and Triage (SAFE-T) and Suicide Behaviors Questionnaire (SBQ-R).

In the US Army, all providers must consider suicide risk for all soldiers evaluated in an emergency department and must administer the C-SSRS if there is a suicide risk concern Also, acute care hospitals, such as Reading Hospital, have integrated the C-SSRS Screener (with additional triage points) as part of a hospital suicide screening protocol and policy. Overall, the C-SSRS has been endorsed or adopted into policies by approximately 30 US states, several countries, and many national and global institutions, and is about to become the primary measure used in all NIMH suicide research (PhenX toolkit).

4.9 Reporting of Adverse Events

The number of empirically validated treatments aimed at reducing suicidal ideation and behaviors remains small. According to Oquendo et al. (2011), there have been fewer than 30 studies that focused on assessing psychosocial and pharmacological interventions that may benefit individuals at risk for suicidal behavior (Oquendo et al. 2011). Intervention research in most of medicine focuses on conditions associated with the greatest morbidity and mortality. Although suicidal patients, a majority of whom have a psychiatric or substance use disorder, constitute such a population there is a dearth of intervention trials in suicidal individuals. Two barriers that may explain the small number of intervention trials for suicidal individuals include ethical issues, such as the decision of whether to enter vulnerable populations into randomized trials, and the expectation of lethal outcomes in treatment trials for conditions with high mortality (Oquendo et al. 2004).

Therefore, the foreseeable occurrence of a fatal or near-fatal event in intervention clinical trials, for which suicide reduction is the outcome of interest, requires a consideration of adverse event (AE) or adverse drug event (ADE) identification and reporting standards. Across different institutions and agencies that conduct and/or supervise intervention trials, definitions of adverse events are often too general and too variable to allow for comparability between studies and meaningful interpretation of study results (Czaja et al. 2006, Santiago et al. 2003). Consequences of the lack of clarity and consistency in defining adverse events include the potential for underreporting during clinical trials, which poses a threat to the safety of trial participants. One clinical- and nonresearch-setting study found that voluntary reporting only yielded 1 in 20 adverse drug events (Cullen et al. 2003), while others have found that medical adverse events were underreported at varying rates, ranging from 50 to 96 % (Barach and Small 2000). This underreporting may originate from a variety of sources that may include, but are not limited to, fear that the study will be terminated, deterrence posed by time-consuming paperwork necessary for reporting an adverse event, and population characteristics (Oquendo et al. 2011) (see also Ratcliff et al., this volume).

Regarding adverse event reporting, Gandhi et al. (2000) identified methods of detecting ADEs that include voluntary reporting, chart review, and computerized monitoring (Gandhi et al. 2000). Common types of voluntary reporting used to detect ADEs include spontaneous voluntary reporting and stimulated voluntary reporting. Spontaneous voluntary reporting has been a common mechanism utilized by institutions to identify ADEs, but this form of reporting identifies only a small portion (approximately 5 %) of ADEs (Cullen et al. 2003). Relatedly, stimulated voluntary reporting, a real-time verbal inquiry, made reporting quick and easy, but a problem arose as ADEs were reported verbally, yet only a small fraction of these ADEs were filed on a reporting system (Weingart et al. 2000). Another common ADE identification method, chart review, looks retrospectively for ADEs documented in an individual's medical chart. Importantly, conducting chart reviews usually requires a substantial amount of training and is costly and time-consuming (Gandhi et al. 2000). Accordingly, research has demonstrated that only a very small percentage of events actually make it to the medical chart (Gandhi et al. 2000) and that there can be significant variation in the review of ADE data (Bates et al. 1998; Sanazaro et al. 1991). Computerized monitoring, which can screen administrative and clinical databases and identify certain events, appears to be promising. Computerized monitoring identified 731 ADEs in an 18month period, an eightfold increase in ADE identification when compared to spontaneous voluntary reporting alone (Classen et al. 1991). However, chart reviews are able to detect 20 % more ADEs when compared to computerized monitoring; of note, computerized monitoring required 11 person-hours per week, while chart reviews required 55 person-hours per week (Jha et al. 1991).

To improve adverse event identification and reporting, unified and consistent definitions and systems of reporting must be developed. Suicide research and terminology has been plagued by a lack of conceptual clarity and a large variability in nomenclature, and developing universally applied definitions can allow for comparability of adverse events across clinical trials and research studies. Furthermore, systematizing adverse event reports into a database can provide researchers and investigators with a method to compare safety results (Califf et al. 1998). Ultimately, developing comprehensive and accurate systems of reporting will allow for prevention opportunities as certain patterns may be noticed.

4.10 Conclusion

Suicide prevention is of high national and international importance and identification of at-risk individuals is the first necessary step toward prevention. Research and clinical practice have been challenged by methodological limitations regarding assessment of suicidal ideation and behavior. Such issues have undermined confidence in epidemiological findings and have had a profound impact on drug safety questions. Systematic assessment for suicidal risk is feasible and provides more reliable outcomes, establishing operationalized criteria for inclusion and exclusion of trial participants, and specifying parameters for triggering referrals, thus decreasing unnecessary referral and burden. Therefore, assessment of suicidal ideation and behavior should be routinely integrated across public health settings. Knowledge of the full range of suicidal ideation and behaviors and key criteria for differentiating suicidal and nonsuicidal events is paramount to the advancement of suicide risk assessment. Brief, feasible, research-supported risk assessment tools can identify individuals at increased risk for suicide.

References

Appleby L et al (1996) General practitioners and young suicides: a preventive role for primary care. The Br J Psychiatr 168(3):330–333

Arias SA et al (2014) Using structured telephone follow□up assessments to improve suicide□related adverse event detection. Suicide Life Threat Behav. doi:10.1111/sltb.12088

Baca-Garcia E et al (2010) Suicide attempts among women during low estradiol/low progesterone states. J Psychiatr Res 44(4):209–214

Barach P, Small SD (2000) Reporting and preventing medical mishaps: lessons from non-medical near miss reporting systems. BMJ 320(7237):759–763

Barber ME et al (1998) Aborted suicide attempts: a new classification of suicidal behavior. Am J Psychiatr 155(3):385–389

Bates DW et al (1998) Effect of computerized physician order entry and a team intervention on prevention of serious medication errors. JAMA 280(15):1311–1316

Beck AT et al (1990) Relationship between hopelessness and ultimate suicide: a replication with psychiatric outpatients. Am J Psychiatr 147(2):190–195

Beck AT et al (1999) Suicide ideation at its worst point: a predictor of eventual suicide in psychiatric outpatients. Suicide Life Threat Behav 29:1–9

Beck AT, Brown GK, Steer RA (1997) Psychometric characteristics of the scale for suicide ideation with psychiatric outpatients. Behav Res Ther 35(11):1039–1046

Beck A, Greenberg R (1971) The nosology of suicidal phenomena: past and future perspectives. Bull Suicidol 8:7

Beck AT, Kovacs M, Weissman A (1979) Assessment of suicidal intention: the scale for suicide ideation. J Consult Clin Psychol 47(2):343–352

Bennett M (2013) Brain networks, hormones and genes implicated in depression. In: Virginia woolf and neuropsychiatry. Springer, Berlin, pp 67–106

Bongiovi-Garcia ME et al (2009) Comparison of clinical and research assessments of diagnosis, suicide attempt history and suicidal ideation in major depression. J Affect Disord 115 (1–2):183–188

Bowman CH, Evans CEY, Turnbull OH (2005) Artificial time constraints on the Iowa gambling task: the effects on behavioural performance and subjective experience. Brain Cogn 57 (1):21–25

Brent DA et al (1993) Psychiatric risk factors for adolescent suicide: a case-control study. J Am Acad Child Adolesc Psychiatr 32(3):521–529

Brown GK et al (2000) Risk factors for suicide in psychiatric outpatients: a 20-year prospective study. J Consult Clin Psychol 68(3):371–377

Brown GK, Steer RA, Henriques GR, Beck AT (2005) The internal struggle between the wish to die and the wish to live: a risk factor for suicide. Am J Psychiatry 162(10):1977–1979

Brown GK, Currier G, Stanley B (2008) Suicide attempt registry pilot project. In: National Institute of Mental Health annual meeting of the Developing Centers for Intervention and Prevention of Suicide, Canandaigua, NY

Buss AH, Durkee A (1957) An inventory for assessing different kinds of hostility. J Consult Psychol 21(4):343–349

Califf RM et al (2003) Toward protecting the safety of participants in clinical trials. Control Clin Trials 24(3):256–271

Centers for Disease Control and Prevention. Injury Prevention & Control: Data & Statistics (WISQARS). Retrieved from http://www.cdc.gov/injury/wisqars/index.html

Classen DC et al (1991) Computerized surveillance of adverse drug events in hospital patients. JAMA 266(20):2847–2851

Conwell Y, Thompson C (2008) Suicidal behavior in elders. Psychiatr Clin North Am 31 (2):333–356

Crosby AO, Ortega L, Melanson C (2011) Self-directed violence: uniform definitions and recommended data elements, Version 1.0. In: Centers for disease control and prevention, Atlanta, GA

Crosby A (2010) Self-directed violence: uniform definitions and data elements. National Center for Injury Prevention and Control, Centers for Disease Control and Prevention, Atlanta

Cullen DJ et al (1995) The incident reporting system does not detect adverse drug events: a problem for quality improvement. The Jt Comm J Qual Improv 21(10):541–548

Currier G, Brown G, Stanley B (2009) Unpublished data: scale for suicide ideation total score by level of C-SSRS severity of ideation, 2009. American Foundation for Suicide Prevention

Czaja SJ et al (2006) Data and safety monitoring in social behavioral intervention trials: the REACH II experience. Clin Trials 3(2):107–118

De Leo D et al (2004) Definitions of suicidal behaviour. In: Leo DD et al (eds) Suicidal behaviour: theories and research findings. Hogrefe & Huber Publishers, Ashland, pp 17–39

Druss B, Pincus H (2000) Suicidal ideation and suicide attempts in general medical illnesses. Arch Intern Med 160(10):1522–1526

Dwivedi Y, Mann JJ, Currier D (2012) Medication in suicide prevention insights from neurobiology of suicidal behavior. CRC Press, Boca Raton

Eaton DK et al (2012) Youth risk behavior surveillance-United States, 2011. MMWR Surveill Summ 61(4):1–162

Ewing JA (1984) Detecting alcoholism: the cage questionnaire. JAMA 252(14):1905–1907

Fawcett J (1992) Suicide risk factors in depressive disorders and in panic disorder. J Clin Psychiatr 53(Suppl):9–13

Fawcett J et al (1990) Time-related predictors of suicide in major affective disorder. Am J Psychiatr 147:1189–1194

Fergusson D et al (2005) Association between suicide attempts and selective serotonin reuptake inhibitors: systematic review of randomised controlled trials. BMJ 330(7488):396

Food and Drug Administration (2012) Suicidal Ideation and behavior: prospective assessment of occurrence in clinical trials, draft guidance. Guidance for Industry

Gandhi T, Seder D, Bates D (2000) Methodology matters. Identifying drug safety issues: from research to practice. Int J Qual Health Care 12(1):69–76

Gibbons RD, Amatya AK, Brown CH, Hur K, Marcus SM, Bhaumik DK et al (2010) Post-approval drug safety surveillance. Annu Rev Public Health 31:419–437

Goldsmith SK et al (eds) (2002) Reducing suicide. The National Academics Press, Washington, DC, p 496

Gould MS et al (2003) Youth suicide risk and preventive interventions: a review of the past 10 years. J Am Acad Child Adolesc Psychiatr 42(4):386–405

Harris EC, Barraclough B (1997) Suicide as an outcome for mental disorders: a meta-analysis. Br J Psychiatr 170(3):205–228

Harris EC, Barraclough BM, Winslow F (1994) Suicide as an outcome for medical disorders. Medicine 73(6):281–296
Hawton K (1987) Assessment of suicide risk. Br J Psychiatr 140:145–153
Hesdorffer DC et al (2013) Suicidal ideation and behavior screening in intractable focal epilepsy eligible for drug trials. Epilepsia 54(5):879–887
Hjelmeland H, Knizek BL (1999) Conceptual confusion about intentions and motives of nonfatal suicidal behavior: a discussion of terms employed in the literature of suicidology. Arch Suicide Res 5(4):275–281
Holi M et al (2008) Detecting suicidality among adolescent outpatients: evaluation of trained clinicians' suicidality assessment against a structured diagnostic assessment made by trained raters. BMC psychiatr 8(1):97
Horwitz AG, Czyz EK, King CA (2014) Predicting future suicide attempts among adolescent and emerging adult psychiatric emergency patients. J Clin Child Adolesc Psychol 28:1–11 (ahead-of-print)
Insel T (2010) The under-recognized public health crisis of suicide. In: National Institute of Mental Health Director's Blog
Isometsa E (1998) Suicide attempts preceding completed suicide. Br J Psychiatr 173(6):531–535
Jha AK et al (1998) Identifying adverse drug events development of a computer-based monitor and comparison with chart review and stimulated voluntary report. J Am Med Inform Assoc 5 (3):305–314
Jiménez E et al (2013) Genetic variability at IMPA2, INPP1 and GSK3β increases the risk of suicidal behavior in bipolar patients. Eur Neuropsychopharmacol 23(11):1452−1462
Joiner TE Jr et al (2003) Worst-point suicidal plans: a dimension of suicidality predictive of past suicide attempts and eventual death by suicide. Behav Res Ther 41(12):1469–1480
Kaplan HB, Pokorny AD (1969) Self-derogation and psychosocial adjustment. J Nerv Ment Dis 149(5):421–434
Katzan I, Viguera A, Burke T, Buchanan J, Posner K (2013) Improving suicide screening at the Cleveland clinic through electronic self-reports: PHQ-9 and the Columbia-suicide severity rating scale (C-SSRS). In: 1st annual meeting of the international academy for suicide research, Montreal, Canada
Keilp JG et al (2006) Aggressiveness, not impulsiveness or hostility, distinguishes suicide attempters with major depression. Psychol Med 36(12):1779–1788
Keilp J et al (2014) Neuropsychological deficits in past suicide attempters with varying levels of depression severity. Psychol Med 1–10
Kerr DC et al (2014) Young adult follow□up of adolescent girls in juvenile justice using the Columbia suicide severity rating scale. Suicide Life Threat Behav 44(2):113−129
Kessler RC, Borges G, Walters EE (1999) Prevalence of and risk factors for lifetime suicide attempts in the National Comorbidity Survey. Arch Gen Psychiatr 56(7):617–626
King CA et al (2009) Adolescent suicide risk screening in the emergency department. Acad Emerg Med 16(11):1234–1241
King C et al (2012) Using the C-SSRS to assess adolescents in psychiatric emergency settings predictive validity across a one-year period, May 2012. In: 52nd annual NCDEU meeting, Phoenix, AZ
Kugler K, Jones WH (1992) On conceptualizing and assessing guilt. J Pers Soc Psychol 62 (2):318–327
Kuo W-H, Gallo JJ, Tien A (2001) Incidence of suicide ideation and attempts in adults: the 13-year follow-up of a community sample in Baltimore, Maryland. Psychol Med 31(07):1181–1191
Laje G et al (2007) Genetic markers of suicidal ideation emerging during citalopram treatment of major depression. Am J Psychiatr 164(10):1530–1538
Lewinsohn PM, Rohde P, Seeley JR (1994) Psychosocial risk factors for future adolescent suicide attempts. J Consult Clin Psychol 62(2):297–305

Liu K (2009) Suicide rates in the world: 1950–2004. Suicide Life Threat Behav 39(2):204–213
Luoma JB, Martin CE, Pearson JL (2002) Contact with mental health and primary care providers before suicide: a review of the evidence. Am J Psychiatr 159(6):909–916
Malone KS, Szanto K, Corbitt E, Mann JJ (1995) Clinical assessment versus research methods in the assessment of suicidal behavior. Am J Psychiatr 152(1):1601
Mann JJ (2003) Neurobiology of suicidal behaviour. Nat Rev Neurosci 4(10):819–828
Mann JJ et al (2005) Family history of suicidal behavior and mood disorders in probands with mood disorders. Am J Psychiatr 162(9):1672–1679
Mann J, Currier D (2010) Stress, genetics and epigenetic effects on the neurobiology of suicidal behavior and depression. Eur Psychiatr 25(5):268–271
Marzuk P et al (1997) The prevalence of aborted suicide attempts among psychiatric in-patients. Acta Psychiatr Scand 96(6):492–496
McCarty CA et al (2011) Adolescents with suicidal ideation: health care use and functioning. Acad Pediatr 11(5):422–426
Meyer RE et al (2010) Suicidality and risk of suicide–definition, drug safety concerns, and a necessary target for drug development: a consensus statement. J Clin Psychiatr 71(8):e1–e21
Mundt JC et al (2013) Prediction of suicidal behavior in clinical research by lifetime suicidal ideation and behavior ascertained by the electronic Columbia-suicide severity rating scale. J Clin Psychiatr 74(9):887–893
Mundt J et al (2011) eC-SSRS assessments of lifetime ideation and behavior are predictive of suicidal behaviors occuring during trial participation. In: Poster session presented at ISCTM 2011 autumn conference, Amelia Island, Florida. Accessed 3–4 Oct 2011
Nock MK et al (2008) Cross-national prevalence and risk factors for suicidal ideation, plans and attempts. Br J Psychiatr 192(2):98–105
Nordström P, Samuelsson M, Åsberg M (1995) Survival analysis of suicide risk after attempted suicide. Acta Psychiatr Scand 91(5):336–340
Oquendo M et al (2004) Prospective study of clinical predictors of suicidal acts after a major depressive episode in patients wtih major depressive disorder or bipolar disorder. Am J Psychiatr 161(8):1433–1441
Oquendo MA et al (2011) Variability in the definition and reporting of adverse events in suicide prevention trials: an examination of the issues and a proposed solution. Arch Suicide Res 15 (1):29–42
Oquendo MA, Halberstam B, Mann JJ (2003) Risk factors for suicidal behavior. Stand Eval Clin Pract 22:103–129
Orbach I et al (1991) A multi-attitude suicide tendency scale for adolescents. Psychol Assess A J Consul Clin Psychol 3(3):398–404
Orbach I et al (2003) Mental pain: a multidimensional operationalization and definition. Suicide Life Threat Behav 33(3):219–230
O'Carrol PW (1989) A consideration of the validity and reliability of suicide mortality data. Suicide Life Threat Behav 19(1):16
O'Carroll PW et al (1996) Beyond the tower of Babel: a nomenclature for suicidology. Suicide Life Threat Behav 26(3):237–252
Pearson J et al (2001) Issues to consider in intervention research with persons at high risk for suicidality. National Institute of Mental Health, Bethesda, MD. http://www.nimh.nih.gov/research/highrisksuicide.cfm
Perlis RH et al (2007) Association between treatment-emergent suicidal ideation with citalopram and polymorphisms near cyclic adenosine monophosphate response element binding protein in the STAR* D study. Arch Gen Psychiatr 64(6):689
Perroud N et al (2009) Genetic predictors of increase in suicidal ideation during antidepressant treatment in the GENDEP project. Neuropsychopharmacology 34(12):2517–2528

Peñta JB, Caine ED (2006) Screening as an approach for adolescent suicide prevention. Suicide Life Threat Behav 36(6):614–637
Pfeffer CR et al (1993) Suicidal children grow up: rates and psychosocial risk factors for suicide attempts during follow-up. J Am Acad Child Adolesc Psychiatr 32(1):106–113
Posner K et al (2007) Columbia classification algorithm of suicide assessment (C-CASA): classification of suicidal events in the FDA's pediatric suicidal risk analysis of antidepressants. Am J Psychiatr 164(7):1035–1043
Posner K et al (2007) Factors in the assessment of suicidality in youth. CNS Spectr 12(2):156
Posner K et al (2011) The Columbia-suicide severity rating scale: initial validity and internal consistency findings from three multisite studies with adolescents and adults. Am J Psychiatr 168(12):1266–1277
Posner K, Greist J, Mundt J, Federico M, Amira L, Goldstein E, Pearlstein S, Buchanan J (2013) The full range of suicidal behaviors, its total number, and suicidal ideation predict short-term risk of suicidal behavior in clinical trials. In: Autumn conference of the International Society for CNS Clinical Trials and Methodology, Philadelphia, Pennsylvania. Accessed Sept 30–Oct 2 2013
Posner K (2012) Columbia suicide severity rating scale: improved precision while redirecting scarce resources, suicide training day for office of mental health. Stonybrook Medicine and VA, Stony Brook, NY
Posner K (2012) Prediction of suicidal behavior in clinical trials using the C-SSRS. Paper presented at the 52nd Annual NCDEU Meeting, Phoenix, Arizona
Posner K (2014) Increasing Understanding and Prediction of Suicide Risk, Improving Care Delivery and Redirecting Scarce Resources with the Columbia Suicide Severity Rating Scale. Presented at Israeli Conference of Suicide Research, Ruppin Academic Center, Israel
Posner K (2009) The value of systematic assessment: initial findings from prospective studies. In: International suicidality capstone meeting, Academia, Government and Industry Forum, New York State Psychiatric Institute, New York, NY
Roy A (1982) Risk factors for suicide in psychiatric patients. Arch Gen Psychiatr 39 (9):1089–1095
Sacks S et al (2005) Substance abuse treatment for persons with co-occurring disorders. Center for substance abuse treatment. Treatment Improvement Protocol (TIP) Series 42. DHHS Publication No. (SMA) 05−3922. Substance Abuse and Mental Health Services Administration, Rockville
Safer D, Zito JM (2007) Do antidepressants reduce suicide rates? Public Health 121(4):274–277
Samet S, Smith M, Endicott J (1996) Psychiatric research interview for substance and mental disorders (PRISM): reliability for substance abusers. Am J Psychaitr 153:1195–1201
Sanazaro PJ, Mills DH (1991) A critique of the use of generic screening in quality assessment. JAMA 265(15):1977–1981
Santiago L, Debanne S, Neuhauser D (2003) Tracking adverse events in RCTs: lack of agreement among regulatory institutions. Qual Saf Health Care 12(3):234
Schill T (1990) A measure of self-defeating personality. Psychol Rep 66(3c):1343–1346
Selzer ML (1971) The Michigan alcoholism screening test: the quest for a new diagnostic instrument. Am J Psychiatr 127(12):1653–1658
Shneidman ES (1993) Suicide as psychache: A clinical approach to self-destructive behavior. Jason Aronson, Northvale
Skinner HA (1982) The drug abuse screening test. Addict Behav 7(4):363–371
Stanford MS et al (2009) Fifty years of the Barratt impulsiveness scale: an update and review. Personality Individ Differ 47(5):385–395
Stanley B (2009) Managing suicide risk in clinical trials. In: International suicidality capstone meeting, Academia, government, and industry forum, New York, NY. Accessed 26–27 Jan 2009

Steer RA et al (1988) Eventual Suicide in Interrupted and Uninterrupted Attempters: A Challenge to the Cry-for-Help Hypothesis. Suicide Life Threat Behav 18(2):119–128

Suominen K et al (2004) Health care contacts before and after attempted suicide among adolescent and young adult versus older suicide attempters. Psychol Med 34(02):313–321

Turecki G et al (2012) The neurodevelopmental origins of suicidal behavior. Trends Neurosci 35 (1):14–23

Vannoy SD et al (2007) The relationship between suicide ideation and late-life depression. Am J Geriatric Psych 15(12):1024–1033

Weingart SN, Ship AN, Aronson MD (2000) Confidential clinician-reported surveillance of adverse events among medical inpatients. J Gen Intern Med 15(7):470–477

Wichstrom L (2000) Predictors of adolescent suicide attempts: a nationally representative longitudinal study of Norwegian adolescents. J Am Acad Child Adolesc Psychiatr 39 (5):603–610

Part II
Risk Factors

Chapter 5
Stress and Vulnerability: A Developing Model for Suicidal Risk

Jorge Lopez-Castroman, Emilie Olié and Philippe Courtet

Abstract A large body of research built over the last few decades examines the interaction between stressful events and vulnerability traits to explain how a person becomes suicidal. This stress-diathesis model has been extremely fruitful to improve our understanding of suicidal behavior, but recent findings suggest that interactions could be more complex than expected. Indeed, environmental insults during pregnancy, childhood, or adolescence induce neurodevelopmental changes that increase the vulnerability for suicidal behavior in later life. In this chapter, we will outline the significance of recent neurodevelopmental findings for the stress-vulnerability factors of suicidal behavior. The coherence and applicability of an integrative neurodevelopmental model of suicidal behavior will be discussed in the light of current research concerning genetics, neuroimaging, and neuropsychology, and the new classification systems.

5.1 Introduction

Despite treatment and prevention advances on major psychiatric disorders, suicidal behavior still constitutes a major public health problem. Research into this behavior has increased exponentially during the last decade, and a complex network of factors, both predisposing and triggering the suicidal acts, is being unraveled. This dynamic network connects mental disorders, life experiences, social and familial interactions, physical illness, and neurobiology into what is known as the suicidal process. However, until a deeper understanding of the relationships between these factors is developed, crucial issues such as yielding an accurate prediction of future suicidal acts or determining the best treatment for suicidal patients remain distant.

J. Lopez-Castroman · E. Olié · P. Courtet (✉)
Département D'urgence et Post-Urgence Psychiatrique, L'Hôpital Lapeyronie,
371, Avenue du Doyen Gaston Giraud, 34295 Montpellier Cedex 5, France
e-mail: philippe.courtet@univ-montp1.fr

K.E. Cannon and T.J. Hudzik (eds.), *Suicide: Phenomenology and Neurobiology*,
DOI 10.1007/978-3-319-09964-4_5

The term 'stress' names the reaction experienced by an individual when facing an environmental condition that is either a threat, a challenge, or a concern. It has a significant impact on mental health and is associated with suicidal acts, which can be triggered by stressful situations even if the individual is not particularly predisposed. Studies on suicidal behavior usually conceptualize stress as negative and discontinuous events during the lifetime, but chronic stress also increases suicidal risk (Fergusson et al. 2000). A number of interaction models linking stress and suicidal risk have been proposed (Dwivedi and van Heeringen 2012). Most of these models include the concept of diathesis, or constitutional vulnerability. Depending on the model, clinical (McGirr and Turecki 2007), cognitive (Jollant et al. 2005), anatomical (Jollant et al. 2011), or neurobiological (Mann and Arango 1992) aspects of the diathesis are emphasized. However, the diathesis itself is not enough to start a suicidal crisis. For instance, subjects with similar biological and experiential background, such as monozygotic twins, may present or not suicidal behavior depending on the stressful situations they are exposed to (Pompili et al. 2006).

5.2 Studies on the Stress-Diathesis Model

The explanatory model proposed by Mann and Arango (1992) integrated for the first time neurobiology and psychopathology in a stress-diathesis model of the suicidal process, and has served as a basis for many studies on suicidal behavior. They posited the existence of common risk factors for suicidal behavior across mental disorders, classifying them as state- (stressor) or trait-dependent (diathesis). For instance, a depressive episode would trigger suicidal acts in subjects with impulsive traits. Stressors would therefore determine the timing of the suicidal acts (Fig. 5.1).

Although cumulative evidence in several domains supports a stress-diathesis model of suicidal behavior, there are also conflicting results that highlight its complexities. Psychosocial stressors such as poor social adjustment, job loss, or declining health have been consistently associated with an increased risk of suicidal behavior (Blackmore et al. 2008). However, the results of prospective studies

Fig. 5.1 The stress-diathesis model of suicidal behavior

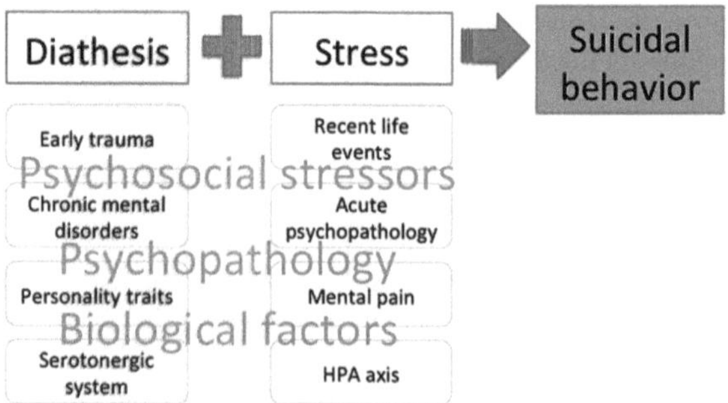

examining the effect of life events on suicidal behavior have not been conclusive (Oquendo et al. 2013). When examining longitudinally the determinants of suicide attempts, Oquendo et al. (2013) found that health- and work-related life events, as well as major depressive episodes, increased by 13-fold the risk of a subsequent suicide attempt among depressed subjects, provided that they did not have comorbid borderline personality disorder. They also found that predisposing features such as female gender or suicidal cognitions were related to the risk and timing of the suicidal act. Yet, among depressed subjects with borderline personality disorder, the effect of life events or major depressive episodes on suicidal behavior appeared to be buffered. Borderline personality disorder, a condition particularly predisposed to suicidal behavior because of its association with pessimism, impulsivity, and early trauma, seemed paradoxically to cope better with negative life events. The authors hypothesized that a lower threshold for stress could explain these findings; "normal" events could be as important as life events for borderline patients.

On the other hand, clinical studies have shown important differences between suicide attempters and non-attempters independently of related mental disorders. Suicide attempters present higher levels of impulsive aggression, hopelessness, and more frequent familial history of suicidal behavior, personal history of childhood adversities, and head injury. All of these factors are part of a diathesis for future suicidal behaviors (Krakowski and Czobor 2004; Lopez-Castroman et al. 2012; Oquendo et al. 2004; Perroud et al. 2008). However, although most subjects with mental disorders never attempt suicide, psychopathology is probably the main risk factor for suicidal behavior, present in 90 % of completed suicides and 80 % of suicide attempts (Nock et al. 2010). In global rates there is a particular contribution of affective disorders to suicidal behavior because of their high prevalence, but anxiety disorders, psychotic disorders, eating disorders, and substance use disorders (particularly use of alcohol or nicotine), as well as borderline personality disorder, also contribute significantly (Bolton and Robinson 2010).

There is also convincing evidence on the influence of biological factors both as predisposing and precipitating agents of suicidal behavior. The most consistent biological finding in suicidal behavior is the implication of the serotonin system, the dysfunction of which represents a constitutional risk factor. The largely replicated findings of an association between low cerebrospinal fluid (CSF) levels of serotonin and suicidal behavior, independently of psychiatric disorder, gave a substantial weight to the existence of a specific biological suicidal vulnerability. A large number of studies using different indicators of serotonergic dysfunction suggest that this dysfunction may act as a vulnerability trait of suicidal behavior (Mann 2003). On the other hand, abnormal stress responses such as hyperactivity of the hypothalamic-pituitary-adrenal axis (HPA), evaluated with the dexamethasone suppression test, are linked with suicidal behavior (Coryell and Schlesser 2001). Lastly, a decrease in cholesterol and brain-derived neurotrophic factor (BDNF) levels, measured in blood serum or plasma, have also been associated with impaired brain plasticity among individuals with suicidal behavior (Lee and Kim 2011).

Mental or "psychic" pain is a concept that describes pervasive negative affect that is experienced by the sufferer as pain (Orbach et al. 2003). Such affect can fluctuate somewhat widely in intensity, and some authors have pointed to mental pain as an effective potential trigger of suicidal acts. Mental pain also seems to increase the propensity to suicidal ideation (Olié et al. 2010), and can be assessed and targeted for prevention (Mee et al. 2011). Interestingly, mental pain might increase the risk of severe suicidal behaviors especially when accompanied by difficulties with social communication and loneliness (Gvion et al. 2014).

The study of the notes left by suicide completers and psychological autopsy studies indicate that suicide victims were nearly always suffering from a psychiatric disorder and submitted to environmental stressors. However, environmental stressors and psychiatric disorders are necessary but non-sufficient conditions for attempting suicide. Long-term prospective studies reveal that suicide attempters are at high risk of committing suicide in their lifetime (about 13 % will) (Tidemalm et al. 2008). The personal history of suicide attempt is the main risk factor for subsequent suicidal behavior, indicating the existence of a vulnerability to suicide. Additionally, individuals suffering from a mental disorder are at particularly high risk during the first years of illness. This suggests that suicidal vulnerability is more easily expressed when subjects are exposed for the first time to major stresses represented by a psychiatric condition. As an example, in a study of patients with unipolar depression, rates of suicidal behavior were 74.4 % for the first episode, 18.8 % for the second one and 6.5 % for subsequent ones (Mann et al. 1999).

Prospective studies bring more evidence supporting the stress-diathesis model. A cohort of adult affective patients after a major depression episode that was followed prospectively for 2 years in New York showed an additive effect of the three most powerful predictors of future suicidal acts (history of suicide attempt, subjective severity of depression, and cigarette smoking) and also of another two predisposing factors: pessimism and impulsive-aggression (Oquendo et al. 2004). Of note, another prospective study by the same group demonstrated that clinical predictors of suicidal acts vary between genders (Oquendo et al. 2007). In a 21-year longitudinal study of a birth cohort of 1,265 New Zealand young adults, those who developed major depression had increased rates of suicidal ideation and suicide attempt. Again, suicidal ideation or suicide attempts appeared in a minority of depressed young adults. Thus, additional factors seemed to modify the vulnerability (or resilience) to suicidal responses, including: familial history of suicide, childhood abuse, personality features, peer affiliations, and school performance (Fergusson et al. 2003).

5.3 Current Directions: Genetics, Neuroimaging and Neuropsychology

Genetic factors play a significant role in suicidal behaviors, and can interact with stressful events to increase the risk of suicidal behavior. In an innovative study, Caspi (2003) revealed that a variant of the serotonin transporter gene was associated with increased risk of suicidal ideation after significant life events. This finding was later replicated in abused depressed patients (Shinozaki et al. 2013), psychiatric inpatients with a history of suicide attempts (Gibb et al. 2006), and substance-dependent patients (Roy et al. 2007). Apart from monoaminergic systems, other gene x environment (GxE) interactions involving glutamatergic, GABAergic and corticotrophin related genes are being investigated, as well as genes involved in neurotrophic processes (particularly the gene encoding BDNF) or in inflammatory processes (Mandelli and Serretti 2013; Perroud et al. 2008). Independently of psychopathology, concordance rates of suicidal behavior ranging from 6 to 35 % have been reported in studies examining monozygotic twins (Pedersen and Fiske 2010). Of note, although the transmission of suicidal behavior across generations seems to be independent of Axis-I disorders, it could be mediated by intermediate phenotypes (endophenotypes), like impulsive aggression or hopelessness (Courtet et al. 2011).

Few studies have connected stress and suicide through neuroimaging. Jollant et al. (2008) compared the neural correlates of implicit emotional processing in euthymic males with a history of depression according to history of suicide attempt. Men with a past history of suicide attempt showed increased sensitivity to anger reflecting others' disapproval, were more likely to act on negative emotions, and paid less attention to mildly positive stimuli. These results support the hypothesis of a predisposition for suicidal acts in negative circumstances (Jollant et al. 2008). More recently, Reisch et al. (2010) used fMRI through the presentation of autobiographical scripts to reactivate the memories of a recent suicide attempt in females. Three conditions were examined: mental pain, suicide action, and neutral activity. The recollection of mental pain was associated with decreased prefrontal activity compared to the recollection of suicide action, which showed an increased activity in the frontal cortex. To explain their findings the authors hypothesized that goal-directed suicidal behavior would be undertaken to reduce the mental pain, which would act as a traumatic stressor.

The pursuit of neurocognitive markers of suicide vulnerability constitutes also a very productive area of research. Suicidal behavior may be viewed as a consequence of an altered decision process when facing stressful situations. Proof of such alteration has been found in several studies mostly using the Iowa Gambling Task among adolescent (Bridge et al. 2012) or adult populations (Jollant et al. 2005, 2010) of suicide attempters in which attempters appear to ignore past experiences when performing a reward/punishment task (Dombrovski et al. 2010). Importantly, the use of computerized association tests is a promising area of research that could be used to identify individuals at risk in stressful situations (Cha et al. 2010). Moreover, ecological momentary assessments through portable devices can be used to obtain real-life longitudinal data of affective variability and suicidal ideation in response to environmental stressors (Palmier-Claus et al. 2012).

5.4 Life Is More Complex: Vulnerability Contributes to Stress

On the one hand, alterations in decision-making, a putative suicidal endophenotype involved in the ability of the individual to make choices in daily life, are correlated to the occurrence of problematic affective relationships (Jollant et al. 2007), threatening individual's social bounds. On the other hand, according to the theory of attachment (Bowlby 1977), the perception of being rejected or neglected, and by extension being abused in childhood or in adulthood, leads to rejection sensitivity and the perception of being unwanted in general (Ehnvall et al. 2008). Being excluded or rejected leads to reactive behaviors, which could be dysfunctional: aggressive, antisocial, or self-injurious behaviors (Williams 2007). To be impulsive/aggressive or to be less prone to approach others due to pessimism/hopelessness exacerbates the risk of social isolation. Social isolation and interpersonal difficulties, both psychosocial stresses relevant to precipitate suicidal acts, may be partially due to suicidal vulnerability factors. Interestingly, contacting people by telephone one month after being discharged from an emergency department for deliberate self-poisoning may help reduce the number of suicide re-attempts over 1 year, independently of the identification of subjects at risk or the implementation of a crisis intervention (Vaiva et al. 2006). This highlights the very powerful effect of perceived social isolation.

Suicidal vulnerability may lead the subjects to consider non-stressful environmental events as stressors because of hypersensitivity to psychological pain or social exclusion. Indeed, using functional MRI, ventromedial prefrontal and cingulate regions associated with suicidal vulnerability (Jollant et al. 2010, 2008) have also been involved in social rejection/distress (Eisenberger et al. 2003) and psychological pain perception (van Heeringen et al. 2010). Thus, the suicidal act relies on a stress-vulnerability model, complicated by the role of vulnerability to emerging stress.

5.5 Connecting Vulnerability-Stress with Neurodevelopment

The interaction of disturbances during development with genetically modulated temperaments may explain the triggering effects of later life stressors through personality and coping styles. In other words, vulnerability traits determined by alterations in neurodevelopment and biological substrates interact dynamically with acute stressors enabling suicidal behavior.

5.5.1 Prenatal and Perinatal Risk Factors

Neurodevelopment starts during pregnancy. Different research teams have described a "birth season" effect in suicide, which may be independent of any associated psychopathology. The largest study to date examined 6.5 millions persons and 80,000 suicides in Hungary and reported that suicide risk was associated with a spring or summer birth: being born in July increased the risk by 14 % compared with a birth in December (Döme et al. 2010).

Several hypotheses have been proposed to explain these surprising findings. Brain insults by infectious agents during development could convey vulnerability for suicidal behavior when interacting with particular genetic conditions. Seasonal variations of serotonin metabolism, inducing decreases in CSF serotonin levels, could also be associated with impulsivity and, secondarily, with an augmentation of suicidal risk (Chotai et al. 2006). Finally, melatonin rates and circadian rhythms vary depending on the season of birth among healthy new-born and the vesperal chronotype is associated with impulsivity, which could lead to suicidal behavior (Chotai 2005). Interestingly, subjects born in risk periods such as spring present more often the "S" allele of the serotonin transporter that is associated with suicidal vulnerability (Gonda et al. 2012).

Two very large cohorts followed prospectively for 30 years in Sweden and Scotland support the influence of perinatal factors on suicidal risk. Future suicide attempts, studied only in the Swedish cohort, were increased in subjects with small birth length, multiparity, low sociocultural level, and young age of the mother (Mittendorfer-Rutz et al. 2004). The risk of completed suicide was associated with low birth weight and young maternal age in both studies, but an association with multiparity and unemployment of the parents was additionally found in the Scottish cohort (Riordan et al. 2006). On the other hand, postnatal growth could also play a significant role. A weak weight gain in the first year after birth was associated with a higher risk of suicide for 15,000 English subjects born between 1911 and 1930. This finding was independent of birth weight, socio-economic level, and the type of diet of the new-born (Barker et al. 1995). Finally, very preterm birth, childhood maltreatment, and personality traits seem to have additive effects that influence the age at onset of the first suicide attempt (Blasco-Fontecilla et al. 2013).

5.5.2 The Role of Childhood Maltreatment

Childhood maltreatment is strongly associated with suicidal behavior in adulthood (Short and Nemeroff, this volume). It is also a prevalent life event that can be reported by a majority of suicide attempters in some populations (Lopez-Castroman et al. 2012). Childhood abuse interacts with family and genetic factors in increasing the risk of early onset suicidal behavior, and higher impulsive aggressive traits (Lopez-Castroman et al. 2012, 2014; Slama et al. 2009). The mechanisms that link childhood maltreatment and suicidal behavior remain unclear. Literature on neurodevelopment has demonstrated that early trauma affects cognitive and affective processes causing less intellectual performance, memory impairments, alterations in executive functions, and emotional dysregulation (Pechtel and Pizzagalli 2010). These impairments may confer an increased risk of adult psychopathology and facilitate the onset of suicidal behaviors. Several authors have also proposed impulsive aggression as a mediating factor between childhood abuse and suicidal behavior. Although causal relations cannot be explored without prospective studies, high impulsive aggression in abused patients is associated with more severe suicidal behaviors (Lopez-Castroman et al. 2014).

5.5.3 Biological Embedding

Biologic transfer mechanisms, particularly changes in gene expression, might explain the impact of negative life experiences, such as childhood abuse, in the multifactorial process of suicidal behavior (See Dwevedi, this volume). The mechanisms that allow early experiences to modulate brain development and determine vulnerability or resilience seem to implicate epigenetic factors. Epigenetic modifications lead to the repression or activation of genetic expression, and have been identified in several genes (related with glucocorticoid receptors, BDNF, arginine vasopressin system, and corticotropin-releasing hormone) in connection with early environmental changes in animal models (review in: Turecki et al. 2012).

Although most of these studies examined post-natal epigenetic regulation, stress during pregnancy may also induce epigenetic changes. Studies with rodents highlight the importance of the timing of epigenetic alterations. Stress during early pregnancy seem to allow an epigenetic reprogramming of the rat genome causing long-term modifications on the HPA axis. The type of stress is also important, minimal stressors could be associated with resilience, while massive or prolonged stress would lead to developmental frailty.

The exact role of vulnerability genes in suicidal behavior warrants further research. For instance, how the “s” allele of the serotonin transporter increases risk? This is paradoxal because this allelic variant is associated with a diminished recapture of serotonin, the mode of action of serotoninergic antidepressants that have shown effectiveness in the prevention of suicide reattempts. Could this genetic polymorphism act through neurodevelopmental means? Studies with knockout mice support this hypothesis. If the mutation is viable, it would induce large modifications with homeostatic consequences on neurodevelopment (Lesch and Mössner 2006). Additionally, the early role of serotonin and its receptors in the course of prenatal development, as well as its influence on the morphogenesis of the brain, suggests that serotonin influences the development and brain maturation of mammals before taking its role as a neurotransmitter. Besides, there seems to be a common genetic background between neurodevelopmental alterations and suicidal behavior (Perroud et al. 2008).

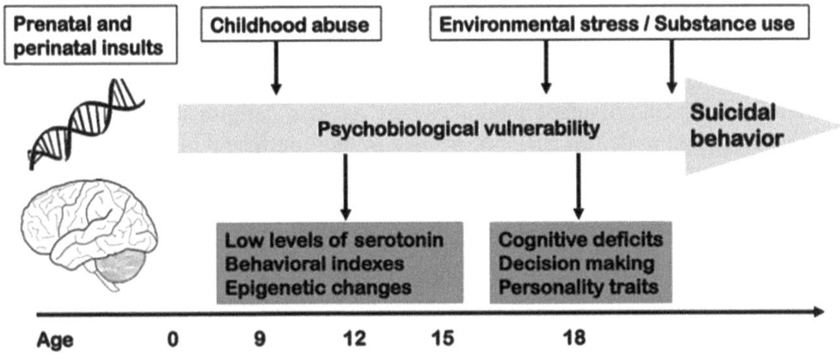

Fig. 5.2 A developmental model of suicidal behavior

5.5.4 Toward a Neurodevelopmental Model of Suicidal Behavior

The neurodevelopment hypothesis was initially used to explain the pathophysiology of schizophrenia. But being nonspecific, it is applicable to other mental disorders, including suicidal behavior. Prospective cohort studies show that impulsive aggression in childhood remains stable until adulthood and is associated with an elevated risk of suicidal behaviors (Pihlakoski et al. 2006). Thus, Caspi et al. (1996) described an increased risk of antisocial personality or depression in adulthood for children of 3 years of age showing lack of self control or behavioral inhibition, respectively. In both cases, the risk of suicidal behaviors was increased (Fig. 5.2).

At a biological level, serotoninergic abnormalities leading to suicidal vulnerability have also been observed among adolescent subjects (Tyano et al. 2006). During adolescence, environmental stressors may exacerbate imbalances in the function of limbic and ventral prefrontal areas, leading to suicidal behavior, a risk that may be mediated by genetic factors (Casey et al. 2010). Biological data for young children is scarce, but points in the same direction (Clarke et al. 1999). The stability of impulsive-aggression traits connected to serotoninergic systems (Oxenstierna et al. 1986) favors the idea of an early onset of psychobiological disturbances that would be later expressed as auto- or hetero- aggressive behaviors. Studies of epidemiological and molecular genetics report similar findings in childhood and adolescence (Dwivedi and Zalsman 2012).

There are also some neuropsychological indexes that support a neurodevelopmental model of suicidal behavior. A large Swedish prospective study found a clear association between low intelligence and later suicide risk, independently of socioeconomic level or mental disorders (Gunnell et al. 2005). Intellectual deficits could be the consequence of alterations in early brain development and explain the risk of suicidal behavior in adulthood. As mentioned before, decision-making constitutes also a cognitive trait of suicide vulnerability that is modulated by the interaction of sexual abuse in childhood and a genotypic variant of the CRH-R1 gene (Guillaume et al. 2013). Recent data suggest that anomalies in decision-making might appear already in adolescence (Oldershaw et al. 2009).

Therefore, certain cognitive anomalies may have an early onset in the course of neurodevelopment under the effect of genetic or environmental factors in childhood or even pregnancy. We do not yet know the precise timing when cognitive alterations appear. Are they present in early development or are they dependent of brain maturation processes, like adolescent "pruning"? Current data suggest that perinatal events increase suicidal risk by inducing stable epigenetic changes that affect the expression of genes coding for neurotrophic factors and proteins involved in stress regulation. These epigenetic modulations would cause subsequently neurobiological alterations such as hyperactivity of the HPA axis, which would in turn be associated with the development of specific emotional or behavioral phenotypes characterized by anxiety or impulsive-aggression.

The neurodevelopmental model of suicidal behavior emphasizes the importance of early development, a period particularly sensitive to negative experiences, in human as in animal models, that could lead to long-term consequences. However, this does not imply that any anomaly would make subjects become suicidal. It rather conveys a dynamic conception where later environmental factors modulate the deleterious effects of early insults. This understanding of suicidal vulnerability could thus allow a better prevention and early screening of subjects at risk that could be targeted by new treatment strategies.

5.6 Significance for New Classification Systems (DSM-5)

The inclusion of suicidal behavior disorder in the last edition of the Diagnostic and Statistical Manual of Mental Disorders (DSM-5) finally recognizes the specificity of suicidal behavior. It is defined by the existence of a suicide attempt, as opposed to suicidal ideation or non-suicidal self-harm, in the last 2 years. This corresponds with the previously discussed idea of suicidal vulnerability conveyed by a recent suicide attempt, which identifies subjects at high risk of recurrence that could be targeted for prevention efforts. The DSM-5 mentions some examples of environmental stressors that should be taken into account when evaluating the suicide risk: "recently learning of a potentially fatal medical diagnosis such as cancer, experiencing the sudden and unexpected loss of a close relative or partner, loss of employment, or displacement from housing" (American Pychiatric Association 2013).

Research in the last 40 years has provided enough evidence of suicidal behavior as a distinct entity, that complies with all the validity criteria for psychiatric nosology proposed by Robins and Guze (1970). In fact, several authors have advocated for its inclusion in diagnostic manuals (Oquendo et al. 2008). These criteria include: 1) a good clinical description and clear borders with differential diagnoses (Posner et al. 2007); 2) the identification of postmortem and in vivo markers, such as serotonin dysfunction, HPA axis hyperactivity, cognitive impairments, or neuroanatomical anomalies described above; 3) the confirmation of prospective increases of suicidal behaviors among patients with these markers (Oquendo et al. 2006); 4) the transmission of risk across generations (Brent and Melhem 2008), which has been confirmed by molecular genetics and G x E studies.

It is to be expected that the specific category of suicidal behavior will favor suicide evaluation, treatment, and prevention. Existing evidence clearly demonstrates that suicide risk is neither adequately evaluated nor sufficiently treated. Until now, practicing psychiatrists or clinicians could not include suicidal behaviors among diagnoses and according to DSM-IV they would only evaluate suicidal risk in some specific mental disorders such as major depression. A patient with schizophrenia hospitalized due to a suicidal crisis is currently discharged with just a diagnosis of schizophrenia, omitting the main condition that motivated the episode of care. Furthermore, the specificity of suicidal behavior disorder as a psychopathological condition emphasizes the need for specific treatment approaches. These treatments exist. For instance, lithium has anti-suicidal properties and selective serotonin reuptake inhibitors reduce impulsive-aggression, independently of their effect on depression (Cipriani et al. 2013).

In summary, the stress-diathesis model provides a framework in which to integrate suicidal behavior disorder, and may facilitate interventions through specific treatment or prevention strategies targeting subjects at risk. The complexity of suicidal behavior demands an adjustment of current treatments considering biological markers and psychosocial factors.

References

American Pychiatric Association (2013) Diagnostic and Statistical Manual of Mental Disorders: DSM 5

Barker DJ, Osmond C, Rodin I et al (1995) Low weight gain in infancy and suicide in adult life. BMJ 311:1203

Blackmore ER, Munce S, Weller I et al (2008) Psychosocial and clinical correlates of suicidal acts: results from a national population survey. Br J Psychiatry 192:279–284

Blasco-Fontecilla H, Jaussent I, Olié E et al (2013) Additive effects between prematurity and postnatal risk factors of suicidal behavior. J Psychiatr Res 47:937–943

Bolton JM, Robinson J (2010) Population-attributable fractions of Axis I and Axis II mental disorders for suicide attempts: findings from a representative sample of the adult, non-institutionalized US population. Am J Public Health 100:2473–2480

Bowlby J (1977) The making and breaking of affectional bonds. I. Aetiology and psychopathology in the light of attachment theory. An expanded version of the Fiftieth Maudsley Lecture, delivered before the Royal College of Psychiatrists, 19 November 1976. Br J Psychiatry 130:201–210

Brent DA, Melhem N (2008) Familial transmission of suicidal behavior. Psychiatr Clin North Am 31:157–177

Bridge JA, McBee-Strayer SM, Cannon EA et al (2012) Impaired decision making in adolescent suicide attempters. J Am Acad Child Adolesc Psychiatry 51:394–403

Casey BJ, Jones RM, Levita L et al (2010) The storm and stress of adolescence: insights from human imaging and mouse genetics. Dev Psychobiol 52:225–235

Caspi A (2003) Influence of life stress on depression: moderation by a polymorphism in the 5-HTT Gene. Science 301:386–389
Caspi A, Moffitt TE, Newman DL, Silva PA (1996) Behavioral observations at age 3 years predict adult psychiatric disorders. Longitudinal evidence from a birth cohort. Arch Gen Psychiatry 53:1033–1039
Cha CB, Najmi S, Park JM et al (2010) Attentional bias toward suicide-related stimuli predicts suicidal behavior. J Abnorm Psychol 119:616–622
Chotai J (2005) Novelty seekers and summer-borns are likely to be low in morningness. Eur Psychiatry 20:307
Chotai J, Murphy DL, Constantino JN (2006) Cerebrospinal fluid monoamine metabolite levels in human newborn infants born in winter differ from those born in summer. Psychiatry Res 145:189–197
Cipriani A, Hawton K, Stockton S, Geddes JR (2013) Lithium in the prevention of suicide in mood disorders: updated systematic review and meta-analysis. BMJ 346:f3646
Clarke RA, Murphy DL, Constantino JN (1999) Serotonin and externalizing behavior in young children. Psychiatry Res 86:29–40
Coryell W, Schlesser M (2001) The dexamethasone suppression test and suicide prediction. Am J Psychiatry 158:748–753
Courtet P, Gottesman II, Jollant F, Gould TD (2011) The neuroscience of suicidal behaviors: what can we expect from endophenotype strategies. Transl Psychiatry 1:e7–7
Dombrovski AY, Clark L, Siegle GJ et al (2010) Reward/Punishment reversal learning in older suicide attempters. Am J Psychiatry 167:699–707
Döme P, Kapitány B, Ignits G, Rihmer Z (2010) Season of birth is significantly associated with the risk of completed suicide. Biol Psychiatry 68:148–155
Dwivedi Y, van Heeringen K (2012) Stress-diathesis model of suicidal behavior. CRC Press, Boca Raton
Dwivedi Y, Zalsman G (2012) Genetics of suicidal behavior in children and adolescents. CRC Press, Boca Raton
Ehnvall A, Parker G, Hadzi-Pavlovic D, Malhi G (2008) Perception of rejecting and neglectful parenting in childhood relates to lifetime suicide attempts for females–but not for males. Acta Psychiatr Scand 117:50–56
Eisenberger NI, Lieberman MD, Williams KD (2003) Does rejection hurt? An FMRI study of social exclusion. Science 302:290–292
Fergusson DM, Beautrais AL, Horwood LJ (2003) Vulnerability and resiliency to suicidal behaviours in young people. Psychol Med 33:61–73
Fergusson DM, Woodward LJ, Horwood LJ (2000) Risk factors and life processes associated with the onset of suicidal behaviour during adolescence and early adulthood. Psychol Med 30:23–39
Gibb BE, McGeary JE, Beevers CG, Miller IW (2006) Serotonin transporter (5-HTTLPR) genotype, childhood abuse, and suicide attempts in adult psychiatric inpatients. Suicide Life Threat Behav 36:687–693
Gonda X, Fountoulakis KN, Csukly G et al (2012) Star-crossed? The association of the 5-HTTLPR s allele with season of birth in a healthy female population, and possible consequences for temperament, depression and suicide. J Affect Disord 143:75–83
Guillaume S, Perroud N, Jollant F et al (2013) HPA axis genes may modulate the effect of childhood adversities on decision-making in suicide attempters. J Psychiatr Res 47:259–265
Gunnell D, Magnusson PKE, Rasmussen F (2005) Low intelligence test scores in 18 year old men and risk of suicide: cohort study. BMJ 330:167
Gvion Y, Horresh N, Levi-Belz Y et al (2014) Aggression-impulsivity, mental pain, and communication difficulties in medically serious and medically non-serious suicide attempters. Compr Psychiatry 55:40–50
Jollant F, Bellivier F, Leboyer M et al (2005) Impaired decision making in suicide attempters. Am J Psychiatry 162:304–310
Jollant F, Guillaume S, Jaussent I et al (2007) Impaired decision-making in suicide attempters may increase the risk of problems in affective relationships. J Affect Disord 99:59–62

Jollant F, Lawrence NL, Olié E et al (2011) The suicidal mind and brain: a review of neuropsychological and neuroimaging studies. World J Biol Psychiatry 12:319–339
Jollant F, Lawrence NS, Giampietro V et al (2008) Orbitofrontal cortex response to angry faces in men with histories of suicide attempts. Am J Psychiatry 165:740–748
Jollant F, Lawrence NS, Olié E et al (2010) Decreased activation of lateral orbitofrontal cortex during risky choices under uncertainty is associated with disadvantageous decision-making and suicidal behavior. NeuroImage 51:1275–1281
Krakowski MI, Czobor P (2004) Psychosocial risk factors associated with suicide attempts and violence among psychiatric inpatients. Psychiatr Serv 55:1414–1419
Lee B-H, Kim Y-K (2011) Potential peripheral biological predictors of suicidal behavior in major depressive disorder. Prog Neuropsychopharmacol Biol Psychiatry 35:842–847
Lesch KP, Mössner R (2006) Inactivation of 5HT transport in mice: modeling altered 5HT homeostasis implicated in emotional dysfunction, affective disorders, and somatic syndromes. Handb Exp Pharmacol 175:417–456
Lopez-Castroman J, Jaussent I, Beziat S et al (2012) Suicidal phenotypes associated with family history of suicidal behavior and early traumatic experiences. J Affect Disord 142:193–199
Lopez-Castroman J, Jaussent I, Beziat S et al (2014) Increased severity of suicidal behavior in impulsive aggressive patients exposed to familial adversities. Psychol Med 26:1–10
Mandelli L, Serretti A (2013) Gene environment interaction studies in depression and suicidal behavior: an update. Neurosci Biobehav Rev 1–23
Mann JJ (2003) Neurobiology of suicidal behaviour. Nat Rev Neurosci 4:819–828
Mann JJ, Arango V (1992) Integration of neurobiology and psychopathology in a unified model of suicidal behavior. J Clin Psychopharmacol 12:2S–7S
Mann JJ, Waternaux C, Haas GL, Malone KM (1999) Toward a clinical model of suicidal behavior in psychiatric patients. Am J Psychiatry 156:181–189
McGirr A, Turecki G (2007) The relationship of impulsive aggressiveness to suicidality and other depression-linked behaviors. Curr Psychiatry Rep 9:460–466
Mee S, Bunney BG, Bunney WE et al (2011) Assessment of psychological pain in major depressive episodes. J Psychiatr Res 45:1504–1510
Mittendorfer-Rutz E, Rasmussen F, Wasserman D (2004) Restricted fetal growth and adverse maternal psychosocial and socioeconomic conditions as risk factors for suicidal behaviour of offspring: a cohort study. Lancet 364:1135–1140
Nock MK, Hwang I, Sampson NA, Kessler RC (2010) Mental disorders, comorbidity and suicidal behavior: results from the National Comorbidity survey replication. Mol Psychiatry 15:868–876
Oldershaw A, Grima E, Jollant F et al (2009) Decision making and problem solving in adolescents who deliberately self-harm. Psychol Med 39:95–104
Olié E, Guillaume S, Jaussent I et al (2010) Higher psychological pain during a major depressive episode may be a factor of vulnerability to suicidal ideation and act. J Affect Disord 120:226–230
Orbach I, Mikulincer M, Gilboa-Schechtman E, Sirota P (2003) Mental pain and its relationship to suicidality and life meaning. Suicide Life-Threat Behav 33:231–241
Oquendo MA, Baca-García E, Mann JJ, Giner J (2008) Issues for DSM-V: suicidal behavior as a separate diagnosis on a separate axis. Am J Psychiatry 165:1383–1384
Oquendo MA, Bongiovi-Garcia ME, Galfalvy H et al (2007) Sex differences in clinical predictors of suicidal acts after major depression: a prospective study. Am J Psychiatry 164:134–141
Oquendo MA, Currier D, Mann JJ (2006) Prospective studies of suicidal behavior in major depressive and bipolar disorders: what is the evidence for predictive risk factors? Acta Psychiatr Scand 114:151–158
Oquendo MA, Galfalvy H, Russo S et al (2004) Prospective study of clinical predictors of suicidal acts after a major depressive episode in patients with major depressive disorder or bipolar disorder. Am J Psychiatry 161:1433–1441
Oquendo MA, Perez-Rodriguez MM, Poh E et al (2013) Life events: a complex role in the timing of suicidal behavior among depressed patients. Mol Psychiatry 1–8

Oxenstierna G, Edman G, Iselius L et al (1986) Concentrations of monoamine metabolites in the cerebrospinal fluid of twins and unrelated individuals–a genetic study. J Psychiatr Res 20:19–29
Palmier-Claus JE, Taylor PJ, Gooding P et al (2012) Affective variability predicts suicidal ideation in individuals at ultra-high risk of developing psychosis: an experience sampling study. Br J Clin Psychol 51:72–83
Pechtel P, Pizzagalli DA (2010) Effects of early life stress on cognitive and affective function: an integrated review of human literature. Psychopharmacology 214:55–70
Pedersen NL, Fiske A (2010) Genetic influences on suicide and nonfatal suicidal behavior: twin study findings. Eur Psychiatry 25:264–267
Perroud N, Courtet P, Vincze I et al (2008) Interaction between BDNF Val66Met and childhood trauma on adult's violent suicide attempt. Genes Brain Behav 7:314–322
Pihlakoski L, Sourander A, Aromaa M et al (2006) The continuity of psychopathology from early childhood to preadolescence: a prospective cohort study of 3-12-year-old children. Eur Child Adolesc Psychiatry 15:409–417
Pompili M, Galeandro PM, Lester D, Tatarelli R (2006) Suicidal behavior in surviving co-twins. Twin Res Hum Genet 9:642–645
Posner K, Oquendo MA, Gould M et al (2007) Columbia classification algorithm of suicide assessment (C-CASA): classification of suicidal events in the FDA's pediatric suicidal risk analysis of antidepressants. Am J Psychiatry 164:1035–1043
Reisch T, Seifritz E, Esposito F et al (2010) An fMRI study on mental pain and suicidal behavior. J Affect Disord 126:321–325
Riordan DV, Selvaraj S, Stark C, Gilbert JSE (2006) Perinatal circumstances and risk of offspring suicide. Birth cohort study. Br J Psychiatry 189:502–507
Robins E, Guze SB (1970) Establishment of diagnostic validity in psychiatric illness: its application to schizophrenia. Am J Psychiatry 126:983–987
Roy A, Hu X-Z, Janal MN, Goldman D (2007) Interaction between childhood trauma and serotonin transporter gene variation in suicide. Neuropsychopharmacology 32:2046–2052
Shinozaki G, Romanowicz M, Passov V et al (2013) State dependent gene-environment interaction: serotonin transporter gene-child abuse interaction associated with suicide attempt history among depressed psychiatric inpatients. J Affect Disord 147:373–378
Slama F, Courtet P, Golmard JL et al (2009) Admixture analysis of age at first suicide attempt. J Psychiatr Res 43:895–900
Tidemalm D, Langstrom N, Lichtenstein P, Runeson B (2008) Risk of suicide after suicide attempt according to coexisting psychiatric disorder: Swedish cohort study with long term follow-up. BMJ 337:a2205–a2205
Turecki G, Ernst C, Jollant F et al (2012) The neurodevelopmental origins of suicidal behavior. Trends Neurosci 35:14–23
Tyano S, Zalsman G, Ofek H et al (2006) Plasma serotonin levels and suicidal behavior in adolescents. Eur Neuropsychopharmacol 16:49–57
Vaiva G, Vaiva G, Ducrocq F et al (2006) Effect of telephone contact on further suicide attempts in patients discharged from an emergency department: randomised controlled study. BMJ 332:1241–1245
van Heeringen K, Van den Abbeele D, Vervaet M et al (2010) The functional neuroanatomy of mental pain in depression. Psychiatry Res 181:141–144
Williams KD (2007) Ostracism. Annu Rev Psychol 58:425–452

Chapter 6
Traumatic Brain Injury (TBI) and Post Traumatic Stress Disorder (PTSD) as Risk Factors for Suicidal Thoughts and Behaviors

Sarra Nazem, Eryn Lonnquist, Lindsey L. Monteith and Lisa A. Brenner

Abstract Posttraumatic stress disorder (PTSD) and traumatic brain injury (TBI) are associated with increased risk for suicidal thoughts and behaviors. This chapter explores possible underlying neurocognitive and neuroanatomical factors related to PTSD and TBI that may contribute to increased susceptibility to suicidal thoughts and behaviors. The neurocognitive working model of suicidal behavior is used as a guiding framework (Jollant et al. 2011). Possible mechanisms involving altered modulation of value attribution, impaired regulation of emotional and cognitive responses, and facilitation of acts in an emotional context are explored within PTSD, TBI, and their co-occurrence. Discussion of clinical implications and limitations of this conceptual model, as well as directions for future research are provided.

S. Nazem (✉) · L.L. Monteith
Veterans Integrated Service Network 19 (VISN 19) Mental Illness Research, Education and Clinical Center (MIRECC), University of Colorado, Anschutz Medical Campus, 1055 Clermont St., Denver, CO 80220, USA
e-mail: Sarra.Nazem@va.gov

E. Lonnquist
VISN 19 MIRECC, Department of Neurology, University of Colorado, Anschutz Medical Campus, Aurora, CO, USA

L.A. Brenner
VISN 19 MIRECC, Departments of Psychiatry, Physical Medicine and Rehabilitation, and Neurology, University of Colorado, Anschutz Medical Campus, Aurora, CO, USA

S. Nazem · L.L. Monteith
Department of Psychiatry, University of Colorado, Anschutz Medical Campus, Aurora, CO, USA

K.E. Cannon and T.J. Hudzik (eds.), *Suicide: Phenomenology and Neurobiology*,
DOI 10.1007/978-3-319-09964-4_6

6.1 Introduction

Suicide rates among members of the United States (U.S.) military have increased substantially since the commencement of Operation Iraqi Freedom (OIF) and Operation Enduring Freedom (OEF). At the same time, posttraumatic stress disorder (PTSD) and traumatic brain injury (TBI) have been identified as "signature wounds" of these conflicts (Brenner, Vanderploeg and Terrio, 2009). These conditions frequently co-occur, and are individually associated with suicidal thoughts and behaviors (Bahraini et al.'s 2013; Bullman and Kang 1994; Ilgen et al. 2010; Brenner et al. 2011b); thus, understanding the neurocognitive and neuroanatomical mechanisms by which they confer risk is critical. To facilitate this process, the neurocognitive working model of suicidal behavior is used (Jollant et al. 2011). We begin with brief overviews on PTSD, TBI (mild, moderate, and severe), and co-occurring PTSD and TBI – describing their epidemiology and their associations with risk for suicidal thoughts and behaviors, with specific attention to military personnel and veteran samples. Subsequently we review Jollant et al. (2011) model and propose how it can be used to understand the association between PTSD and/or moderate to severe TBI with suicidal behaviors. The chapter concludes with clinical implications and recommendations for future research.

6.2 Posttraumatic Stress Disorder

6.2.1 Definition

In the *Diagnostic and Statistical Manual of Mental Disorders, Fifth Edition* (*DSM-5*), Posttraumatic Stress Disorder (PTSD) is defined as a trauma- and stressor-related disorder that can occur following exposure to a traumatic event (American Psychiatric Association 2013). DSM-5 criteria includes 20 potential symptoms, which fall into four different clusters: intrusive symptoms; avoidance; negative alterations in cognitions and mood; and alterations in arousal and reactivity. To be diagnosed with PTSD, an individual must experience the onset or exacerbation of symptoms for at least one month following exposure to the trauma, and the symptoms must cause significant distress and/or impairment.

6.2.2 Epidemiology

The lifetime prevalence of combat-related PTSD among U.S. Veterans and military personnel ranges from 6 to 31 %, with a point prevalence of 2–17 % (Richardson et al. 2010). In OEF/OIF service members, a population-based study estimated the prevalence of current PTSD to be 13.8 % (Tanielian and Jaycox 2008). This is consistent with recent findings among previously deployed OEF/OIF service members and veterans, in which estimates of PTSD in non-treatment-seeking samples ranged from 5 to 20 % (Ramchand et al. 2010). In treatment-seeking samples, estimates range from 4 to 50 % (Ramchand et al. 2010). These are significantly higher than those among the general U.S. population. Among a nationally representative sample of U.S. adults, the lifetime prevalence of PTSD was 6.8 % (Kessler et al. 2005a), and the 12-month prevalence of PTSD was 3.5 % (Kessler et al. 2005b).

6.2.3 Association with Suicide

6.2.3.1 Suicidal Ideation

Several recent reviews on PTSD and suicide risk—including two meta-analyses (Krysinska and Lester 2010; Panagioti et al. 2012) and one systematic review (Pompili et al. 2013)—have found PTSD to be associated with increased risk for suicidal ideation (SI). Among OEF/OIF veterans, those who screened positive for PTSD were 4.45 times more likely to report SI (Jakupcak et al. 2009). Subthreshold PTSD symptoms are also associated with SI (Marshall et al. 2001).

6.2.3.2 Suicide Attempt

PTSD is also associated with suicide attempt (SA). A recent review of PTSD and suicidal self-directed violence (SDV) concluded that approximately 24–40 % of veterans diagnosed with PTSD had attempted suicide (Panagioti et al. 2009). Of note, these rates were based primarily on samples of Vietnam-era veterans with chronic PTSD; in contrast, research on the association between PTSD and SAs among OEF/OIF veterans has been limited. Nonetheless, extant research suggests that PTSD is significantly associated with a history of SA. Although comorbid psychiatric diagnoses—such as major depression—further compound suicide risk, the association between PTSD with SI and SAs remains significant after controlling for other psychiatric diagnoses (Krysinska and Lester 2010; Panagioti et al. 2009, 2012).

6.2.3.3 Suicide

In contrast to the robust literature on PTSD and increased risk for SI and SA, research on PTSD and suicide death is limited (Panagioti et al. 2012). Bullman and Kang (1994) found that, among male Vietnam veterans, those with PTSD were significantly more likely to die by suicide (relative risk = 3.97; 95 % confidence interval = 2.20–7.03) than those without PTSD. Ilgen et al. (2010) obtained similar findings with a sample of veterans who used Veterans Health Administration (VHA) services. Veterans with a diagnosis of PTSD were 1.93 times more likely to die by suicide (95 % confidence interval for hazard ratios: 1.79–2.08), compared to veterans without PTSD.

Three recent studies with varying populations and methodological approaches did not find PTSD to be significantly associated with suicide (Desai et al. 2005; LeardMann et al. 2013; Zivin et al. 2007). Desai et al. (2005) examined suicide risk factors among veterans discharged from VA psychiatric inpatient units with a diagnosis of PTSD, schizophrenia, bipolar affective disorder, or major affective disorder. Veterans with a PTSD diagnosis at discharge had significantly lower suicide rates, compared to veterans without PTSD. Zivin et al. (2007) conducted a retrospective cohort study of suicide risk factors in depressed veterans, using data from the VA National Registry for Depression. Unexpectedly, veterans with comorbid PTSD and depression had lower rates of suicide than depressed veterans without PTSD; the authors speculated that this may be due to veterans with PTSD receiving more mental health treatment than veterans without comorbid PTSD. Most recently, LeardMann et al. (2013) conducted a prospective cohort study with former and current military personnel using data from the Millennium Cohort Study. PTSD (i.e., a positive PTSD screen or self-reported lifetime diagnosis of PTSD) was not significantly associated with suicide in unadjusted or adjusted (i.e., age and sex) analyses.

Although these three studies did not find PTSD to be significantly associated with suicide, several important factors should be considered. For example, increased suicide risk associated with PTSD may differ based on population and methodological approaches (e.g., inpatient population, depressed sample, length of follow-up time). Furthermore, PTSD may not confer additional risk for suicide when considered in relation to other disorders or when comorbid with disorders.

6.2.4 Summary

In sum, PTSD appears to be associated with SI and SAs (Krysinska and Lester 2010; Panagioti et al. 2009, 2012). In some circumstances, PTSD is associated with suicide (Bullman and Kang 1994; Ilgen et al. 2010); however, this association has not been found when examining veterans in more acute settings (Desai et al. 2005) or with pronounced psychiatric comorbidity, suggesting that the association between PTSD and suicide is likely complex and influenced by the presence of other psychiatric disorders (Desai et al. 2005; Zivin et al. 2007). More research is needed to identify potential moderators of the association between PTSD and suicide.

6.3 Traumatic Brain Injury

6.3.1 *Definition*

Using Department of Defense criteria, traumatic brain injury (TBI) is defined as a "traumatically induced structural injury and/or physiological disruption of brain function as a result of an external force that is indicated by […]: any period of loss or a decreased level of consciousness (LOC); any loss of memory for events immediately before or after the event; any alteration in mental state at the time of the injury […]; neurological deficits […] that may or may not be transient; or intracranial lesion" (Department of Veterans Affairs and Department of Defense 2009). Severity of injury can be determined by duration of LOC, duration of posttraumatic amnesia, and severity of Glasgow Coma Scale at initial evaluation.

Blast exposure is the most common mechanism for TBI among OEF/OIF service members, though traditional mechanisms of injury (e.g., falls, vehicular accidents) have also been reported (Terrio et al. 2009). Although significant work is being conducted to increase understanding of underlying mechanisms of blast injury, it is believed that with traditional mechanisms, the brain is pushed against the sides of the cranium, resulting in direct injury at the site of the impact and indirect injury across from the site of the blow (Bigler 2001). Based on the hard, inflexible nature of the skull, the brain is particularly susceptible to direct injury along the frontal and temporal lobes, where the sphenoid bone divides the anterior and middle fossas, resulting in commonly seen frontotemporal deficits in TBI (Bigler 2007). However, shear injury can occur from rotational forces sustained during the injury. These rotational forces cause Diffuse Axonal Injury (DAI), which consists of multifocal injury to white matter tracts in the brainstem, parasagittal white matter of the cerebral cortex, corpus callosum, and the gray-white junctions of the cerebral cortex (Meythaler et al. 2001). Vascular compromise, edema, and a cascade release of excitotoxic chemicals (Bigler 2001) may also contribute to cognitive, physical, and emotional dysfunction (Van Der Naalt et al. 1999).

6.3.2 *Course*

Typically, most people who sustain a mild TBI (mTBI) return to baseline functioning within one year. Between 7 and 33 % of individuals with mTBI continue to have symptoms one year after injury (Belanger and Vanderploeg 2005). However, in moderate to severe TBI, symptoms are more persistent with one study showing recovery to preinjury levels at only 40 % in cognitive competency, leisure, and recreation (Dikmen et al. 2003). Moreover, Draper and Ponsford (2008) found that patients showed significant impairment on measures of processing speed, memory, and executive function, with severity of injury being correlated with more affected test performance. Executive dysfunction is strongly linked to cognitive, behavioral, and functional outcomes, including community integration (Hanks et al. 1999).

6.3.3 Epidemiology

Approximately 8–22.8 % of military personnel deployed to Iraq or Afghanistan report a history consistent with mTBI (Hoge et al. 2008; Schneiderman et al. 2008; Terrio et al. 2009). Within OEF/OIF service members from 2000 to 2012, the majority of TBIs sustained are mild (77 %), as opposed to moderate (17 %) or severe (2 %) (Fischer 2013). In a sample of veterans from all eras seeking VHA mental health services, Brenner et al. (2013) found that the prevalence of probable TBI (based on a TBI screen) was 45 %. A subset of participants were interviewed and reported that the severity of their worst lifetime TBI was 57 % mild, 16 % moderate, and 27 % severe (Brenner et al. 2013).

6.3.4 Association with Suicide

6.3.4.1 SI

Research on TBI and subsequent SI has been limited. An initial systematic review on suicidal thoughts and behaviors following TBI was conducted by Simpson and Tate (2007), who concluded that individuals with TBI report high rates of SI, ranging from 3 to 33 % with the majority of studies obtaining rates above 10 %. More recently, Bahraini et al. (2013) conducted an update to Simpson and Tate's (2007) review. They identified two new studies which reported rates of SI among those with TBI (mild, moderate, or severe) as ranging from 28.3 % in a community sample (Tsaousides et al. 2011) to 72.7 % among veterans with post-TBI psychiatric hospitalization (Gutierrez et al. 2008).

6.3.4.2 SA

In their systematic review, Simpson and Tate (2007) reported a wide range of SA prevalence rates among individuals with TBI, ranging from 1 to 60 %, and attributed the variability to methodological issues. Bahraini et al. (2013) identified two new studies that reported on rates of SA among individuals with TBI. In a sample of veterans evaluated by an interdisciplinary TBI team, 7.1 % had a SA documented in their VA medical record in the 2 years following their TBI (mild, moderate, or severe; Breshears et al. 2010). A much higher rate of post-TBI SA (27.3 %) was observed in a sample of veterans with a history of TBI (primarily moderate or severe) and post-TBI psychiatric inpatient admissions. However, these findings were based on a small sample ($n = 22$; Gutierrez et al. 2008). In regard to these samples, Bahraini et al. (2013) noted concerns regarding potential biases.

6.3.4.3 Suicide

Findings regarding TBI and death by suicide are more robust. Both systematic reviews on TBI and suicide (Bahraini et al. 2013; Simpson and Tate 2007) found evidence for an increased risk of suicide among TBI survivors. In a seminal Danish study, civilians with TBI (varying levels of severity) had a higher incidence of suicide when compared to the general population (Teasdale and Engberg 2001). Using a retrospective cohort design, Brenner et al. (2011b) found that veterans in the VHA with any history of TBI (i.e., collapsing all levels of injury severity) were 1.55 times more likely to die by suicide, compared to veterans with no TBI history, adjusting for demographics and psychiatric diagnoses (including PTSD).

6.3.5 Summary

TBI does appear to have a clear association with suicide. Further research is required to confirm initial findings which suggest associations between TBI and SI and SA.

6.4 Co-occurring PTSD and TBI

6.4.1 Epidemiology

As trauma exposure can entail both psychological and biomechanical trauma, PTSD and TBI can also co-occur. Estimates of PTSD among military personnel and veterans with TBI vary widely. One recent review reported rates ranging from 12 to 89 % (Bahraini et al. 2014); however as methodological factors can impact estimations of co-occurrence, research on the prevalence of co-occurring PTSD and TBI should be interpreted cautiously. Despite existing challenges, Carlson et al. (2011) noted "strikingly consistent" (p. 110) findings among three large studies with military personnel who served in OEF/OIF (Hoge et al. 2008; Schneiderman et al. 2008; Tanielian and Jaycox 2008). That is, 5–7 % of individuals screened positive for both mTBI and PTSD (Carlson et al. 2011). Furthermore, among individuals who screened positive for probable mTBI, 33–39 % also screened positive for probable PTSD (Carlson et al. 2011). In terms of symptoms, individuals with co-occurring PTSD and mTBI report more severe post-concussive and PTSD symptoms (Barnes et al. 2012; Brenner et al. 2010; Ragsdale et al. 2013; Schneiderman et al. 2008).

6.4.2 Association with Suicide

6.4.2.1 SI

When examining the impact of TBI on SI among those with PTSD, TBI has not been found to be a significant predictor. Two retrospective cross-sectional studies were conducted with veterans and military personnel with PTSD; both found that those with a history of mTBI were no more likely to report SI than those without mTBI (Barnes et al. 2012; Romesser et al. 2011). Several methodological concerns severely limit the validity of these findings, including the use of single-item measures of SI, inconsistent or unclear criteria for establishing the absence of TBI, and not sufficiently controlling for potential confounders (Bahraini et al. 2013). Additionally, the study by Barnes et al. (2012) was not sufficiently powered to detect small effects, and it was unclear whether lifetime mTBI history was assessed in the control group (Bahraini et al. 2013).

6.4.2.2 SA

In regard to the association of co-occurring PTSD and TBI on SA, PTSD significantly predicts past SA, irrespective of TBI history. Brenner et al. (2011a) found that veterans with both PTSD and TBI (i.e., mild, moderate, or severe) were 3.29 times more likely than veterans with TBI only to have a history of SA. Additionally, veterans with comorbid PTSD and TBI were 2.54 times more likely than veterans with neither TBI nor PTSD to have a prior SA.

6.4.2.3 Suicide

No studies were identified that examined the impact of co-occurring PTSD and TBI on suicide.

6.4.3 Summary

The co-occurrence of PTSD and TBI appears to be highly variable and population dependent. Studies of SI in those with co-occurring TBI and PTSD have not been significantly powered and have had methodological problems, limiting available knowledge in this area. However, studies have found a positive association among

PTSD, TBI, and SAs. Taken together, the findings noted above suggest that further investigation regarding the co-occurrence of TBI history and PTSD on SI, SA, and suicide is warranted.

6.5 Jollant et al. (2011) Three-Step Suicidal Process and Underlying Impairment

Jollant et al. (2011) suggest that the suicidal process can be understood as a sequence of three steps from triggering of automatic negative emotions, to intense and prolonged negative emotional states; to the suicidal act. Moreover, the authors highlight the importance of understanding potential cognitive and neuroanatomic factors that may facilitate each of the distinct steps. In order to develop a neuro-cognitive working model of common factors underlying the three-step process, Jollant et al. (2011) conducted a review of studies focused on SDV and cognitive and neuroanatomical dysfunctions. Neuropsychological and imaging studies published prior to 2010 were identified and reviewed. Areas of cognitive dysfunction identified included: *high attention to specific emotional stimuli* ("five positive studies including one fMRI study"); *impaired decision making* ("four positive and two correlational studies"); *lower problem-solving abilities* ("numerous positive studies"); *reduced verbal fluency* ("three positive and one negative study"); *non-emotional attention* ("two positive and two negative studies"); *and reversal learning* ("two positive, three negative and one positive correlational studies") (p. 321). In terms of neuroimaging, the authors suggest that the most robust findings emerged from comparisons between patients who had attempted suicide and those who had not. Areas implicated included the: *ventrolateral prefrontal cortex* (PFC) ("two structural, two functional and two correlational studies"); *anterior cingulate gyrus* ("two functional", "one pharmacological" and "two correlational studies"); *dorsomedial PFC* ("one functional and two correlational studies"); *dorsolateral PFC* ("one structural and one correlational study"); and potentially to a lesser degree the *amygdala and medial temporal cortex* ("one structural and one functional study") (p. 321).

Based upon neuropsychological and neuroanatomical findings, Jollant et al. (2011) hypothesize that three areas of cognitive dysfunction may be implicated in facilitating suicidal crises during periods of stress. These include: altered modulation of value attribution; reduced regulation of emotional and cognitive responses; and facilitation of acts in emotional contexts (Fig. 6.1). Clinically, these areas of cognitive function can be observed as: (1) value attribution—increased sensitivity to others and the environment; (2) reduced regulation of emotional and cognitive responses—poor problem-solving skills, lack of cognitive flexibility; and (3) facilitation of acts in emotional contexts—impulsivity or challenges associated with disinhibiting behavior (Homaifar et al. 2012b; Jollant et al. 2011). As will be explored below, each of these areas has also been studied vis-à-vis PTSD and/or TBI.

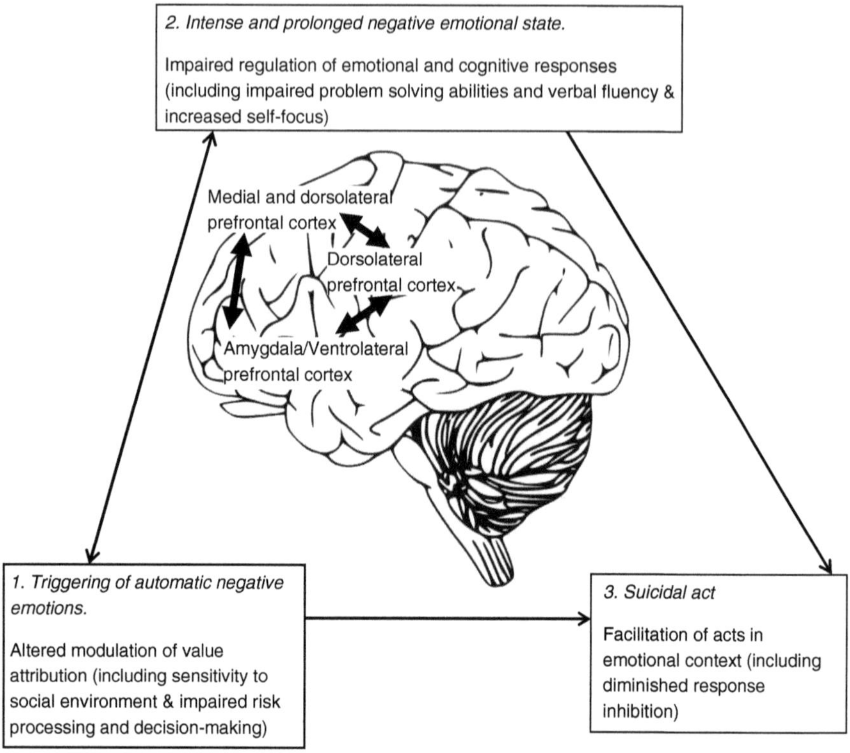

Fig. 6.1 Jollant et al. (2011) Model

6.6 Altered Modulation of Value Attribution and Underlying Neuroanatomical Dysfunction

6.6.1 PTSD

The hallmark symptoms of PTSD can be attributed to both underlying emotional and cognitive processes. Furthermore, these two processes are thought to interact with one another to both explain the emergence and maintenance of the disorder. For example, Brown and Morey (2012) have proposed an emotion-cognition interaction model which is based on two networks of altered brain activation (i.e., trauma-disrupted network and a fear learning network). Evidence for deficits within these two networks could potentially explain predisposition, or susceptibility, for suicidal behavior among individuals with PTSD.

As commonly seen in the clinical presentation of the disorder, individuals with PTSD often struggle with the ability to accurately assign value to external events. This inability is reflected by struggles with re-experiencing, hyperarousal, and avoidance symptoms. Behavioral processes of fear conditioning and extinction are often used to explain how PTSD may impact the ability to accurately assign value to external stimuli. For example, several studies and reviews have found evidence for enhanced fear conditioning (Hayes et al. 2012) in individuals with PTSD. Imaging results suggest greater activation in the amygdala in PTSD (Etkin and Wager 2007; Liberzon and Sripada 2007; Shin et al. 2005, 2006; Shvil et al. 2013), which is important given that the amygdala is involved in the assessment of threat-related stimuli. Studies suggest that individuals with PTSD show greater activation in the amygdala when presented with both trauma-related stimuli and affective stimuli (Shin et al. 2006; Shvil et al. 2013). The hyperresponsivity of the amygdala likely intensifies processes associated with risk-detection, especially as it relates to hyperarousal and vigilance (Liberzon and Sripada 2007), thus making it more likely that the individual is inaccurately assessing value of external events. This initial inability to perceive the environment accurately plays an integral role in processes to follow, such as those that underlie attention, memory, and problem solving.

Across a variety of different paradigms (e.g., emotional stroop), evidence suggests that individuals with PTSD suffer from attentional biases. These biases appear to relate primarily to an individual's inability to disengage from negative stimuli (Hayes et al. 2012) and have been found to be positively associated with intrusive symptoms (Weber 2008). Together these findings suggest a feedback loop in which difficulty disengaging from negative stimuli increases the likelihood of intrusive symptoms, which in turn facilitates continued attentional bias. These attentional biases also have direct implications for memory encoding processes, as greater resources may be directed toward encoding emotional information (Hayes et al. 2012) at the cost of neutral information.

The brain structures (e.g., amygdala, dorsal anterior cingulate cortex (ACC), insula, ventromedial PFC) thought to be implicated in the previously described deficits seen in PTSD do not completely overlap with brain areas thought to be associated with altered value attribution seen in individuals with a history of suicidal behavior (Jollant et al. 2011); however, findings do suggest similar underlying processes related to suicide risk. The hyperactivation of the amygdala, a key defining feature of the fear network, could present susceptibility of both increased negative emotions (e.g., anger) and biased perceptual processes. Due to elevation of threat perceptions in the environment with subsequent difficulty disengaging from negative stimuli, an individual with PTSD is likely to engage in disadvantaged decision making, which appears to be associated with a predisposition to suicidal behavior (Jollant et al. 2011).

6.7 Impaired Regulation of Emotional and Cognitive Responses and Underlying Neuroanatomical Dysfunction

6.7.1 PTSD

The triggering of automatic negative emotions and attentional biases, especially over prolonged periods of time, likely contributes to intense and prolonged negative states. In fact, several authors suggest that the emotional and cognitive resources that are dedicated to threat perception leave fewer resources available to oversee the regulation of responses (Hayes et al. 2012; Weber 2008). Intense negative states with poor emotional and cognitive regulation could likely present greater susceptibility to suicidal behaviors, especially via processes related to hopelessness and rumination.

Neuroimaging studies have provided evidence that hyperactivity in emotion processing networks (e.g., amygdala, ventrolateral PFC, medial PFC) and hypoactivation in the dorsal executive functioning processing networks are associated with impaired maintenance of information in working memory (Hayes et al. 2012). Impaired maintenance of information within working memory due to emotional distraction likely has important implications for emotional and cognitive regulation. For example, these deficits could impact concentration ability, mental flexibility, and memory encoding, all aspects necessary to regulatory mechanisms.

In addition to deficits in working memory, individuals with PTSD consistently show bias for both episodic and autobiographical memories (Weber 2008). For example, individuals with PTSD show greater memory bias for traumatic information, and studies have found that individuals with PTSD perform worse when asked to recall personal memories compared to individuals without PTSD (Hayes et al. 2012). Findings suggest that recall often lacks detailed information and shows consistent "gist-like" performance across both traumatic memories and neutral/positive events (Hayes et al. 2012). Implications for this type of biased memory could facilitate reduced problem-solving abilities, especially given the deficit in memory for autobiographical events. As discussed by Jollant et al. (2011), poor recall, or biased recall, for autobiographical events, likely creates even greater difficulty when attempting to generate solutions for emotional regulation based on prior experience.

The hypoactivation of the mPFC may be a large contributor to difficulties in emotional and cognitive regulation. In addition to providing inhibitory control over the amygdala, the mPFC is believed to play a role in the contextualizing of stimuli, which helps guide the selection of appropriate responses based on environmental factors (Liberzon and Sripada 2007). Diminished functioning of the mPFC, which is tasked with regulation of affect and integration of emotional and cognitive information, then, is likely less effective in larger executive control processes, especially when affective content is triggered (Brown and Morey 2012). Furthermore, deficits in the mPFC are likely associated with diminished habituation of amygdala responses (Shin et al. 2005). Together, the lack of inhibitory control, poorer extinction/habituation processes, and overall diminished functioning of the mPFC, contribute to greater demands on the fear network. These greater demands tax emotional and cognitive regulatory abilities, especially when activated within an emotional context and could prolong the negative emotional state and reduce problem-solving abilities, both factors that may contribute to suicide risk.

6.8 Facilitation of Acts in Emotional Context Underlying Neuroanatomical Dysfunction

6.8.1 PTSD

The ability to engage in complex goal-directed behavior requires the synthesis of many of the aforementioned processes, especially those involving attention, working memory, flexibility, and planning. Given that many of these processes are impacted when PTSD is present, overall executive control of behavior is likely challenged. Poor regulation of attention and responses to stimuli likely play a large role in the development of potentially maladaptive coping mechanisms (Aupperle et al. 2012). Regardless of whether these coping mechanisms are either directly or indirectly associated with suicidal behaviors, the presence of maladaptive coping mechanisms, especially due to underlying difficulties with response inhibition, could present another view of neurobiological susceptibility for suicidal behaviors.

Several researchers have suggested a possible functional relationship between the amygdala and mPFC (Hayes et al. 2012; Shin et al. 2005, 2006). This functional relationship may help to conceptualize how the aforementioned areas of susceptibility for risk interact with one another to facilitate additional suicidal risk. Neuroimaging studies suggest that there may be a functional exchange between hyperactivation of prefrontal areas and the hypoactivation of inhibition areas (Aupperle et al. 2012). Hyperactivation promotes biased perception of increased negativity, while hypoactivation leads to the inability to manage incoming information within the context of competing contextual stimuli. For example, studies using several paradigms (e.g., continuous performance tasks, Go/No-go, attention network tasks) consistently find that individuals with PTSD have difficulty with the inhibition of automatic responses (Aupperle et al. 2012). Additional findings suggest that individuals with PTSD also have difficulty disengaging from emotional stimuli, which as previously described effects memory and working memory, but also overall executive function. If unable to disengage from emotional stimuli, behavioral responses (including those aimed at regulatory function) could likely be characterized by more emotional valence (Etkin and Wager 2007). Furthermore, inability to disengage or inhibit responses to a stimulus that is emotionally taxing promotes avoidance behavior, which further reinforces the pattern of maladaptive coping. Heightened emotional coping and/or avoidance are key factors that maintain PTSD symptoms. These same behaviors, however, could also serve as catalysts to more severe forms of inadequate coping, such as suicidal behaviors.

6.9 PTSD and Suicide: Overall Conclusion

Although the disruptions of emotional and cognitive processes in PTSD do not completely overlap with those described by Jollant et al. (2011), the nature of these disrupted processes do share similarities with the proposed model. First, hyperactivation of the amygdala results in increased opportunities for negative emotional triggers. These triggers are predominated by threat characterization and effect the ways in which the individual responds to the environment. These increased affective triggers dominate the neurocognitive profile, making problem solving increasingly difficult, leading to poorer emotional and cognitive control, with fewer resources devoted to response inhibition. This increased susceptibility may help to explain why individuals with PTSD may be at greater risk for suicidal behaviors.

6.10 Altered Modulation of Value Attribution and Underlying Neuroanatomical Dysfunction

6.10.1 Moderate to Severe TBI

Focal injuries to the frontal and temporal lobes are common after a TBI (Bigler 2001). As a result, those with moderate to severe injury often present with dysexecutive, behavioral, affective, and cognitive problems (Bigler 2001; Zappala et al. 2012; Stuss 2011). In turn, those with a history of TBI can have a dramatic change in personality, impulse control problems, lack of social awareness, disinhibition, and attention modulation deficits. Each of these areas of deficit is likely to interact with one another to facilitate increased risk for suicidal behavior. Moreover, they correspond with aspects of the Jollant et al. (2011) model.

While value attribution as defined by Jollant et al. (2011) has not been directly studied in TBI, many related topics have been, such as the executive dysfunction seen in rumination. This has a strong relationship with hopelessness, depression, and impaired problem-solving ability as well as with SI and suicidal behavior (Morrison and O'Connor 2008). Increased rumination may impact the ability to accurately assign value to external and internal events. Rumination has been localized to the anterior and posterior medial PFC, areas known to be frequently damaged in TBI (Bigler 2001). Disruption of these areas by TBI may lead to problems in regulating the amount of rumination occurring in those with SI.

6.11 Impaired Regulation of Emotional and Cognitive Responses and Underlying Neuroanatomical Dysfunction

6.11.1 Moderate to Severe TBI

Impaired regulation of emotional and cognitive responses is one of the hallmarks of TBI, including emotional instability or lability, depression, and dysphoria. Problems with emotional regulation have an impact on cognitive flexibility and the ability to problem solve, both executive functions that have been implicated in suicide risk by other authors (Homaifar et al. 2012b). One such executive function, emotional regulation, is thought to predominately occur in the ACC (Bush et al. 2000), an area frequently damaged in TBI due to its location. Coding of negative moral feelings including guilt, embarrassment, and shame also take place in the medial prefrontal cortex (Takahashi et al. 2004). Without the ability to regulate emotional and cognitive responses after a TBI, individuals are left more vulnerable to suicidal thoughts and behaviors.

In addition to having problems with regulating emotion, working memory is also affected in TBI. These working memory difficulties and need for more brain area to accomplish tasks may also place larger demands on emotional and cognitive regulation leading to greater prolonged negative emotional states. fMRI has shown blood flow abnormalities in the frontal lobes in those with moderate and severe TBI when compared to normal subjects, suggesting greater quantity of brain areas are required for completing the same working memory task (Christodoulou et al. 2001). This need for increased activation when completing tasks has been seen in mTBI as well (Jantzen et al. 2004). This working memory difficulty may contribute to the increased problems with rumination previously discussed. With both increased rumination and difficulty regulating emotional and cognitive responses, having poor working memory likely contributes to worsening of these problems, possibly increasing the magnitude of each and contributing to the increased risk for suicidal thoughts and behaviors in TBI.

In addition to the more medial problems discussed above in the frontal lobe as a result of TBI, dysexecutive syndromes can also occur with damage more laterally to the frontal lobe, specifically to the dorsolateral and ventrolateral PFC. Organization, planning, reasoning, set-shifting, and monitoring can all be affected in this syndrome. Impulsivity and decision-making problems have been found in those with TBI on the Immediate and Delayed Memory Task (Dougherty et al. 2004) and the Iowa Gambling Test (Bechara et al. 1994), respectively. One study investigating executive dysfunction found that individuals with SAs had more perseverative errors on the Wisconsin Card Sort Test (Heaton et al. 1993) than individuals without SAs (Homaifar et al. 2012a). This suggests that the executive dysfunction in TBI may play a role in being unable to cease perseveration over suicidal thoughts and may impede attending to goal-directed behavior. This ‘cognitive rigidity’ has been seen in suicide attempters with reduced problem-solving ability and likely contributes to the increased suicide risk in TBI. Unfortunately, many of these studies are small and do not adequately take into account comorbidities known to occur in TBI, such as depression, pointing to the need for further research in this area.

6.12 Facilitation of Acts in Emotional Context Underlying Neuroanatomical Dysfunction

6.12.1 Moderate to Severe TBI

Besides problems with emotional regulation, TBI is also characterized by disinhibition and impulsivity. For example, behavioral syndromes are characterized by aggressive or abusive behavior, selfishness, lability, impulsivity, environmental dependency, and a lack of empathy and can be best understood as a problem with impulse control and an inability to integrate feedback into one's behavior in a meaningful way. This syndrome results from damage to the orbitofrontal region, which mediates comportment and social intelligence. Certainly, disinhibition and impulsiveness contribute to Jollant et al. (2011) characterization of facilitation of acts in an emotional context as the final step in the model. This disinhibition can result in violence toward self or others. Studies have supported claims of increased aggression toward others in those with a history of TBI compared to those with other injuries (Tateno et al. 2003). In addition, other observational studies showed that those with frontal injury had higher rates of aggression compared to those with injury in other locations (Tateno et al. 2003). Other studies have shown that those with a history of TBI have a diminished capacity for empathy (Wood and Williams 2008). Many other factors play into future violence after TBI, such as premorbid conditions, but as stated by Wortzel et al. (2013), injury to the orbitofrontal cortex may lower the individual's ability to inhibit such behaviors. SDV, such as suicide, may follow the same pattern of a lowered ability to inhibit behavior due to alterations in impulse control, increased aggression, and increased disinhibition. This area of the brain is also activated by social exclusion as well as other situations involving self-blame and social rejection, emphasizing a possible interplay with the previously described deficits in value attribution and emotional regulation (Eisenberger et al. 2003). This diminished ability to inhibit SDV may enable a suicidal act in an individual who may already have a tendency toward increased perseveration about the external environment or other triggers.

6.13 TBI and Suicide: Overall Conclusions

Although the cognitive and emotional problems in TBI do not overlap exactly with Jollant et al. (2011) model, the idea of an inability to regulate cognitive and emotional responses combined with facilitation of acts due to the frontotemporal injuries commonly seen in TBI could be a useful way to conceptualize the reasons that suicidal thoughts and behaviors are increased with TBI. With the medial frontal lobe affected, individuals are unable to accurately assign value and appropriate valance to emotion. The lateral PFC damage then causes difficulty in 'set-shifting' and contributes to increased rumination and inability to creatively problem solve compounding the mPFC's difficulties with working memory and emotional regulation. Finally, damage to the orbitofrontal region contributes to impulsivity and a higher rate of aggression. These factors may all work in concert within the Jollant et al. (2011) model to increase the risk for SDV in those with moderate and severe TBI.

6.14 Three-Step Suicidal Process and Underlying Neuroanatomical Dysfunction Among Those with Co-occurring Moderate to Severe TBI and PTSD

As previously discussed, knowledge regarding co-occurring moderate to severe TBI and PTSD is limited. Although there are common brain areas implicated in both conditions, resulting outcomes are likely affected by both individual and systematic factors (Brenner 2011). Additionally, the overlap in symptoms and areas of impairment complicate our understanding of which underlying condition may be implicated, limiting findings using neuropsychological measures (Brenner et al. 2009a). Furthermore, how the neuroanatomical dysfunction of both conditions confer risk for suicidal behavior is complicated by the fact that some researchers suggest that TBI may increase risk for PTSD (Bryant et al. 2010; Matthews et al. 2011). Despite these challenges, the overlap in implicated brain areas suggests that the co-occurrence of TBI and PTSD may present vulnerabilities to suicidal behavior.

Underlying neuroanatomical dysfunctions in the co-occurrence of TBI and PTSD include the amygdala and PFC. Because tracts connecting the amygdala and the mPFC are vulnerable to disruption due to TBI (Stein and McAllister 2009), it may be possible that TBI increases PTSD vulnerabilities related to assigning value to external events, thus increasing sensitivity to negative emotions and stimuli. Additionally, TBI and PTSD deficits within the PFC (Brenner 2011) may also impair emotion regulation abilities, further compounding effects of rumination, working memory, and recall deficits seen in each condition alone.

In addition to brain areas of overlap between the two conditions, research suggests that the two conditions may work in concert with one another to confer risk for suicidal behavior. For example, the presence of TBI may affect the cognitive resources that would typically be employed when engaging in problem-solving and emotion regulation, thus exacerbating the effects of PTSD symptoms (Stein and McAllister 2009). Similarly, TBI may exacerbate PTSD symptoms by diminishing the ability to self-regulate and inhibit behavioral responses (Nelson et al. 2009). The overlap in the conditions, especially within the dorsolateral PFC (Stein and McAllister 2009), may increase deficits in the ability to self-monitor (Matthews et al. 2012), facilitating suicidal behavior. Thus, when examining how the co-occurrence of TBI and PTSD may confer risk for suicidal behaviors, it is important to consider how the occurrence of one condition (e.g., TBI) likely reduces the cortical reserve available, making the effects of a second condition (e.g., PTSD) possibly more pronounced (Stein and McAllister 2009).

6.15 Clinical Implications

Based on the existing literature, as well as the conceptual model as proposed in this chapter, there are important clinical implications to consider. As described throughout the chapter, there are several areas of possible underlying susceptibility that may be implicated in suicidal behavior. When working with individuals who have PTSD or have experienced a TBI, it is important to assess for these underlying susceptibilities. Although formal neuropsychological or neuroimaging techniques could be used, it is also possible to assess for vulnerabilities during a clinical interview. Homaifar et al. (2012b) recommend several basic assessment strategies that can be used to identify deficits in executive dysfunction. Corresponding with the deficits outlined in the Jollant et al. (2011) model, these areas include impulsivity/inhibition, insight/lack of self-awareness, and thinking processes. If deficits are noted, it is important to screen for SI. This screening should be carried out regularly, especially when individuals report changes in psychological or cognitive symptoms.

Identified deficits associated with each of the components of the Jollant et al. (2011) model could also be used when performing safety planning with an individual who is at risk for suicidal behaviors. Safety plans involve the identification of warning signs, coping strategies, supports, and emergency resources that an individual can use if they find themselves in crisis. In addition to the assessment recommendations described above, Homaifar et al. (2012b) also suggest areas of intervention that correspond with the vulnerabilities outlined in the Jollant et al. (2011) model, which can be easily adapted to the safety planning process. For example, the provider can work with the individual to identify coping strategies to promote immediate gratification, improve awareness to warning signs, and build problem-solving skills by brainstorming steps to take during a crisis (Homaifar et al. 2012b).

If an individual is at risk for suicidal behaviors, means restriction, another aspect of the safety plan, would be especially important as this would limit ability to carry out suicidal acts as described in the third component of the Jollant et al. (2011)

model. This process would involve working with the individual to identify ways to make the environment safe. Examples include limiting direct access to firearms by using gun locks/cabinets, and/or having a third party control access to firearms by keeping keys or gun cabinet combinations. Other critical means restriction methods may involve blister packaging to limit overdosing on medications and removing or limiting access to alcohol/drugs/knives. Adding reminders of reasons for living to the environment (e.g., photos of loved ones, mementos of accomplishments) may be another successful strategy to improve decision-making during a heightened emotional state, especially if the individual is susceptible to prolonged negative emotional states.

6.16 Limitations and Future Research

To our knowledge this is the first application of the Jollant et al. (2011) model to conceptualize how TBI and PTSD are associated with increased risk for suicidal behaviors. This chapter reflects novel thinking in this understudied area and is intended to promote interest in future research on the topic; however, the following limitations should be considered.

It is important to note that research on the Jollant et al. (2011) model is preliminary. Although the model was built upon empirical literature, articles reviewed when developing the model were limited and there have been no subsequent studies to verify model components. Second, the current chapter did not utilize a systematic review in its inclusion of studies. Thus, quality of research design and data were not evaluated for inclusion. This approach was utilized to consider a broader realm of the available literature to assist in the conceptual application of the Jollant et al. (2011) model. Future reviews would likely benefit from the use of a systematic review to better scrutinize the strengths and weaknesses of the relevant literature.

Future researchers may want to examine the role that mediators and moderators play in each component of the model and subsequent suicidal behaviors. Research designs that activate a component of the model could also improve the sensitivity and specificity of model components. For example, a design that could trigger altered value attribution to elicit emotional and cognitive regulation could assist in better understanding underlying mechanisms and aspects of vulnerability.

As noted throughout the chapter, there are significant limitations in the current research on PTSD, TBI, and suicidal behaviors. Some of these limitations are inherent to the conditions themselves, affecting outcomes of studies and the ability to make conclusions across studies. For example, heterogeneity of the conditions are common; based on associated symptomology, each individual with TBI and PTSD can present differently. Literature on TBI, especially mTBI, is not well understood at this time. Although significantly more research exists on PTSD, the current literature is now limited due to changes in DSM criteria. Finally, because research on the co-occurrence between TBI and PTSD is limited, difficulties in interpreting how the two conditions may confer risk for suicidal behaviors persist. It is unknown whether the two conditions combine to establish greater susceptibility to suicidal behaviors or whether there are other mechanisms at play.

Much like the heterogeneity involved in TBI and PTSD, the Jollant et al. (2011) model also provides possible profiles of risk that are heterogeneous. Furthermore, the model presents a continuum of possible risk within each component. It is unclear at which point deficits would confer greatest risk and how this would impact the relationship among the three components. Finally, it is worth noting that an application of a network/tract- based model may be most helpful in understanding how impairment across areas of the brain is implicated in risk rather than a neuroanatomical approach that looks at each brain structure separately, as is common in the current literature and reflected in the Jollant et al. (2011) model.

The use of a broader range of methodological designs could assist in addressing some of these limitations. First, research that explores both overall neurobiology as well as the neuroanatomy of specific symptoms could prove especially useful in understanding neuroanatomical functioning of each condition. Second, improved functional imaging that takes into account other relevant variables (psychiatric comorbidity, duration of symptoms, etc.) could help improve models by drawing awareness to the relevance of additional factors related to each condition. Finally, it is recommended that studies take into account the co-occurring fact of low exposure and low outcome (i.e., death by suicide) within this domain and use appropriate methodological designs that improve the ability to detect differences between groups.

References

American Psychiatric Association (2013) Diagnostic and statistical manual of mental disorders, 5th edn. American Psychiatric Publishing, Arlington (Print)

Aupperle RL et al (2012) Executive function and PTSD: disengaging from Trauma. Neuropharmacology 62(2):686–694

Bahraini NH et al (2014) Traumatic brain injury and posttraumatic stress disorder. Psychiatr Clin North Am 37(1):55–75

Bahraini NH et al (2013) Suicidal ideation and behaviours after traumatic brain injury: a systematic review. Brain Impairment 14(1):99–112

Barnes SM, Walter KH, Chard KM (2012) Does a history of mild traumatic brain injury increase suicide risk in veterans with PTSD? Rehabil Psychol 57(1):18–26

Bechara A et al (1994) Insensitivity to future consequences following damage to human pre-frontal cortex. Cognition 50(1–3):7–15

Belanger HG, Vanderploeg RD (2005) The neuropsychological impact of sports-related concussion: a meta-analysis. J Int Neuropsychol Soc 11(4):345–357

Bigler ED (2001) The lesion(s) in traumatic brain injury: implications for clinical neuropsychology. Arch Clin Neuropsychol 16(2):95–131

Bigler ED (2007) Anterior and middle cranial fossa in traumatic brain injury: relevant neuroanatomy and neuropathology in the study of neuropsychological outcome. Neuropsychology 21(5):515–531

Brenner LA (2011) Neuropsychological and neuroimaging findings in traumatic brain injury and post-traumatic stress disorder. Dialogues Clin Neurosci 13(3):311–323

Brenner LA et al (2011a) Posttraumatic stress disorder, traumatic brain injury, and suicide attempt history among veterans receiving mental health services. Suicide Life-Threat Behav 41 (4):416–423

Brenner LA, Ignacio RV, Blow FC (2011b) Suicide and traumatic brain injury among individuals seeking veterans health administration services. J Head Trauma Rehabil 26(4):257–264

Brenner LA et al (2013) Prevalence and screening of traumatic brain injury among veterans seeking mental health services. J Head Trauma Rehabil 28(1):21–30

Brenner LA et al (2009a) An exploratory study of neuroimaging, neurologic, and neuropsychological findings in veteran with traumatic brain injury and/or posttraumatic stress disorder. Mil Med 174(4):347–352

Brenner LA, Rodney DV, Heidi T (2009b) Assessment and diagnosis of mild traumatic brain injury, posttraumatic stress disorder, and other polytrauma conditions: burden of adversity hypothesis. Rehabil Psychol 54(3):239–246

Brenner LA et al (2010) Traumatic brain injury, posttraumatic stress disorder, and postconcussive symptom reporting among troops returning from Iraq. J Head Trauma Rehabil 25(5):307–312

Breshears RE et al (2010) Predicting suicidal behavior in veterans with traumatic brain injury: the utility of the personality assessment inventory. J Pers Assess 92(4):349–355

Brown VM, Morey RA (2012) Neural systems for cognitive and emotional processing in posttraumatic stress disorder. Front Psychol 3:1–14

Bryant RA et al (2010) The psychiatric sequelae of traumatic injury. Am J Psychiatry 167 (3):312–320

Bullman TA, Kang HK (1994) Posttraumatic stress disorder and the risk of traumatic deaths among vietnam veterans. J Nerv Ment Dis 182(11):604–610

Bush G, Luu P, Posner MI (2000) Cognitive and emotional influences in anterior cingulate cortex. Trends Cogn Sci 4(6):215–222

Carlson KF et al (2011) Prevalence, assessment, and treatment of mild traumatic brain injury and posttraumatic stress disorder: a systematic review of the evidence. J Head Trauma Rehabil 26 (2):103–115

Christodoulou C et al (2001) Functional magnetic resonance imaging of working memory impairment after traumatic brain injury. J Neurol Neurosurg Psychiatry 71(2):161–168

Department of Veterans Affairs and The Department of Defense (2009) VA/DoD clinical practice guideline for management of concussion/mild traumatic brain injury. http://mhs.osd.mil/Content/docs/pdfs/policies/2007/07-030.pdf

Desai RA, Dausey DJ, Rosenheck RA (2005) Mental health service delivery and suicide risk: the role of individual patient and facility factors. Am J Psychiatry 162(2):311–318

Dikmen SS et al (2003) Outcome 3 to 5 years after moderate to severe traumatic brain injury. Arch Phys Med Rehabil 84(10):1449–1457

Dougherty DM et al (2004) Laboratory measured behavioral impulsivity relates to suicide attempt history. Suicide Life-Threat Behav 34(4):374–385

Draper K, Ponsford J (2008) Cognitive functioning ten years following traumatic brain injury and rehabilitation. Neuropsychology 22(5):618–625

Eisenberger NI, Lieberman MD, Williams KD (2003) Does rejection hurt? an FMRI study of social exclusion. Science 302(5643):290–292

Etkin A, Wager TD (2007) Functional neuroimaging of anxiety: a meta-analysis of emotional processing in PTSD, social anxiety disorder, and specific phobia. Am J Psychiatry 164 (10):1476

Fischer H (2013) United States military casualty statistics: operation iraqi freedom and operation enduring freedom. Library of Congress Washington DC Congressional Research Service

Gutierrez PM, Brenner LA, Huggins JA (2008) A preliminary investigation of suicidality in psychiatrically hospitalized veterans with traumatic brain injury. Arch Suicide Res 12 (4):336–343

Hanks RA et al (1999) Measures of executive functioning as predictors of functional ability and social integration in a rehabilitation sample. Arch Phys Med Rehabil 80(9):1030–1037

Hayes JP, VanElzakker M, Shin LM (2012) Emotional and cognitive interactions in ptsd: a review of neurocognitive and neuroimaging studies. Front Integr Neurosci 6:1–14
Heaton RK et al (1993) Wisconsin card sorting test: computer version 2. Psychological Assessment Resources, Odessa
Hoge CW et al (2008) Mild traumatic brain injury in US soldiers returning from Iraq. New Engl J Med 358(5):453–463
Homaifar BY et al (2012a) Traumatic brain injury, executive functioning, and suicidal behavior: a brief report. Rehabil Psychol 57(4):337–341
Homaifar BY et al (2012b) Executive functioning as a component of suicide risk assessment: clarifying its role in standard clinical applications. J Mental Health Couns 34(2):110–120
Ilgen MA et al (2010) Psychiatric diagnoses and risk of suicide in veterans. Arch Gen Psychiatry 67(11):1152–1158
Jakupcak M et al (2009) Posttraumatic stress disorder as a risk factor for suicidal ideation in Iraq and Afghanistan war veterans. J Trauma Stress 22(4):303–306
Jantzen KJ et al (2004) A prospective functional MRI imaging study of mild traumatic brain injury in college football players. Am J Neuroradiol 25(5):738–745
Jollant F et al (2011) The suicidal mind and brain: a review of neuropsychological and neuroimaging studies. World J Bio Psychiatry 12(5):319–339
Kessler RC et al (2005a) Lifetime prevalence and age-of-onset distributions of DSM-IV disorders in the national comorbidity survey replication. Arch Gen Psychiatry 62(6):593–602
Kessler RC et al (2005b) Prevalence, severity, and comorbidity of 12-month DSM-IV disorders in the national comorbidity survey replication. Arch Gen Psychiatry 62(6):617–627
Krysinska K, Lester D (2010) Post-traumatic stress disorder and suicide risk: a systematic review. Arch Suicide Res 14(1):1–23
LeardMann CA et al (2013) Risk factors associated with suicide in current and former US military personnel. JAMA 310(5):496–506
Liberzon I, Chandra SS (2007) The functional neuroanatomy of PTSD: a critical review. Prog Brain Res 167:151–169
Marshall RD et al (2001) Comorbidity, impairment, and suicidality in subthreshold PTSD. Am J Psychiatry 158(9):1467–1473
Matthews SC et al (2012) Combat-exposed war veterans at risk for suicide show hyperactivation of prefrontal cortex and anterior cingulate during error processing. Psychosom Med 74 (5):471–475
Matthews SC et al (2011) A multimodal imaging study in U. S. veterans of operations Iraqi and enduring freedom with and without major depression after blast-related concussion. Neuroimage 54(1):S69–S75
Meythaler JM et al (2001) Current concepts: diffuse axonal injury–associated traumatic brain injury. Arch Phys Med Rehabil 82(10):1461–1471
Morrison R, O'Connor RC (2008) A systematic review of the relationship between rumination and suicidality. Suicide Life-Threat Behav 38(5):523–538
Nelson LA et al (2009) Relationship between processing speed and executive functioning performance among OEF/OIF veterans: implications for postdeployment rehabilitation. J Head Trauma Rehabil 24(1):32–40
Panagioti M, Gooding PA, Tarrier N (2012) A meta-analysis of the association between posttraumatic stress disorder and suicidality: the role of comorbid depression. Compr Psychiatry 53(7):915–930
Panagioti M, Gooding P, Tarrier N (2009) Post-traumatic stress disorder and suicidal behavior: a narrative review. Clin Psychol Rev 29(6):471–482
Pompili M et al (2013) Posttraumatic stress disorder and suicide risk among veterans: a literature review. J Nerv Mental Dis 201(9):802–812
Ragsdale KA et al (2013) Posttraumatic stress disorder in OEF/OIF veterans with and without traumatic brain injury. J Anxiety Disord 27(4):420–426
Ramchand R et al (2010) Disparate prevalence estimates of PTSD among service members who served in Iraq and Afghanistan: possible explanations. J Trauma Stress 23(1):59–68

Richardson LK, Frueh BC, Acierno R (2010) Prevalence estimates of combat-related post-traumatic stress disorder: critical review. Aust NZJ Psychiatry 44(1):4–19

Romesser J et al (2011) A preliminary study of the effect of a diagnosis of concussion on PTSD symptoms and other psychiatric variables at the time of treatment seeking among veterans. Mil Med 176(3):246–252

Schneiderman AI, Braver ER, Kang HK (2008) Understanding sequelae of injury mechanisms and mild traumatic brain injury incurred during the conflicts in Iraq and Afghanistan: persistent postconcussive symptoms and posttraumatic stress disorder. Am J Epidemiol 167 (12):1446–1452

Shin LM, Rauch SL, Pitman RK (2006) Amygdala, medial prefrontal cortex, and hippocampal function in PTSD. Ann NY Acad Sci 1071(1):67–79

Shin LM et al (2005) A functional magnetic resonance imaging study of amygdala and medial prefrontal cortex responses to overtly presented fearful faces in posttraumatic stress disorder. Arch Gen Psychiatry 62(3):273–281

Shvil E et al (2013) Neural, psychophysiological, and behavioral markers of fear processing in PTSD: a review of the literature. Curr Psychiatry Rep 15(5):1–10

Simpson G, Tate R (2007) Suicidality in people surviving a traumatic brain injury: prevalence, risk factors and implications for clinical management. Brain Inj 21(13–14):1335–1351

Stein MB, McAllister TW (2009) Exploring the convergence of posttraumatic stress disorder and mild traumatic brain injury. Am J Psychiatry 166(7):768–776

Stuss DT (2011) Traumatic brain injury: relation to executive dysfunction and the frontal lobes. Curr Opin Neurol 24(6):584–589

Takahashi H et al (2004) Brain activation associated with evaluative processes of guilt and embarrassment: an Fmri study. Neuroimage 23(3):967–974

Tanielian TL, Jaycox LH (eds) (2008) Invisible wounds of war: psychological and cognitive injuries, their consequences, and services to assist recovery, vol 720. Rand Corporation

Tateno A, Jorge RE, Robinson RG (2003) Clinical correlates of aggressive behavior after traumatic brain injury. J Neuropsychiatry Clin Neurosci 15(2):155–160

Teasdale TW, Engberg AW (2001) Suicide after traumatic brain injury: a population study. J Neurol Neurosurg Psychiatry 71(4):436–440

Terrio H et al (2009) Traumatic brain injury screening: preliminary findings in a US army brigade combat team. J Head Trauma Rehabil 24(1):14–23

Tsaousides T, Cantor JB, Gordon WA (2011) Suicidal ideation following traumatic brain injury: prevalence rates and correlates in adults living in the community. J Head Trauma Rehabil 26 (4):265–275

Van Der Naalt J et al (1999) Computed tomography and magnetic resonance imaging in mild to moderate head injury: early and late imaging related to outcome. Ann Neurol 46(1):70–78

Weber DL (2008) Information processing bias in post-traumatic stress disorder. Open Neuroimaging J 2:29–51

Wood RL, Williams C (2008) Inability to empathize following traumatic brain injury. J Int Neuropsychol Soc 14(02):289–296

Wortzel HS, Brenner LA, Arciniegas DB (2013) Traumatic brain injury and chronic traumatic encephalopathy: a forensic neuropsychiatric perspective. Behav Sci Law 31(6):721–738

Zappala G, Thiebaut de Schotten M, Eslinger PJ (2012) Traumatic brain injury and the frontal lobes: what can we gain with diffusion tensor imaging? Cortex 48(2):156–165

Zivin K et al (2007) Suicide mortality among individuals receiving treatment for depression in the veterans affairs health system: associations with patient and treatment setting characteristics. Am J Public Health 97(12):2193–2198

Chapter 7
Genetic Risk Factors for Suicidal Behavior

Marco Sarchiapone and Marianna D'Aulerio

Abstract Suicidal behavior comprises a range of heterogeneous entities, from completed suicide to suicide attempts to suicidal ideation (Mann 1998). While the causes of suicide are complex and no simple explanations of the phenomenon exist, it is clear that there is a diathesis component, whereby converging factor such as an acute stressor as well as present and past life circumstances can operate on a backdrop of biological susceptibility. This chapter summarizes the principal research addressing genetic susceptibility to suicide. Even if only the biological vulnerability can be explained, it is acknowledged that the origin and causes of suicidal behavior are a multifactorial act, in which biological aspects are always related to the influence of the environment.

7.1 Introduction

Several researchers have addressed the issue of the origin of suicidal behavior. One of the most useful theoretical models to explain suicidal behavior is the stress-diathesis model. Mann (1998) focused his attention particularly on the role of genetic contribution to suicidal behavior, asserting that genetic make-up as well as acquired susceptibility contributes to a person's constitutional predisposition or diathesis (Wasserman 2000).

The word diathesis, or predisposition, refers to the individual tendency or susceptibility to disease as a result of interaction between genetic vulnerabilities and environmental stress. According to this model, people possessing this predisposition have a greater chance of developing psychological disorders when presented with particular stressful life events. In contrast, people with higher resiliency or low biological vulnerability for a particular disorder need high levels of stress to trigger symptoms of that disorder. According to Mann, the risk for suicidal acts is determined

M. Sarchiapone (✉) · M. D'Aulerio
Medicine and Health Sciences Department, University of Molise, Via De Santis, 86100 Campobasso, Italy
e-mail: Marco.sarchapone@me.com

K.E. Cannon and T.J. Hudzik (eds.), *Suicide: Phenomenology and Neurobiology*,
DOI 10.1007/978-3-319-09964-4_7

not only by a psychiatric illness (the stressor) but also by a diathesis. This diathesis consists of tendencies for greater depression and suicidal ideation, less reason for living, higher rates of lifetime aggression and impulsivity, comorbid borderline personality disorder, substance use disorder or alcoholism, family history of suicidal acts, head injury, smoking, and childhood abuse history (van Heeringen 2012). In particular, Mann (1998) described a predisposition to suicidal acts to be part of a more fundamental predisposition to both externally and self-directed aggression. Aggression and impulsivity are key characteristics, which may be the result of genetic factors or early life experiences.

In a second example of a clinical stress-diathesis model, McGirr and Turecki (2007) suggested that people who attempt or commit suicide have a certain individual predisposition, part of which is given by personality traits, in particular, impulsive-aggressive behaviors. Impulsive-aggressive traits increase suicide risk among a subset of suicides. In this subset, suicide risk does not appear to be a consequence of psychiatric disorder and seems to play a larger role among younger suicides and may mediate familial transmission of suicidal behavior.

7.2 Family, Twin, and Adoption Studies

Family, twin, and adoption studies have demonstrated that the predisposition to suicide includes genetic factors (Petersen et al. 2014) and support the view that the etiology of the familial transmission of suicidal behavior is at least in part genetic, and may be mediated by the transmission of intermediate phenotypes such as impulsive aggression. In addition, there may be environmental causes for familial transmission of intermediate phenotypes and the intergenerational transmission of family adversity (Brent and Melhem 2008).

An association between positive family history and risk of suicide by violent means has been reported (Linkowski et al. 1985), and a large community twin study demonstrated that genetic risk factors accounted for approximately 45 % of the variance in suicidal thoughts and behavior (Statham et al. 1998). Adoption studies also reported increased rates of suicide in the biological rather than adopting relatives of adoptees (Wender et al. 1986).

7.2.1 Family Studies

A number of family studies have implicated familial aggregation in suicidal behavior. Several studies showed a higher rate of suicidal behavior in relatives of suicide victims or attempters compared to relatives of nonsuicidal controls (Brent et al. 1996; Johnson 1998; Malone et al. 1995; Pfeffer et al. 1994; Tsuang 1983). In one of the major studies on the familial transmission of suicide, Roy (1983a, b) demonstrated that almost half (48.6 %) of 243 patients examined with a family history of suicide and with a wide variety of diagnoses (schizophrenia, unipolar and bipolar affective disorders, depressive neurosis, and personality disorders) had attempted suicide. Runeson and Åsberg (2003) investigated all suicides in Swedish subjects born between 1949 and 1969 (N = 8,396). They found that the rate of suicide was significantly higher in the families of suicide victims than in the families of comparison subjects. In addition, the strongest risk factor for suicide in the families was mental disorder as defined by previous psychiatric inpatient care.

In an effort to further understand the familial transmission of suicide Murphy and Wetzel (1982) collected the family history of suicidal behaviors (suicide, attempted suicide, and suicide threats) in 127 patients hospitalized following a suicide attempt. Patients with personality disorders, frequently reported a family history of these behaviors, most notably attempted suicide. More specifically, 16 % of patients with a diagnosis of primary affective disorder had a family history of suicide and 17 % had a family history of suicide attempts.

7.2.2 Twin Studies

Twin studies aim to evaluate the magnitude by which genetic and environmental factors influence a phenotype in a population. Generally, twin studies investigate the risk of a twin exhibiting suicidal behavior given that the co-twin completed suicide. These studies also compare the suicide risk between monozygotic twin (MZ) pairs to dizygotic twin (DZ) pairs, while assuming that environment factors are similar between MZ and DZ (Zai et al. 2012). Roy and Segal (2001) found an increased concordance for suicide in monogyzotic (MZ) versus dizygotic twins (DZ) (14.9 % vs. 0.7 %), which was consistent with Tsuang's original observations (Tsuang 1977). Moreover, Roy et al. found an even higher concordance rate for suicide attempt in the surviving monozygotic twin of the co-twin's suicide in MZ versus DZ twins (38 % vs. 0 %), supporting the view that the clinical phenotype for concordance included both completed suicide and suicide attempts (Roy et al. 1995).

Voracek and Loibl (2007) conducted a comprehensive and up-to-date review of twin studies in order to evaluate the genetic contributions to suicide risk. The authors collected data from 32 studies, published between 1812 and 2006 in six languages and from 13 different countries. The results showed that concordance for complete suicide was significantly more frequent among monozygotic than zygotic twin pairs. A greater concordance for suicidal behavior for monozygotic twins respect to dizygotic twins was also found by Roy et al. (1997).

7.2.3 Adoption Studies

One recent and important adoption study was conducted on a random sample of 1933 adoptees from the Danish Adoption Register, a register of nonfamilial adoptions of Danish children (i.e., the adoptive parents are biologically unrelated to the adoptee). The rate of attempted suicide in full siblings of adoptees who attempted suicide before age 60 years was higher than in full siblings of adoptees who had not attempted suicide (incidence rate ratios [IRR] = 3.45; 95 % confidence interval [CI] = 0.94–12.7). After adjustment for history of psychiatric admission of siblings, the increased rate was statistically significant (IRR = 3.88; 95 % CI—1.42–10.6) (Petersen et al. 2014). In their retrospective cohort study on 8,391 adoptees (2,516 with biological parents died from or hospitalized for suicidal behavior and 5,875 with biological parents with a psychiatric hospitalization but never for suicide attempt), Wilcox et al. (2012) reported that exposure to the hospitalization of an adoptive mother because of a psychiatric disorder amplified an adoptee's risk for suicide attempt.

Von Borczyskowski et al. (2006) conducted a study on suicidal behavior in adolescent and young adult international adoptees. A total of 6,065 international adoptees was compared to 7,340 national adoptees and 1,274,312 nonadopted study subjects, all born between 1963 and 1973 and followed up until 2002 using the National Swedish Register. The results demonstrated an increased risk for suicide attempt and suicide death among international adoptees. On the other hand, national adoptees had lower risks than international adoptees, but had increased risks compared to non-adoptees. It seems that biological parents' morbidity explained approximately one-third of the increased risk for national adoptees. Despite the heroic effort of research and the important results obtained with these kind of studies to demonstrate the existence of genetic risk factors for suicidal behavior, it is currently not possible to identify what are these genetic factors which are being transmitted due to several methodological limitations in these approaches (Brent and Mann 2005; Lester 2002).

7.3 Serotonin Pathway

Identifying specific diathesis-related genes has presented many challenges, although the association between mental disorders and suicide is very clear. More than 90 % of suicide completers have a psychiatric disorder, in particular, mood-related disorders (Arsenault-Lapierre et al. 2004; Cavanagh et al. 2003). Patients suffering from bipolar disorder and schizophrenia have greatly increased rates of suicide with approximately 10 % of patients dying of suicide (Hawton et al. 2005a, b).

In particular, the strong association with depression led researchers to focus their attention on the serotonin system. Studies suggested a role of serotonin in suicide. Indeed, a low cerebrospinal fluid (CSF) concentration of 5-hydroxyindoleacetic acid (5-HIAA), the main metabolite of serotonin, was associated with increased impulsiveness, impaired control of aggressive behaviors, and suicide attempts (Asberg et al. 1976; Linnoila and Virkkunen 1992; Perroud et al. 2010; Virkkunen et al. 1995). Altered serotonergic function is implicated in the etiology and pathogenesis of several major psychiatric conditions, such as suicidal behavior (Arango et al. 2003). Furthermore, Kim et al (2007a, b) reported data among the overlap of genes in common among suicide, bipolar disorder and schizophrenia, suggesting the presence of disorder-specific pathways.

7.3.1 Tryptophan Hydroxylases (TPH1 and TPH2)

Tryptophan is an essential amino acid for serotonin synthesis and tryptophan hydroxylase (TPH) is the initial and rate-limiting enzyme in the biosynthesis of serotonin. In humans, there are two TPH isoenzymes encoded by two different genes. TPH1 was the first gene to be identified and is located on the short arm of chromosome 11 (11p15.3-p14). The second gene (TPH2) is located on the long arm of chromosome 12 (12q21.1).

Using DNA sample from 56 impulsive and 14 nonimpulsive, alcoholic, violent offenders, and 20 healthy volunteers, Nielsen et al (1994) studied the association between suicidal behavior and TPH1 polymorphism. In the highly impulsive group, the authors observed a significant association between TPH genotype and cerebrospinal fluid 5-HIAA concentration. This association suggests that a genetic variant of the TPH gene may influence 5-HIAA concentration in the cerebrospinal fluid and predisposition to suicidal behavior in some individuals.

Galfalvy et al. (2009) genotyped 343 subjects (Caucasian, African–American, Hispanic) presenting with a Major Depressive Episode for polymorphisms A218C in intron 7 and A-6526G in the promoter region of TPH1. They found that both the AA genotype on intron 7 and the AA genotype on the promoter predicted suicide attempts during the 1-year follow-up and were associated with past attempts of high medical lethality.

In their review, Antypa et al. (2013) confirmed the association between variation on the TPH1 gene and 5-HTTLPR gene and violent suicidal behavior in Caucasian populations. Findings on endophenotypes of suicidality, such as aggression and impulsivity traits, showed positive associations for the TPH1, HTR2A, and MAOA genes, but these studies need further replication, since negative associations were also occasionally reported. Studying the A779C polymorphism of the TPH gene, Arango et al. (2003) found that the less common U or A allele variants were associated with suicide attempt. Other studies have found the U allele to be associated with aggression and lower serotonergic function in vivo.

Zill et al. (2004) first reported an association between TPH2 gene polymorphisms and completed suicide. They identified a second tryptophan hydroxylase isoform (TPH2) in mice, which was exclusively present in the brain. Significant association was detected between one single nucleotide polymorphism and suicide and also haplotype analysis produced support for this association.

Ke et al. (2006) selected the A–G single nucleotide polymorphism (SNP) at the position 40237 relative to 5′-end of TPH2 gene in order to evaluate its association with suicide behavior. The authors recruited 102 MD patients with suicidal behavior (attempters) and 123 MD patients without suicidal behavior (nonattempters). Their results demonstrated that the A allele was significantly less frequent in attempters than in nonattempters ($p = 0.0067$). In addition, individuals with the A/A genotype showed a significantly lower risk of suicide behavior than those with the A/G or G/G genotype (OR = 0.35). These findings suggested that the A–G polymorphism of TPH2 may confer susceptibility to suicidal behavior in MD patients.

While the tryptophan hydroxylase genes represent major candidates in numerous genetic association analyses of suicidal behavior, the results thus far have been inconclusive and occasionally conflicting (Zill et al. 2004).

7.3.2 Serotonin Transporter (5-HTT)

The serotonin transporter (5-HTT) regulates serotonergic transmission by removal of serotonin from the synaptic gap. Several studies reported an association between suicidal behavior and serotonin transporter (5-HTT). Mann et al. (2000) found that binding to 5-HTT was lower in the ventral PFC of suicides compared with nonsuicides in postmortem brains from 220 individuals. Anguelova et al. (2003) conducted a meta-analysis on studies investigating 5-HT receptors and the 5-HTT in suicidal behavior. From this meta-analysis, 26 articles met the inclusion criteria and six different 5-HT receptor loci and the 5-HTT promoter 44 bp insertion/deletion polymorphism were investigated. The combined evidence supports an association between suicidal behavior and a promoter 44 bp insertion/deletion polymorphism of the 5-HTT gene and no such association with 102 T/C polymorphism in the 5-HT2A gene.

Li and He (2007) conducted a separate meta-analysis that analyzed cumulative data from European and Asian population. The findings from this meta-analysis suggested a significant association (*P*-value of 0.0068) between the 5-HTTLPR polymorphism and suicidal behavior, further supporting the hypothesis of the involvement of the brain 5-HTT in the pathogenesis of suicidal behavior.

Several researchers are focused on the association between serotonin transporter (5-HTT) gene and suicidal behavior. Even though some of these studies support this hypothesis, other researchers have failed to demonstrate an association which maybe a result of inadequate statistical power and the use of different populations (Li and He 2006). Further studies are necessary in order to better understand the role of 5-HTT in suicidal behavior.

7.3.3 Serotonin Receptors (5HTR1A, 5HTR1B, 5HTR2A, 5HTR2C)

A number of studies have investigated the link between serotonin receptors and suicidal behavior and have resulted in conflicting results. González-Castro et al. (2013) performed a meta-analysis on the association of 5HTR1A gene with suicidal behavior and found that the rs6295 polymorphism was not associated with suicidal behavior. Similarly, no significant association for polymorphisms rs6295 and rs878567 was found in the case-control study. Similar results were found by Kia-Keating et al. (2007). The combined evidence from 789 case and 1,247 control subjects/participants suggested that there was no significant association between the HTR1B G861C polymorphism and suicidal behavior.

On the other hand, Turecki et al. (1999) and Saiz et al. (2008) have suggested a correlation between 5-HT2 receptors and suicidal behavior. Turecki analyzed postmortem data from 56 subjects who had committed suicide and 126 controls and found that 5-HTR2A binding was greater in the prefrontal cortex of suicidal subjects. Saiz and colleagues compared 193 cases of attempted suicide with 420 control cases in order to examine the association between four serotonergic polymorphisms, A-1438G (rs6311) and T102C (rs6313) of the serotonin 2A receptor gene, and STin2 VNTR and 5-HTTLPR of the SLC6A4 gene, and suicidal behavior. The results demonstrated an excess of the −1438A allele both in impulsive suicide attempts and in suicide attempts with high clinical lethality compared the control group, suggesting that the −1438A allele may predispose for nonimpulsive suicidal behavior.

7.4 Other Pathways

7.4.1 Dopaminergic System

Relatively few studies examining the role of dopamine in suicidal behavior have been published (Arango et al. 2003; Wasserman 2000).

7.4.1.1 Homovanillic Acid

Low level of homovanillic acid (HVA) in cerebrospinal fluid (CSF) were found in suicide attempters that were diagnosed with major depression, and the dopamine system seems to be hypofunctional in major depression (Mann 2003). However, as suggested by Mann (2003), the data are too few to actually understand the role of dopaminergic system in suicidal behavior.

The role of CSF dopamine metabolites in suicidal behavior was reported by Roy et al. (1992), who examined 24-hour urinary outputs of HVA in relation to suicidal behavior in depression. Patients with depression who had attempted suicide had significantly smaller urinary outputs of homovanillic acid, dihydroxyphenylacetic acid (DOPAC), and total body output of dopamine (sum dopamine) than patients with depression who had not attempted suicide. Patients with depression who reattempted suicide during 5-year follow-up had significantly smaller urinary outputs of HVA and sum dopamine than patients who did not reattempt suicide, patients who never attempted suicide, and normal control subjects, and had significantly smaller outputs of DOPAC than patients who never attempted suicide or control subjects. These data add to accumulating evidence for low levels of HVA in cerebrospinal fluid and the suggestion that diminished dopaminergic neurotransmission may play a part in suicidal behavior in depression.

7.4.1.2 Dopamine D2 Receptors

Few studies examining the role of the dopamine receptor DRD2 gene (11q22-q23) in suicide have been published. Finckh et al. (1997) analyzed the polymorphism in exon 8 (E8) of the dopamine D2 receptor gene locus (DRD2) (DRD2 E8). The DRD2 (E8) A/A genotype was associated with increased anxiety and depression scores in alcoholics during the follow up after clinical detoxification treatment. In addition, E8 A/A was associated with increased suicide attempts.

Suda et al. (2009) examined associations between suicide attempts and two kinds of functional polymorphisms in the DRD2 gene: TaqIA and −141C Ins/Del. In this study, 120 suicide attempters and 123 unrelated volunteers were examined. Suda et al. demonstrated significant differences in genotypic and allelic frequencies of −141C Ins/Del and TaqIA polymorphisms between suicide attempters and healthy controls (−141C Ins/Del, $p = 0.01$; TaqIA, $p = 0.036$). The Ins allele of −141C Ins/Del was significantly more frequent in suicide attempters ($p = 0.011$), as well as the A2 allele of TaqIA ($p = 0.017$) suggesting that DRD2 gene polymorphisms may be involved in the biological susceptibility to suicide.

The study on 141C Del variant of the DRD2 asserted that this variant might be a protective factor against the development of alcohol withdrawal symptoms. In addition, this variant might also be a risk factor in a highly burdened subgroup of alcoholics with a paternal and grand paternal history of alcoholism and may contribute to the substantially higher likelihood of suicide in alcoholics (Johann et al. 2005).

7.4.1.3 Tyrosine Hydroxylase

Catacholaminergic dysfunction due to abnormalities in the tyrosine hydroxylase (TH) gene has been implicated in the pathogenesis of suicidal behavior and in mood disorders. Recent evidence suggests that TH gene variants may also increase the risk of suicide attempts in schizophrenic patients, although the interaction with established clinical risk factors is unclear (Hu et al. 2013).

Ordway et al. (1994) studied the concentration of tyrosine hydroxylase in the noradrenageric cell bodies of the locus coeruleus of nine age-matched pairs (antidepressant-free suicide victims and controls). This study found higher concentrations of the enzyme in the samples from suicide victims, thus raising the possibility that the expression of tyrosine hydroxylase in locus coeruleus may be relevant in the pathophysiology of suicide.

In their study, Persson et al. (1997) examined a tetranucleotide repeat polymorphism in the first intron of the tyrosine hydroxylase (TH) locus in 118 adult suicide attempters with diagnosis according to DSM-III-R criteria (major depression, anxiety disorders, adjustment disorders, psychoactive substance abuse disorders, psychotic disorders) and in 78 control adult subjects. The authors reported a high prevalence of carriers of TH-K3 allele in suicide attempters with adjustment disorders and low prevalence of carriers of TH-K1 among all suicide attempters.

These findings suggested that the alleles may reflect predisposition for a common phenotype with altered vulnerability for psychiatric disorders.

7.4.1.4 Catechol-O-Methyltransferase

Catechol-O-methyltransferase (COMT) plays an important role in genetics of suicide risk, because it inactivates dopamine and norepinephrine by the addition of a methyl group from S-adenosylmethionine (Zai et al. 2012). A functional polymorphism on the human COMT gene has been shown to influence aggressive and anger-related traits in various clinical populations. The results found by Baud et al. showed that the high activity genotype (Val/Val) was more frequent in suicide attempters than in normal controls. Moreover, the Val/Val genotype markedly affected the scores on two STAXI subscales—Trait Anger and Anger Control—in female suicide attempters, thus suggesting a possible gender effect of the COMT genotype on a stable personality trait (Baud et al. 2007).

The functional polymorphism (COMT Val108/158Met) affects COMT activity, with the valine (Val) variant associated with higher and the methionine (Met) variant with lower COMT activity. This polymorphism is associated with aggressive and suicidal behavior, although the findings on this relationship have not always been consistent.

Nedic et al. (2011) recruited 312 male and 81 female medication-free patients with alcohol dependence and 487 male and 122 female unrelated, nonsuicidal medication-free Caucasian healthy subjects. Their findings demonstrated that male alcoholic suicide attempters had the higher frequency of Met/Met genotype or Met allele and significantly higher aggression and depression scores compared to male nonattempters. These results confirmed the associations between Met allele and aggressive behavior or violent suicide attempts in various psychiatric diagnoses, and suggested that Met allele of the COMT Val108/158 Met might be used as an independent biomarker of suicidal behavior across different psychopathologies.

7.4.2 *Brain-Derived Neurotrophic Factor*

Brain-derived neurotrophic factor (BDNF), the most abundant neurotrophin in the brain, influences the pathophysiology of anxiety and depression. However, to date the role of BDNF in suicide has not been well investigated.

Plasma BDNF levels in 32 major depressive disorder (MDD) patients who had recently attempted suicide, 32 nonsuicidal MDD patients, and 30 normal controls were examined (Kim et al. 2007a, b). BDNF levels were significantly lower in suicidal MDD patients than nonsuicidal MDD patients or normal controls. These results suggested that a reduction of plasma BDNF level may be related to suicidal behavior in major depression and that BDNF level may be a biological marker of suicidal depression (Kim et al. 2007a, b). BDNF levels were decreased in the postmortem brain and plasma samples from suicide subjects (Keller et al. 2010). Postmortem brain samples from suicide subjects showed a statistically significant increase of DNA methylation in Wernicke's area at specific CpG sites in BDNF promoter/exon IV compared with nonsuicide control subjects (Keller et al. 2010).

The association between the BDNF gene Val66Met polymorphism and mood disorders was confirmed also by the study of Nedic et al. (2011). They found that the genotype and allele frequencies for the BDNF gene Val66Met polymorphism did not differ when comparing across depression groups (total, bipolar disorder or major depression) and control subjects. Furthermore, it was shown that this BDNF polymorphism was not associated with age of onset or suicidal history in mood disorder patients. In a sample of 813 Caucasian suicide attempters, childhood sexual abuse was associated with violent suicide attempts in adulthood only among BDNF Val/Val individuals and not among BDNF Val/Met or BDNF Met/Met individuals. The result suggested that BDNF Val66Met may modulates the effect of childhood sexual abuse on the violence of suicidal behavior (N. Perroud et al. 2008).

Dwivedi et al. (2003) analyzed whether the expression of BDNF and/or Trk B isoforms were altered in postmortem brain in subjects who commit suicide (hereafter referred to as suicide subjects) and whether these alterations were associated with specific psychopathologic conditions. The sample consisted of 27 suicide subjects and 21 nonpsychiatric control subjects and Brodmann area 9 and hippocampus were the brain areas examined. This study found that BDNF and Trk B were significantly reduced in both prefrontal cortex and hippocampus in suicide subjects as compared with those in control subjects.

Given the importance of BDNF in mediating physiological functions, including cell survival and synaptic plasticity, the reduced expression of BDNF and Trk B in postmortem brain in suicide subjects suggest that these molecules may play an important role in the pathophysiological aspects of suicidal behavior.

7.5 Hypothalamic-Pituitary-Adrenal Axis

Well-established environmental risk factors for suicidal behavior are events causing significant psychological stress, which are particularly difficult to cope with effectively. High stress levels may cause also unfavorable effects in different brain functions, in partilcular on the hypothalamic-pituitary-adrenal (HPA) axis, involved for the regulation of body's response to stress and has complex interactions with brain serotonergic, noradrenergic, and dopaminergic systems. Indeed, the HPA axis is responsible of modulation of cortisol levels, the major stress hormone, and stress plays a major role in the various pathophysiological processes associated with mood disorders and suicidal behavior. Several studies reported association between abnormalities in the HPA axis and suicidal behaviors (Wasserman et al. 2010).

Adrenal steroid hormones are essential to human life and play a central role in maintaining survival in times of stress. Several lines of evidence suggest an association between HPA axis dysregulation, affective disorders, and suicidal behavior

(Arató et al. 1986). As early as 1965, Bunney and Fawcett (1965) reported high levels of urinary 17-hydroxycorticosteroids in depressed suicidal patients.

Leszczyńska-Rodziewicz et al. (2013) studied the polymorphisms of genes involved in the HPA axis (CRHR1, NR3C1, and AVPBR1). This study was performed on 597 patients, 225 of whom had a history of suicide attempts. Even if the haplotype analysis of the AVPR1b gene revealed an association between the GCA haplotype and suicide attempts, this association was not significant after correcting for multiple testing. Nonetheless, the inconsistencies with the previously published results indicate the importance of the further investigation of these polymorphisms with respect to the risk of suicide attempts.

Moreover, the stress response is mediated by corticotrophin-releasing hormone (CRH), which is known to be a regulator of the HPA pathway. Alterations in the HPA system have been related to impulsivity, aggression, and suicidal behavior, common features in schizophrenia (De Luca et al. 2010).

7.6 Genome-Wide and Epigenetic Studies of Suicide

In the last years, genome-wide association studies (GWA study, or GWAS) has been a great contribution to the understanding of suicidal behavior. GWAS aims to study several genetic variants in different individuals and examine the genome for small variations (single nucleotide polymorphisms or SNPs) that occur more frequently in people with a particular disease than in people without the disease. Recent studies provide evidence that epigenetic mechanisms could deliver the missing link between the heritability of suicidal behavior and the interaction between environment and the genome (Bani-Fatemi et al. 2014). These epigenetic mechanisms, which alter gene expression via alternative mechanisms to the coding DNA sequence, result from environmental effects acting on the genome. Studies in rodents indicate that variation in the early environment will trigger these epigenetic modifications and recent data suggest the same may be true in humans. The expression of a number of genes which are involved in normal brain functions have been shown to be under epigenetic control and seem to be dysregulated in suicide (Labonte and Turecki 2010).

The genome-wide linkage survey for genetic loci that influence the risk of suicidal behavior in the context of mood disorders has been reported by Zubenko et al. (2004). Six linkage peaks with maximum multipoint ΔLOD scores that reached genome-wide adjusted levels of significance (2p, 5q, 6q, 8p, 11q, and Xq) were identified and four of these (2p, 6q, 8p, and Xq) exceeded the criterion for "highly significant linkage." The highest ΔLOD score that emerged from this linkage analysis, 5.08, occurred for ARPs with Depression Spectrum Disorder at D8S1145 at cytogenetic location 8p22-p21. These findings provide evidence for suicide risk loci.

Labonté et al. (2013) used a genome-wide approach to investigate the extent of DNA methylation alterations in the brains of suicide completers. The authors identified 366 promoters that were differentially methylated in suicide completers relative to comparison subjects (273 hypermethylated and 93 hypomethylated). The results demonstrated that promoter DNA methylation levels were significantly greater for several genes in suicide completers relative to control group. Moreover, a significant number of hypomethylated sequences in the promoters of suicide completers were reported, suggesting that DNA methylation patterns may be altered in the brains of suicide completers.

7.7 Conclusions

Suicide is a complex phenomenon. Its multidimensionality, linked to association between social, biological, and psychological factors requires that the understanding of the predisposition to suicide cannot totally explained only by the presences of mental health disorders, even if closely associated to suicidal behavior. Several researchers have established the role of genetic basis of suicidal behavior. However, some of the studies have produced inconsistent findings, often due to difficulties in methods used and difficulties to select the sample. Currently, the more credible studies to explain the role of genetic risk factors for suicidal behaviors are those based on the serotonergic system. The canditate genes (most studied genes are SCL6A4, HTR2A, HTR2C, HTR1A, HTR1B, TPH-1, and TPH-2) pertaining to the serotonergic system have proved to be an important key about the association between suicide behavior and its biological correlates.

References

Anguelova M, Benkelfat C, Turecki G (2003) A systematic review of association studies investigating genes coding for serotonin receptors and the serotonin transporter: II. Suicidal behavior. Mol Psychiatry 8(7):646–653. doi:10.1038/sj.mp.4001336

Antypa N, Serretti A, Rujescu D (2013) Serotonergic genes and suicide: a systematic review. Eur Neuropsychopharmacol J Eur Coll Neuropsychopharmacol 23(10):1125–1142. doi:10.1016/j.euroneuro.2013.03.013

Arango V, Huang Y, Underwood MD, Mann JJ (2003) Genetics of the serotonergic system in suicidal behavior. J Psychiatr Res 37(5):375–386

Arató M, Banki CM, Nemeroff CB, Bissette G (1986) Hypothalamic-pituitary-adrenal axis and suicide. Ann N Y Acad Sci 487(1):263–270. doi:10.1111/j.1749-6632.1986.tb27905.x

Arsenault-Lapierre G, Kim C, Turecki G (2004) Psychiatric diagnoses in 3275 suicides: a meta-analysis. BMC Psychiatry 4:37. doi:10.1186/1471-244X-4-37

Asberg M, Träskman L, Thorén P (1976) 5-HIAA in the cerebrospinal fluid. A biochemical suicide predictor? Arch Gen Psychiatry 33(10):1193–1197

Bani-Fatemi A, Howe AS, De Luca V (2014) Epigenetic studies of suicidal behavior. Neurocase. doi:10.1080/13554794.2013.826679

Baud P, Courtet P, Perroud N, Jollant F, Buresi C, Malafosse A (2007) Catechol-O-methyltransferase polymorphism (COMT) in suicide attempters: a possible gender effect on anger traits. Am J Med Genet Part B Neuropsychiatr Genet 144B(8):1042–1047. doi:10.1002/ajmg.b.30541

Brent DA, Mann JJ (2005) Family genetic studies, suicide, and suicidal behavior. Am J Med Genet Part C Semin Med Genet 133C(1):13–24. doi:10.1002/ajmg.c.30042

Brent DA, Melhem N (2008) Familial transmission of suicidal behavior. Psychiatr Clin North Am 31(2):157–177. doi:10.1016/j.psc.2008.02.001

Brent DA, Bridge J, Johnson BA, Connolly J (1996) Suicidal behavior runs in families. A controlled family study of adolescent suicide victims. Arch Gen Psychiatry 53(12):1145–1152

Bunney WE Jr, Fawcett JA (1965) Possibility of a biochemical test for suicidal potential: an analysis of endocrine findings prior to three suicides. Arch Gen Psychiatry 13:232–239

Cavanagh JTO, Carson AJ, Sharpe M, Lawrie SM (2003) Psychological autopsy studies of suicide: a systematic review. Psychol Med 33(3):395–405

De Luca V, Tharmalingam S, Zai C, Potapova N, Strauss J, Vincent J, Kennedy JL (2010) Association of HPA axis genes with suicidal behaviour in schizophrenia. Journal of Psychopharmacology (Oxford, England), 24(5), 677–682. doi:10.1177/0269881108097817

Dwivedi Y, Rizavi HS, Conley RR, Roberts RC, Tamminga CA, Pandey GN (2003) Altered gene expression of brain-derived neurotrophic factor and receptor tyrosine kinase B in postmortem brain of suicide subjects. Arch Gen Psychiatry 60(8):804–815. doi:10.1001/archpsyc.60.8.804

Finckh U, Rommelspacher H, Kuhn S, Dufeu P, Otto G, Heinz A, Rolfs A (1997) Influence of the dopamine D2 receptor (DRD2) genotype on neuroadaptive effects of alcohol and the clinical outcome of alcoholism. Pharmacogenetics 7(4):271–281

Galfalvy H, Huang Y-Y, Oquendo MA, Currier D, Mann JJ (2009) Increased risk of suicide attempt in mood disorders and TPH1 genotype. J Affect Disord 115(3):331–338. doi:10.1016/j.jad.2008.09.019

González-Castro TB, Tovilla-Zárate CA, Juárez-Rojop I, Pool García S, Genis A, Nicolini H, López Narváez L (2013) Association of 5HTR1A gene variants with suicidal behavior: case-control study and updated meta-analysis. J Psychiatr Res 47(11):1665–1672. doi:10.1016/j.jpsychires.2013.04.011

Hawton K, Sutton L, Haw C, Sinclair J, Deeks JJ (2005a) Schizophrenia and suicide: systematic review of risk factors. Br J Psychiatry J Mental Sci 187:9–20. doi:10.1192/bjp.187.1.9

Hawton K, Sutton L, Haw C, Sinclair J, Harriss L (2005b) Suicide and attempted suicide in bipolar disorder: a systematic review of risk factors. J Clin Psychiatry 66(6):693–704

Hu J, Chan LF, Souza RP, Tampakeras M, Kennedy JL, Zai C, De Luca V (2013) The role of tyrosine hydroxylase gene variants in suicide attempt in schizophrenia. Neurosci Lett. doi:10.1016/j.neulet.2013.11.025

Johann M, Putzhammer A, Eichhammer P, Wodarz N (2005) Association of the -141C Del variant of the dopamine D2 receptor (DRD2) with positive family history and suicidality in German alcoholics. Am J Med Genet Part B Neuropsychiatr Genet Off Publ Int Soc Psychiatr Genet 132B(1):46–49. doi:10.1002/ajmg.b.30085

Johnson SH (1998) End-of-life decision making: what we don't know, we make up; what we do know, we ignore. Law Rev 31(1):13–47

Ke L, Qi ZY, Ping Y, Ren CY (2006) Effect of SNP at position 40237 in exon 7 of the TPH2 gene on susceptibility to suicide. Brain Res 1122(1):24–26. doi:10.1016/j.brainres.2006.09.007

Keller S, Sarchiapone M, Zarrilli F et al (2010) INcreased bdnf promoter methylation in the wernicke area of suicide subjects. Arch Gen Psychiatry 67(3):258–267. doi:10.1001/archgenpsychiatry.2010.9

Kia-Keating BM, Glatt SJ, Tsuang MT (2007) Meta-analyses suggest association between COMT, but not HTR1B, alleles, and suicidal behavior. Am J Med Genet Part B Neuropsychiatr Genet 144B(8):1048–1053. doi:10.1002/ajmg.b.30551

Kim S, Choi K-H, Baykiz AF, Gershenfeld HK (2007a) Suicide candidate genes associated with bipolar disorder and schizophrenia: An exploratory gene expression profiling analysis of post-mortem prefrontal cortex. BMC Genom 8(1):413. doi:10.1186/1471-2164-8-413

Kim Y-K, Lee H-P, Won S-D, Park E-Y, Lee H-Y, Lee B-H, Choi S-H (2007b) Low plasma BDNF is associated with suicidal behavior in major depression. Prog Neuropsychopharmacol Biol Psychiatry 31(1):78–85. doi:10.1016/j.pnpbp.2006.06.024

Labonte B, Turecki G (2010) The epigenetics of suicide: explaining the biological effects of early life environmental adversity. Arch Suicide Res Off J Int Acad Suicide Res 14(4):291–310. doi:10.1080/13811118.2010.524025

Labonté B, Suderman M, Maussion G, Lopez JP, Navarro-Sánchez L, Yerko V, Turecki G (2013) Genome-wide methylation changes in the brains of suicide completers. Am J Psychiatry 170 (5):511–520. doi:10.1176/appi.ajp.2012.12050627

Lester D (2002) Twin studies of suicidal behavior. Arch Suicide Res 6(4):383–389. doi:10.1080/13811110214530

Leszczyńska-Rodziewicz A, Szczepankiewicz A, Pawlak J, Dmitrzak-Weglarz M, Hauser J (2013) Association, haplotype, and gene-gene interactions of the HPA axis genes with suicidal behaviour in affective disorders. Sci World J 207361. doi:10.1155/2013/207361

Li D, He L (2007) Meta-analysis supports association between serotonin transporter (5-HTT) and suicidal behavior. Mol Psychiatry 12(1):47–54. doi:10.1038/sj.mp.4001890

Linkowski P, de Maertelaer V, Mendlewicz J (1985) Suicidal behaviour in major depressive illness. Acta Psychiatr Scand 72(3):233–238. doi:10.1111/j.1600-0447.1985.tb02600.x

Linnoila VM, Virkkunen M (1992) Aggression, suicidality, and serotonin. J Clin Psychiatry 53 (Suppl):46–51

Malone KM, Haas GL, Sweeney JA, Mann JJ (1995) Major depression and the risk of attempted suicide. J Affect Disord 34(3):173–185

Mann JJ (1998) The neurobiology of suicide. Nat Med 4(1):25–30

Mann JJ (2003) Neurobiology of suicidal behaviour. Nat Rev Neurosci 4(10):819–828. doi:10.1038/nrn1220

Mann J, Huang Y, Underwood MD et al (2000) A serotonin transporter gene promoter polymorphism (5-httlpr) and prefrontal cortical binding in major depression and suicide. Arch Gen Psychiatry 57(8):729–738. doi:10.1001/archpsyc.57.8.729

Mann JJ, Arango VA, Avenevoli S, Brent DA, Champagne FA, Clayton P, Wenze A (2009) Candidate endophenotypes for genetic studies of suicidal behavior. Biol Psychiatry 65 (7):556–563. doi: 10.1016/j.biopsych.2008.11.021

McGirr A, Turecki G (2007) The relationship of impulsive aggressiveness to suicidality and other depression-linked behaviors. Curr Psychiatry Rep 9(6):460–466

Murphy GE, Wetzel RD (1982) Family history of suicidal behavior among suicide attempters. J Nerv Ment Dis 170(2):86–90

Nedic G, Nikolac M, Sviglin KN, Muck-Seler D, Borovecki F, Pivac N (2011) Association study of a functional catechol-O-methyltransferase (COMT) Val108/158Met polymorphism and suicide attempts in patients with alcohol dependence. Int J Neuropsychopharmacol 14 (03):377–388. doi:10.1017/S1461145710001057

Nielsen DA, Goldman D, Virkkunen M, Tokola R, Rawlings R, Linnoila M (1994) Suicidality and 5-hydroxyindoleacetic acid concentration associated with a tryptophan hydroxylase polymorphism. Arch Gen Psychiatry 51(1):34–38

Ordway GA, Smith KS, Haycock JW (1994) Elevated tyrosine hydroxylase in the locus coeruleus of suicide victims. J Neurochem 62(2):680–685. doi:10.1046/j.1471-4159.1994.62020680.x

Perroud N, Salzmann A, Saiz PA, Baca-Garcia E, Sarchiapone M, Garcia-Portilla MP, … European Research Consortium for Suicide (EURECA) (2010) Rare genotype combination of the serotonin transporter gene associated with treatment response in severe personality disorder. Am J Med Genet Part B Neuropsychiatr Genet 153B(8):1494–1497. doi:10.1002/ajmg.b.31118

Perroud N, Courtet P, Vincze I, Jaussent I, Jollant F, Bellivier F, Malafosse A (2008) Interaction between BDNF Val66Met and childhood trauma on adult's violent suicide attempt. Genes Brain Behav 7(3):314–322. doi:10.1111/j.1601-183X.2007.00354.x

Persson M-L, Wasserman D, Geijer T, Jönsson EG, Terenius L (1997) Tyrosine hydroxylase allelic distribution in suicide attempters. Psychiatry Res 72(2):73–80

Petersen L, Sørensen TIA, Kragh Andersen P, Mortensen PB, Hawton K (2014) Genetic and familial environmental effects on suicide attempts: a study of Danish adoptees and their biological and adoptive siblings. J Affect Disord 155:273–277. doi:10.1016/j.jad.2013.11.012

Pfeffer CR, Normandin L, Kakuma T (1994) Suicidal children grow up: suicidal behavior and psychiatric disorders among relatives. J Am Acad Child Adolesc Psychiatry 33(8):1087–1097. doi:10.1097/00004583-199410000-00004

Roy A (1983a) Family history of suicide. Arch Gen Psychiatry 40(9):971–974. doi:10.1001/archpsyc.1983.01790080053007

Roy A (1983b) Family history of suicide. Arch Gen Psychiatry 40(9):971–974

Roy A, Segal NL (2001) Suicidal behavior in twins: a replication. J Affect Disord 66(1):71–74

Roy A, Karoum F, Pollack S (1992) Marked reduction in indexes of dopamine metabolism among patients with depression who attempt suicide. Arch Gen Psychiatry 49(6):447–450. doi:10.1001/archpsyc.1992.01820060027004

Roy A, Segal NL, Sarchiapone M (1995) Attempted suicide among living co-twins of twin suicide victims. Am J Psychiatry 152(7):1075–1076

Roy A, Rylander G, Sarchiapone M (1997) Genetics of suicide. Ann N Y Acad Sci 836 (1):135–157. doi:10.1111/j.1749-6632.1997.tb52358.x

Runeson B, Åsberg M (2003) Family history of suicide among suicide victims. Am J Psychiatry 160(8):1525–1526. doi:10.1176/appi.ajp.160.8.1525

Saiz PA, García-Portilla MP, Paredes B, Arango C, Morales B, Alvarez V, Bobes J (2008) Association between the A-1438G polymorphism of the serotonin 2A receptor gene and nonimpulsive suicide attempts. Psychiatr Genet 18(5):213–218. doi:10.1097/YPG.0b013e3283050ada

Statham DJ, Heath AC, Madden PA, Bucholz KK, Bierut L, Dinwiddie SH, Martin NG (1998) Suicidal behaviour: an epidemiological and genetic study. Psychol Med 28(4):839–855

Suda A, Kawanishi C, Kishida I, Sato R, Yamada T, Nakagawa M, Hirayasu Y (2009) Dopamine D2 receptor gene polymorphisms are associated with suicide attempt in the Japanese population. Neuropsychobiology 59(2):130–134. doi:10.1159/000213566

Tsuang MT (1977) Genetic factors in suicide. Dis Nerv Syst 38(7):498–501

Tsuang MT (1983) Risk of suicide in the relatives of schizophrenics, manics, depressives, and controls. J Clin Psychiatry 44(11):396–400

Turecki G, Brière R, Dewar K, Antonetti T, Lesage AD, Séguin M, Rouleau GA (1999) Prediction of level of serotonin 2A receptor binding by serotonin receptor 2A genetic variation in postmortem brain samples from subjects who did or did not commit suicide. Am J Psychiatry 156(9):1456–1458

Van Heeringen K (2012) Stress–diathesis model of suicidal behavior. In: Dwivedi Y (ed) The neurobiological basis of suicide. CRC Press, Boca Raton (FL). http://www.ncbi.nlm.nih.gov/books/NBK107203/

Virkkunen M, Goldman D, Nielsen DA, Linnoila M (1995) Low brain serotonin turnover rate (low CSF 5-HIAA) and impulsive violence. J Psychiatry Neurosci JPN 20(4):271–275

Von Borczyskowski A, Hjern A, Lindblad F, Vinnerljung B (2006) Suicidal behaviour in national and international adult adoptees: a Swedish cohort study. Soc Psychiatry Psychiatr Epidemiol 41(2):95–102. doi:10.1007/s00127-005-0974-2

Voracek M, Loibl LM (2007) Genetics of suicide: a systematic review of twin studies. Wien Klin Wochenschr 119(15–16):463–475. doi:10.1007/s00508-007-0823-2

Wasserman D (2000) Suicide: an unnecessary death. Martin Dunitz, London

Wasserman D, Wasserman J, Sokolowski M (2010) Genetics of HPA-axis, depression and suicidality. Eur Psychiatry J Assoc Eur Psychiatr 25(5):278–280. doi:10.1016/j.eurpsy.2009.12.016

Wender PH, Kety SS, Rosenthal D, Schulsinger F, Ortmann J, Lunde I (1986) Psychiatric disorders in the biological and adoptive families of adopted individuals with affective disorders. Arch General Psychiatry 43(10):923–929

Wilcox HC, Kuramoto SJ, Brent D, Runeson B (2012) The interaction of parental history of suicidal behavior and exposure to adoptive parents' psychiatric disorders on adoptee suicide attempt hospitalizations. Am J Psychiatry 169(3):309–315. doi:10.1176/appi.ajp.2011.11060890

Zai CC, de Luca V, Strauss J, Tong RP, Sakinofsky I, Kennedy JL (2012) Genetic factors and suicidal behavior. In: Dwivedi Y (ed) The neurobiological basis of suicide. CRC Press, Boca Raton (FL). http://www.ncbi.nlm.nih.gov/books/NBK107191/

Zill P, Büttner A, Eisenmenger W, Möller H-J, Bondy B, Ackenheil M (2004) Single nucleotide polymorphism and haplotype analysis of a novel tryptophan hydroxylase Isoform (TPH2) gene in suicide victims. Biol Psychiatry 56(8):581–586. doi:10.1016/j.biopsych.2004.07.015

Zubenko GS, Maher BS, Hughes HB, Zubenko WN, Scott Stiffler J, Marazita ML (2004) Genome-wide linkage survey for genetic loci that affect the risk of suicide attempts in families with recurrent, early-onset, major depression. Am J Med Genet Part B Neuropsychiatr Genet 129B(1):47–54. doi:10.1002/ajmg.b.30092

Chapter 8
Is Suicide Clinically Preventable? What Is the Evidence?

Jan Fawcett

Abstract Suicide is a major public health problem and cause of death, as well as years of life lost. The US suicide rate is at its highest level in over 15 years, and has become an epidemic in both our military forces and veterans of military service. (American Foundation for Suicide prevention). At present there is no evidence that suicide is clinically *predictable* in an individual, even though the standard of care requires that suicide risk be assessed in psychiatric patients, who show an elevated risk in general, and clinical efforts be made to reduce risk. Clinical prediction may be improved in a number of suggested ways, which could lead to more effective short-term prevention. While at present, there is no evidence that short term (2–3 months) treatment can prevent suicide, there is evidence from long-term studies that maintaining maintenance medication can reduce suicide in high risk patients.

8.1 Suicide and Treatment of Mental Disorders

Studies have shown that up to 90 % of suicide victims have evidence of a diagnosable mental illness (Conwell et al. 1996). We have made significant strides in the treatment of depression and other psychiatric disorders that are associated with suicide. The best evidence we have at present shows that psychotherapies such as Dialectal Behavior Therapy (DBT) and Cognitive Therapy (CT) will result in a reduction of suicidal behavior, but so far there is ŋo evidence that these treatments will reduce suicide. Meta-analytic studies of treatment with antidepressants given over 8–12 weeks reduce suicidal ideation, but show no significant difference in suicide rates between pooled antidepressant medication trials and placebo (Sher et al. 2012; Khan et al. 2003)

J. Fawcett (✉)
UPC Clinic, Department of Psychiatry, University of New Mexico,
2400 Tucker Ave NE, 87131 Albuquerque, NM, Mexico
e-mail: jfawcett@salud.unm.edu

K.E. Cannon and T.J. Hudzik (eds.), *Suicide: Phenomenology and Neurobiology*,
DOI 10.1007/978-3-319-09964-4_8

Two studies, to be discussed later, have shown a significant reduction of suicides associated with a continuation of antidepressants, lithium, and antipsychotic medications for at least 6 months over a 34–38 year follow-up in one study (Angst et al. 2002), a with a propensity to be taking antidepressant medications in another follow-up study of 16–20 years (Leon et al. 2011). Also there are a number of studies showing a significant reduction of suicides and attempts in patients taking maintenance lithium carbonate compared to placebo (Cipriani 2013).

Suicide occurs despite treatment. Studies have shown that 42 % of patients had a psychiatric care visit and a review has shown that 33 % of patients were seen in a mental health care setting within a month of their suicide (Robins 1981; Luoma et al. 2002). Luoma's review found that 45 % of patients who commited suicide after having seen a primary care physician within 1 month.

8.2 The Importance of Suicide Risk Detection

For these reasons, it would seem that clinicians treating patients would be in a position to clinically detect the risk of suicide and intervene. It is a standard of care that a mental health clinician conduct an evaluation of their patients for suicide risk and clinically intervene to try to prevent suicide in patients found to be at high acute risk.

Two studies have shown that educating primary care physicians in detecting and treating depression and assessing suicide risk, actually results in an increase in the prescription of antidepressant medications, and a decrease in suicide rates as long as the medication is continued (Hennriksson and Isacsson 2006). Yerevanian et al. (2004) found that the discontinuation of antidepressant medications in patients with depressive disorders was associated with a greater than 5-fold increase in risk for suicidal behavior ($P < 0.0001$). Another more recent study of Veterans showed that suicide associated with a 70 % omission of a suicide risk assessment for suicidal ideation in the clinical record for their last visit before suicide (Smith et al. 2013). However, this same study reported that 85 % of suicides denied suicidal ideation when assessed and 73 % denied suicidal ideation when assessed within 0–7 days prior to suicide. This plus the studies to be reviewed below show how much a clinician can rely on a denial of suicidal ideation or intent.

8.3 The Current Data for Prediction of Suicide

The data cited above point to the importance of a suicide risk assessment in reducing suicide. There have been authoritative studies that have questioned the predictability of suicide by any scaled symptoms list and by clinical features. A classic prospective study of 4,800 hospitalized veterans followed for a mean of 5 years by Pokorny (1983), concluded from the review of prior papers and an analysis of his sample in which 67 suicides occurred, 42 of these within 1 year of hospital discharge, that no clinical factor or set of factors was predictive of suicide. He later published a reanalysis of his data set using more advanced statistical methods such as logistic regression, once again concluding that no set of factors predicting suicide could be found, with any likely factors showing high false positive and false negative rates (Pokorny 1993).

Pokorny went as far as to focus on a high risk group by selecting a group of patients with major depression, schizophrenia, alcoholism, or drug abuse, that were non-black males, with a marital status other than married to concentrate risk factors. With this new "formula" he was able to correctly identify 15 out of 67 suicides with 279 "false-positive" predictions.

He also tried to overcome the problem of the relatively low base rate of suicide by progressively reducing the size of the "other samples" and running predictors. In doing this with the smallest sample of others for comparison, he reached full prediction of suicide for the sample, but also identified the comparison of non-suicides as all suicidal. Pokorny (1993) did reanalyze these data using logistic regression techniques, and was still not able to find clinical predictors of suicide. He concluded that predictors, who have greater sensitivity (will not miss many positive risks—with high false negative predictions) and greater specificity (will not identify a high proportion of high risk patients), are needed.

What did show up in Pokorny's study was a very high rate of suicide in his sample in time periods after hospital discharge up to 1 year, a frequent finding.

Another more recent study by Large and colleagues (2011) (Large et al. 2011) has challenged the predictability of suicide in a large meta-analysis of studies of suicide up to 1 year of discharge from a psychiatric hospital. Unlike the Pokorny study, this meta-analysis was not of prospective studies, but a review of 13 studies of retrospectively determined suicidal outcomes, with only 2 studies included having less than 50 suicides. Across these studies 1594 suicides were reviewed. A prior history of suicide attempt or self-harm and depressive symptoms were found to be moderately associated with suicide (Odds ratios of 3.15 and 2.70, respectively) Factors weakly associated with suicide (Odds Ratios of 1.5–2.5) were male sex, recent social difficulties, a diagnosis of major depressive disorder, present suicidal ideation, and an unplanned discharge.

Demographic factors not associated with suicide within 1 year of discharge were the patients age, marital status, living alone, employment status, ethnicity, and level of education. Other factors not associated with suicide were a prior history of criminal conduct or violence, a family history of mental illness, and co-occurring physical illness. Clinical features not associated with suicide were alcohol abuse, use of other substances, a dual diagnosis of a substance abuse disorder and mental illness, a diagnosis of bipolar disorder of schizophrenia, or a long duration of illness.

The authors cite an overlap of risk factors for patients while inpatients with those within 1 year of discharge. They cite an increased risk of suicide in the hospital in schizophrenics, but not during the year after discharge. An intriguing finding was that being categorized as high risk for suicide in the hospital correlated strongly

(OR 10.9) with inpatient suicide, but not as strongly with suicide (OR 3.94) after discharge.

The authors of this study conclude that no single factor or combination of factors, are strongly associated with suicide in the year following discharge. While about 3 % categorized as high risk are likely to commit suicide, about 60 % of suicides are likely to be categorized as low risk. They further conclude that unpredictable intervening events, which cannot be factored into a suicide assessment, might be more likely after a hospital discharge and allow that it is possible that studies have not examined all the factors associated with post-hospitalization suicides.

8.4 What Risk Factors Can Clinicians Rely on? Suicidal Ideation

Where does this leave the clinician? What about asking the patient about suicidal intent? Inquiring about suicidal thoughts, specific plans and means that are considered a standard for a suicide assessment. An affirmative answer to these questions is certainly important and should be explored in detail.

Patients who make "contingent" suicide threats ("If you don't admit me to the hospital, I'll commit suicide"), may be a different matter. The Lambert (1996, 2002) studies of patients making "contingent" suicide threats that were not admitted from a VA hospital emergency room are instructive. Following these patients and comparing their outcomes with depressive patients evaluated over a 7 month and 10 year period showed that no suicides had occurred in with group at 7 months and at 10 years no suicides were found in the contingent group of patients, but the suicide rate in the depressed group was 10 % at 10 year follow-up. Lambert found most of the contingent threat patients to be diagnosed as drug abusers and homeless.

What about a denial of suicide intent? Our brains seem programed to assume that if an affirmative answer about suicide intent indicates high risk, that a denial of intent might reassure us that the presence of suicide risk is low. But a denial of suicidal intent with no other clinical information is meaningless. This is also true with a patient "contracting" for safety. Isometsa et al. (1995) published 500 cases of suicide, 100 of which committed suicide the same day seen by a therapist. Only 22 % of this sample admitted to suicidal ideation. In a study of inpatient suicides, Busch et al. (2003) reported that 76 % of inpatient suicide patients were charted as reporting no suicidal ideation to a nurse as their last communication before their suicide, 28 % of this sample of suicides had a no suicide or no harm contract recorded in their chart.

8.5 Reaction to a Negative Event

A review of suicide cases suggests that in a high proportion of cases, the patient has sustained a negative event that compounds their illness. Frequently, the patient may downplay or fail to report the event that may push them over-the-edge. This failure to report makes it difficult to study the full effects of negative events and may mislead a clinician.

The following case is illustrative. A patient with poor response to a series of medications to control bipolar disorder tells his psychiatrist that he had purchased a shotgun, loaded it and held it against his chest. He was admitted to an inpatient unit, and since many medications had failed was given a course of ECT. He showed moderate improvement after six treatments and was discharged to home and work. In an outpatient visit he showed improvement of mood, admitted mild suicidal ideation with no plan, which this patient had experience over the past 20 years, told of a planned trip to Afghanistan as part of his work in the coming week and joked about getting to finally use his humanities background, teaching cultural cooperation to consultants, on the trip.

Three hours after his appointment, he went home and hanged himself with an elaborate system he had installed in his apartment over the past 4 days. He left letters for his parents in Europe and many of his acquaintances. A former girl friend called to tell me about his 4-day preparation for the suicide and the fact that they had recently broken up. The treating psychiatrist had assumed that the patient was still married, but found he had recently been divorced and had not mentioned this, as well as his recent break-up. One still wonders what question might have been asked to uncover his elaborate suicide plan. His recent loss of two relationships was a clue that he had elected not to disclose, and it may well have been the event that precipitated his suicide.

In another case a female patient with a mood disorder became severely agitated and depressed. She had suicidal ideation and was admitted to the hospital for several days only to relapse with suicidal ideation and agitation after discharge. She was treated with olanzapine to reduce her severe agitation, and only then told her psychiatrist that she became suicidal after having been raped in a parking lot a few weeks prior. She had been unable to share this with her male therapist, until he had seen her three times and reduced her agitation with olanzapine.

Many times patients in crisis will minimize or leave out of the conversation a precipitating event. It important in doing a suicide risk assessment to ask about the occurrence of a major life stress or anticipated loss in different ways to cue the patient to remember and report the situation. Sometimes making this inquiry in different times during the interview will yield very important information. Hurrying the process will make it more likely that crucial events are left out. Once a stress is identified—a detailed discussion of how the patient is dealing with it or feeling overwhelmed by the situation is necessary to adequately assess suicide risk. This information is perhaps the greatest potential loss in doing a perfunctory interview.

Follow-up questions like "everybody worries—what are you worrying about?", or "how's your love life?" or "any health worries?" depending on the patient, can spark a realization—and provide new information that can be crucial to the identification of a high risk state.

What is proposed is the *repetition of questions about major stresses of losses*, experienced or anticipated throughout the assessment interview as a way of increasing the chances of the patient disclosing this information. Personal clinical experience suggests that when patients present with anxiety symptoms or profound demoralization they often deny any precipitating event until the question is reasked in different ways. Then they frequently will say—"I had forgotten all about that-" Studies of short term risk factors for suicide would not be likely to uncover this type of risk factor—only a careful clinical interview would have the chance to do so.

8.6 The Presence of Lethal Means: Handguns

"Any thoughts of ways to kill yourself?—Like a handgun. Do you own one?"

There are endless ways for any of us to kill ourselves. It is just that most of us are not thinking about it that way. A patient preoccupied with suicide may be thinking of all the possible ways—they are "in" the market. The presence of a handgun to someone "in the suicide market" is extremely dangerous. Many people own handguns. We should ask about this—and if a patient struggling with suicidal thoughts or increased impulsivity, owns a handgun, or other lethal weapon, we should ask them to give it to someone for self keeping until the crisis is past—and record in our notes whether they agreed or not. The patient who recites the many ways he or she could kill themselves should be asked why they are so preoccupied with death.

Why should a patient be asked about a handgun when there are so many other means of suicide? The handgun is the most common method of suicide, and it is symbolic of a suicide weapon. Several years ago, a resident was treating a schizophrenic young male who was severely depressed. He attributed his depression to the "fact" that since he had put the antibiotic Bacitracin on a sore, he was losing his hearing. The patient had read on the internet that Bacitracin (given systemically not topically) could cause hearing loss. He refused treatment for his severe depression because he had also found on the internet, the claim that SSRI antidepressants could cause hearing loss. The patient was asked if he was willing to try a non-SSRI antidepressant, mirtazapine. He grudgingly agreed. The resident wrote a prescription and scheduled the patient back in two weeks. The patient went home and shot himself in the head. In this last interview before the patient's death, he was queried about whether he had a gun. The patient responded "no". Of course, a positive response would have engendered a request to get the firearms out of the house until the patient had recovered.

8.7 Anxiety Severity: Agitation

One of the most important symptom, dimensions which may be an important short term risk factor for suicide, is severity of anxiety. Clinicians often do not consciously assess the severity of anxiety symptoms in their patient. It may be because anxiety is such a common comorbid symptom in mood disorders that it is not carefully assessed.

In 1983, our group assessed the presence and *severity* of anxiety in patients diagnosed as having major depression by the SADS-C, a rating instrument that not only recorded the presence of symptoms, but also their severity. This required time from the clinical interviewer and the expense of establishing the reliability of clinical raters across symptoms. It is probably these reasons, the time required and the expense that the SADS is rarely used in a clinical research environment. DSM-5 and the SCID DSM rating substitute the number of symptoms present as a proxy of severity instead of trying to rely on an assessment of symptom severity because of reliability issues across clinicians. In 1983, we published data showing that in 200 patients diagnosed with MDD, that 62 % of the patients had at least moderate severity co-morbid anxiety and 32 % had severe anxiety recorded (Fawcett and Kravitz 1983).

The SADS-C, psychic anxiety scale is very useful for clinicians (Endicott and Spiitzer 1978). This scale scores anxiety severity on the basis of the patient's report of experienced severity and the amount of time during the patients waking period that the anxiety is experienced. If the patient experiences the coming and going of moderately severe anxiety they would be rated as a 3 on this scale. Severe anxiety, experienced much of the time would be rated as a 4. If the patient reports severe anxiety most of the time, that interferes with other day to day functions, working, paying bills etc., the rating would be severe anxiety (a 5 rating on the SADS-C psychic anxiety scale. I have found that asking the patient if a positive encounter with a loved one, such as a grandchild, or a puppy does not distract them from the anxiety, even for a short time, and the anxiety is omni-present and severe, the appropriate rating would be a 5 for "psychic anxiety" on the SADS-C. This is a significant level with regard to suicide in a study that we will review later. This can be a useful way for a clinician to assess the severity of a patient's anxiety symptoms. This assessment is also is important in assessing treatment targets in patients with treatment resistant depression.

Another study that conveys both the frequency and the wide range of severity of anxiety in depression is the work of Clayton et al. (1991). This study presented a subgroup of 320 patients diagnosed with major depression by the SADS from the NJMH Collaborative Depression Study (CDS) and presented the sum of their scores on six different types of anxiety scales, (including somatic anxiety, psychic anxiety, worry etc.) The plot published illustrated the frequency and severity of anxiety symptoms in patients with primary depression (meaning the diagnosis of MDD preceded any other diagnosis (including anxiety disorders) and suggesting that anxiety appeared with the onset of the depression as opposed to before this onset.

This figure showed that anxiety symptoms were very common across all the cases, but that only about 10 % of patients presented with the most severe ratings of anxiety symptoms.

In 1990, Fawcett et al. published data from the CDS prospective study showing that over a 10 year follow-up, severe psychic anxiety, severe (global) insomnia, panic attacks, severity of loss of interest and pleasure, indecisiveness, and recent increase in alcohol abuse were significantly more severe in patients (n = 13) who committed suicide in the first year after discharge, while "standard" risk factors such as suicidal ideation severity, prior (past and recent) suicide attempts, and severity of hopelessness were not more common in the suicide group. These standard risk factors were significantly associated with suicide in years 2–10 following discharge. This study raised the issue of acute risk factors (related to suicide occurring in days, weeks, or months) as opposed to chronic risk factors for suicide occurring over years later. Acute risk factors for suicide should be of greatest interest to the clinician looking to intervene to prevent a suicide.

It appears that severity of anxiety, severity of insomnia, increase in alcohol abuse were not included in the single prior prospective study of Pokorny as well as the retrospective studies of Large reviewed above, which found no acute or short term predictor clinical variables for suicide.

Obviously, not every patient at risk for suicide will present with anxiety. A chart review study of anxiety-agitation in inpatients who committed suicide found that 79 % of these patients had several day periods of severe anxiety—agitation rated from the chart notes using the SADS-C rating for psychic anxiety, (Busch et al. 2003). Another study of suicide attempts with a severity level sufficient to provoke hospital admission found that 90 % of suicide attempting patients scored their anxiety levels as high (based on SADS-C, psychic anxiety ratings) in the month prior to their attempt (Hall et al. 1999). While these finding regarding anxiety have not been replicated in another prospective study (none have been funded), other studies support the finding that severe anxiety is a risk factor for suicide in addition to the two studies just reviewed.

Stordal et al. (2008) in Norway published an unusual study designed as massive study of health (the HUNT study) In this study over 60,000 subjects rated their mood on the Hospital Anxiety and Depression scale, over several years, on a monthly basis (except for July). This sample contained a subsample of 10,670 males and 3,833 females who died by suicide. Those committing suicide were found to do so when their rating peaked at the same time for both depression and anxiety severity ($r = 0.72$, $p = 0.01$). Suicides occurred peaked in June and a smaller peak on October. Depression tended to vary ($p = 0.001$), while anxiety scores less variation over time.

Another study by Pfeiffer et al. 2009 presented outcomes for 887,000 veterans followed with depression. This study found a significantly elevated odds ratio (OR = 1.2) for suicide associated with the diagnoses with generalized anxiety disorder, anxiety disorder, panic disorder, but not PTSD or other anxiety disorders. Most interesting was the increased odds ratio for suicide (OR = 1.7) in those patients receiving anxiolytic medications (benzodiazepines or buspirone) and a further elevated odds ratio (OR = 2.4) in a sub-group taking high dose anxiolytic medications. This study shows evidence of an association of suicide with more severe anxiety symptoms, but also raises questions about the efficacy of benzodiazepines for treating severe comorbid anxiety to reduce suicide risk.

Some studies have not reported a relationship between a history of suicide attempts and comorbid anxiety disorders as diagnosed by the SCID (Nakagawa et al. 2008). However, these studies, did not address suicide or the severity of anxiety, only past attempts and suicidal ideation and they focused on the diagnosis of generalized anxiety disorder, while many patients with mood disorders develop anxiety symptoms with the onset of their disorder.

8.8 Other Risk Factors: Active Substance or Alcohol Use

Comorbid substance abuse/alcohol abuse is common as a comorbid complication of mental illness. They also increase the risk of suicide. It is clear that aggressive impulsivity is a trait that promotes suicidal behavior (Nock et al. 2009), and it is also clear that substance or alcohol abuse promotes impulsivity. It is very difficult, if not impossible to successfully treat other psychiatric disorders in the active presence of substance/alcohol abuse. One study found that the presence of alcohol abuse alone was associated with suicide across diagnostic categories. (Flansborg-Madsen et al. 2009) and other studies have found alcohol abuse as a risk factor (Beck et al. 1989).

Personality Disorders, especially borderline and antisocial personality disorder, both of which are also associated with the presence of impulsive behavior have been associated with suicidal behavior, but not in a time-related sense. It is of interest that it has been shown that the presence of anxiety is associated with higher levels of impulsivity, Nock et al. 2009, in a study of the occurrence of suicide attempts across 21 countries, has shown that suicidal ideation alone does not predict suicidal behavior, but suicidal ideation associated with increased anxiety or impulsivity does lead to suicidal behavior.

8.9 Suicide May not Be Predictable: A Suicide Risk Assessment Is the Standard of Care

We have no evidence that suicide is predictable in a short time frame. We have reviewed evidence that suicide may be more likely when a patient is depressed, severely anxious, of overwhelmed by life stress or anticipated negative events. A recent study showed that 70 % of patients who committed suicide had no charted evidence of a suicide assessment in the last visit prior to their suicide (Smith et al. 2013).

8.10 What Is the Evidence that Treatment Can Prevent Suicide?

Another chapter in this book has covered in depth the evidence that certain types of psychotherapy can reduce suicidal behavior. With respect to medication, an important meta-analysis by Khan has shown that in 8–12 week courses of antidepressants or antipsychotic medications do not result in less suicides (in a group of patients selected not to be at high suicidal risk) than placebo. There is evidence of a decrease of suicidal ideation on patients receiving SSRIs (Sher et al. 2012), but no evidence of a reduction in suicide over 2–3 months of treatment.

However, there are two long-term follow-up studies that find that sustained treatment with medication reduce suicide, A study by Angst et al. in a 34–38 year follow up of 220 patient hospitalized for MDD, and 200 followed for bipolar disorder, find that if a patient stays on medications for a minimum of 6 months despite being more severely ill, they have a 2.5x less likelihood of suicide. The suicide rate was still higher than normal for the treated group. This study showed that the more the medications taken by the patient are, the better will be their outcome.

A more recent analysis of CDS patients over a 16–20 year follow-up by Leon et al. 2011, has shown that a higher propensity for taking antidepressant medications resulted in a 20 % decrease in suicide and suicide attempts. So, thus far, there is evidence from long-term studies that if patients stay on medication they are less likely to commit suicide. This shows that promoting adherence to maintenance medication has evidence for a reduction of suicide.

We have no evidence of short-term reduction in suicide from treatment thus far. Of course this evidence may be difficult to find as well as an ethical challenge. We need more effective ways to determine high suicide risk as well as more effective treatment to reduce suicide risk. There is evidence that severity of anxiety/agitation can be reduced by atypical antipsychotic medications such as quetiapine and olanzapine (Nishiyama and Matsumoto 2013; Bandelow et al. 2014; Montgomery et al. 2014). This may be a way of treating severe anxiety and agitation that may reduce the risk for suicide. This seems the best approach available at present when one considers the high rate of suicide associated with the presence and even high dosage of benzodiazepines reported above in the Pfeiffer et al. study. If benzodiazepines must be used to treat comorbid anxiety because of tolerance issues, the author recommends clonazepam because of its longer half-life.

The finding that ketamine, infused intravenously, in some patients can eliminate ideas of suicidal preoccupation after 40 min to several hours in responders, let us know that it is possible to reverse suicidal thinking. Unfortunately, this effect lasts a short time and at present we do not understand the mechanism sufficiently to maintain this anti-suicide effect. However, we have a proof of concept that encourages a continued search for treatment that can reverse suicidal risk (Larkin and Beautrais 2011; Zigman and Blier 2013; Gloannis and De Leo 2014).

Directions for the future in terms of being more effective in preventing suicide depend on the discovery of more robust acute risk factors and methods to clinically access this information. The deployment of more effective suicide risk assessments as well as the development of more effective treatments such as those suggested by the initial studies of ketamine, could increase our ability to prevent suicide more often.

8.11 Summary

The evidence concerning whether suicide is clinically preventable has been reviewed. At present there is no evidence that suicide is clinically predictable in an individual, even though the standard of care requires that suicide risk be assessed in psychiatric patients, who show an elevated risk in general, and clinical efforts be made to reduce risk. We know of clinical factors that are weakly associated with increased risk, but knowing when that risk is about to be acted on is not presently possible. It may be that studies of risk have not considered all risk factors, such as severe anxiety, which is often reversible with treatment. The clinical approach to the assessment of risk may become more effective with improved clinical approaches to suicide assessment. Improved methods of clinical assessment of suicide risk could lead to more effective short-term prevention. At present, there is no evidence that short term (2–3 months) treatment can prevent suicide, but there is evidence that maintaining maintenance medication can reduce suicide in high risk patients from long-term studies, and that stopping effective medications result in increased rates of suicide in clinical samples.

There is recent evidence of the potential for pharmacologic intervention to reduce suicide risk over the short-term. Improving and expanding our ability to clinically assess short-term risk factors for suicide and finding more effective pharmacologic treatments that recent evidence suggests is possible could significantly increase our capacity to reduce suicide in high risk patients, which constitute a large proportion of suicides. More successful means of encouraging effective treatment of depression through physician education and enlisting more high-risk people into getting effective treatment will be required as well.

References

Angst F, Stassen HH, Clayton PJ et al. (2002) Mortality of patents with mood disorders: follow-up over 34–38 years. J Affect Disord 68(2–3):67–81

Bandelow B, Bauer M, Vieta E et al (2014) Extended release quetiapine fumarate as adjunct to antidepressant therapy in patients with major depressive disorder: pooled analysis of patients with anxious depression versus low levels of anxiety at baseline. World J Biol Psychiatr 15 (2):155–166

Beck AT et al (1989) Alcohol abuse ans eventual suicide: a 5- to 10-year prospective study of alcohol-abusing suicide attempters. J Stud Alcohol 50(3):202–209
Busch KA, Fawcett J, Jacobs D (2003) Clinical correlates of inpatient suicide. J Clin Psychiatr 64 (1):14–19
Cipriani A (2013) Review: lithium reduces the risk of suicide compared with placebo in people with depression and bipolar disorder. Evid Based Mental health 16(4):112
Clayton PJ, Grove WM, Coryell W et al. (1991) Follow-up and family study of anxious depression. Am J Psychiatr 148(11):1512–1517
Conwell Y, Duberstein PH, Cox C et al (1996) Relationships of age and axis I diagnoses in victims of completed suicide: a psychological autopsy study. Am J Psychiatr 153(8):1001–1008
De Gloannis, DeLeo D (2014) Oral ketamine augmentation for chronic suicidality in treatment resistant depression. Audt-NZ J Psychiatr 48:686, 22 Jan 2014
Endicott J, Spiitzer R (1978) A diagnostic interview: the schedule for affective disorders and schizophrenia. Arch Gen Psychiatr 35(7):837–844
Fawcett J, Kravitz HM (1983) Anxiety syndromes and their relationship to depressive illness. J Clin Psychiatr 44(8):8–11
Fawcett J, Scheftner WA, Fogg L et al (1990) Time-related predictors of suicide in major affective disorder. Am J Psychiatr 147(9):1189–1194
Flansborg-Madsen T, Knop J, Mortensen EL et al (2009) Alcohol use disorders increase the risk of completed suicide- irrespective of other psychiatric disorders. A longitudinal cohort study. Psychiatry Res 167(1–2):123–130
Hall RC, Platt DE, Hall RC (1999) Suicide risk assessment: a review of risk factors for suicide in 100 patients who made severe suicide attempts. Evaluation of suicide risk in a time of managed care. Psychosomatics 40(1):18–27
Hennriksson S, Isacsson G (2006) Increased antidepressant use and fewer suicides in Jamtland County, Sweden, after a primary care educations programme on the treatment of depression. Acta Psychiatrica Scand 114:159–167
Isometsa ET, Heikkinen ME, Marttunen MJ et al (1995) The last appointment before suicide: is suicide intent communicated? Am J Psychiatr 152(6):919–922
Khan A, Khan S, Kolts R, Brown WA (2003) Suicide rates in clinical trials of SSRIs, other antidepressants, and placebo: analysis of FDS reports. Am J Psychiatr 160(4):790–792
Lambert MT (2002) Seven year outcomes of patients evaluated for suicidality. Psychiatric Serv 53 (1):92–94
Lambert MT, Bonner J (1996) Characteristics and six month outcome of patients sho use suicide threats seek hospital admission. Psychiatr Serv 47(8):871–873
Large M, Sharma S, Cannon E et al. (2011) Risk factors for suicide within a year of discharge from a psychiatric hospital: a systematic analysis. Aust- NZ Psychiatr 45(8):619–628
Larkin GL, Beautrais SL (2011) A preliminary naturalistic study of low-dose ketamine for depression and suicide ideation in the emergency department. Int J Neuropsychopharmacol 14 (8):1127–1131
Leon AC, Solomon DA, Li C et al (2011) Antidepressants and risk of suicide and suicide attempts: a 27-year observational study. J Clin Psychiatr 72(5):580–586
Luoma JB, Martin CE, Pearson JL (2002) Contact with mental health and primary care providers before suicide: a review of the evidence. Am J Psychiatr 159(6):909–916
Montgomery SA, Jocklear JC, Svedsafer H et al. (2014) Efficacy of once-daily extended release quetiapine fumarate in patients with different levels of severity of generalized anxiety disorder. Int Clin Psychopharmacol 3 Jan 2014
Nakagawa A et al (2008) Bipolar Disord 10:530–538
Nishiyama A, Matsumoto H (2013) Quetiapine reduces irritability and risk of suicide in patients with agitated depression. Tokai J Exp Clin Med 38(2):93–96
Nock MK, Hwang J, Sampson N et al (2009) Cross-national analysis of the association among mental disorders and suicidal behavior: findings for the WHO World Mental Health Surveys. PLOS Med 6(8):1371

Pfeiffer PN, Ganoczy D, Ilgen M (2009) Comorbid anxiety as a suicide risk factor among depressed veterans. Depress Anxiety 26(8):752–757
Pokorny AD (1983) Prediction of suicide in psychiatric patients: report of a prospective study. Arch Gen Psychiatr 49(3):249–257
Pokorny AD (1993) Suicide prediction revisited. Suicide Life Threat Behav 23(1):1–10
Robins E (1981) The final months, pp 424–425. Oxford University Press, Oxford
Sher L, Stanley BH, Posner K et al (2012) Decreased suicidal ideation in depressed patients with or without comorbid stress disorder treated with selective serotonin reuptake inhibitors: an open study. Psychiatry Res 190(2–3):261
Smith EG, Kim HM, Ganoczy D et al (2013) Suicide risk assessment received prior to suicide death by Veterans health administration patients with a history of depression. J Clin Psychiatr 74(3):226–232
Stordal E, Morken C, Mykietun A et al (2008) Monthly variation in prevalence rates of comorbid anxiety and depression in the general population at 63–65 degrees North: the HUNT study. J Affect Disord 106(3):273–278
American Foundation for Suicide Prevention. www.ASFP.org
Yerevanian BL, Koek RJ, Feusner JD et al. (2004) Antidepressants and suicidal behavior in unipolar depression. Acta Psychiatr Scand 110:452–458
Zigman D, Blier P (2013) Urgent ketamine infusion rapidly eliminated suicidal ideation for a patient with major depressive disorder: a case report. J Clin Psychopharmacol 33(2):270–272

Chapter 9
Neurological Disease and Suicidal Behavior

Thomas J. Hudzik and Gerard J. Marek

Abstract Neurological disease both results from and produces imbalances in the functions of brain circuitry, with resultant alterations in behavior, cognition, and social interactions, among others aspects. These issues can contribute heightened risk for suicidal behavior under a diathesis consistent with such behavior. In this chapter, risk for suicide is addressed for a number of neurological disorders, including Autism Spectrum Disorder (ASD), Parkinson's Disease, epilepsy, and Tourette's Disorder. Neurologic disease is very frequently comorbid with psychiatric disease, although it can be difficult to separate symptoms of the primary neurological disorder from what might be an independent psychiatric disorder. However, given the high incidence of psychiatric symptoms in neurological disorders, especially anxiety and depression, some of these patient populations can be at especially high risk, and should be carefully monitored as a result.

9.1 Introduction

Considering the emergence and maturation of biological psychiatry over the last decade, it seems unusual from the perspective of a neuroscientist to be considering neurological disease as separate from psychiatric disease, especially from the standpoint of risk factors. Indeed, psychiatric symptoms are more often than not present in neurologic patients as well as neurologic symptoms being present in psychiatric patients. However, if one considers that primary neuropathology in

T.J. Hudzik (✉)
Preclinical Safety, AbbVie Global Pharmaceutical Research and Development,
One North Waukegan Road, North Chicago, IL 60064, USA
e-mail: thomas.hudzik@abbvie.com

G.J. Marek
Global Medical Science, CNS and Pain, Astellas Pharma Global Development,
1 Astellas Way, N6.107, Northbrook, IL 60062, USA
e-mail: gerard.marek@astellas.com

K.E. Cannon and T.J. Hudzik (eds.), *Suicide: Phenomenology and Neurobiology*,
DOI 10.1007/978-3-319-09964-4_9

neurology is defined with greater certainty than is often the case in psychiatry, perhaps the distinction remains useful.

Neurological diseases encompass a wide range of disorders with symptoms spanning from the relatively subtle and stable as with essential tremor to those that are progressive, degenerative, and devastating to quality of life of both patients and their caregivers. While the relationship between primary psychiatric diseases with suicidal behavior is often relatively clear, anxiety, depression, or loss of impulse control secondary to or comorbid with neurological disease may not be as clearly understood. For example, symptoms of depression in an Alzheimer's dementia patient may be masked by the symptoms of the primary disease, or a Parkinson's patient may not even recognize changes in their impulse control or mood to report these to their physician (Brand et al. 2007). Even if psychiatric symptoms are recognized in a patient with neurological disease, there may be an assumption on the part of the physician that treatment of the primary disease will positively affect psychiatric symptoms which are secondary. That of course may or may not be true, depending upon the treatment and the patient.

Some special consideration within, but not limited to neurology patient populations are the degree of verbal fluency and fidelity, degree (or ability) of agreement between self-report, caregiver report, physician's assessment, disease severity and progression, instruments used to garner information, and age. Additionally, there is a growing awareness of the bi-directional impact of disease comorbidity, that is, patients with neurological disease are at greater risk of developing major depressive disorder (MDD), (Rickards 2005, 2006) which can then lead to suicidal behavior, and likewise, patients with lifelong MDD are likely more prone to develop other diseases including neurological diseases over the course of their lives. Untreated psychiatric symptoms in patients with neurological disorders are associated with poorer prognosis and obviously poorer quality of life (Agrawal and Rickards 2011, Rickards 2005). Therefore, ensuring that symptoms are recognized and effectively treated will result in overall better outcomes for the patient.

While the scope of the present chapter cannot encompass all neurological diseases, we intended to focus on some of the more common, as well as several which not have received much prior attention. Additionally, Traumatic Brain Injury is extremely well-covered in another chapter (Nazem et al. 2008, This Volume). Given the diversity of neurological diseases, the risk factors may be weighted very differently among different sets of neurology patients.

9.2 Autism Spectrum Disorder

Autism Spectrum Disorder (ASD) is characterized fundamentally as a disorder in social interaction which can range from the social awkwardness inherent in Asperger's to the near-total isolation of a severely affected autistic patient. Prevalence estimates have been increasing over the last few decades, and the CDC now estimate that more than 1 % of the pediatric population have ASD (CDC 2012). Contributing factors to social dysfunction include impaired cognition, attention, verbal, and nonverbal communication, and a restricted behavioral repertoire (DSM 5). The neurobiological underpinnings of autism have been the focus of a great deal of research over the last 100 years, and while etiology has remained elusive, there do appear to be structural abnormalities in the brains of patients (Brambilla et al. 2003). Among the brain regions which have been most consistently described as abnormal are increased total brain volume, increased cerebellar, amygdala and caudate volume, and reduced corpus callosum volume (Verhoeven et al. 2010; Stanfield et al. 2008). Structural differences imply functional differences, and indeed application of functional imaging has demonstrated that autistic patients appear to in some cases recruit different brain regions during the processing of cognitive tasks than normal (Brambilla et al. 2003). Overall, despite what can be very marked consequences of the disorder, the neuropathology is relatively subtle and variable, which suggests in turn that connectivity among brain regions may be of primary importance rather than malfunction of any collection of brain regions. Further, it is clear that neuropathic changes do evolve over time, and how that can be reflected in behavioral changes if of particular interest. Standard of care is highly tailored to the degree of impairment and can range from custodial to no treatment.

In a sample of 350 children with autism 6–16 years of age, mothers reported depressed mood in 54 % of children with high-functioning autism and 42 % with low-functioning autism (Mayes et al. 2011; Murray et al. 2011). Anxiety disorders are also well-known to co-occur in ASD in a much higher rate than in the general population, and is considered to be a primary contributing factor to behavioral disturbances in the population (Kim et al. 2000; Muris et al. 1998).

Given that social isolation is a strong risk factor in suicidal behavior and is a primary characteristic of ADS, it would seem that ASD patients would be at an especially high risk, assuming a certain level of social awareness in this population. Social awareness will vary with disease severity, age, and level of intervention. Diagnosis is most commonly done in early childhood, and it may be useful to consider the youth population separately from those in adolescence and then in later adulthood. In a study of 102 youths aged 7–12 years of age (Storch et al. 2013), identified an 11 % incidence of suicidal ideation and behaviors, which is comparable or even lower that to age-matched peers (Carter et al. 2008). Depression and posttraumatic stress disorder were associated with suicidal thoughts and behaviors (Storch et al. 2013). In a larger (N = 791) study (Mays and Gillon 1993), evaluated a primarily high-functioning (IQ >= 80) population of autistic youths and found a 14 % overall incidence of ideation and behavior, with greatest risk factors being black or Hispanic ethnicity, lower socioeconomic status, male gender, and comorbid depression. In patients with all four risk factors, the incidence increased to as high as 70 %.

It is well known that the incidence of suicidal behavior and of depression can spike in early adulthood, but overall, there is a strong trend for increased probability of appearance with age. This is reflected in observations that the proportion of the population over age 50 have a much higher incidence of MDD and of suicidal behavior than that under age 50 (See Szanto, this volume). Whether this is true in ASD has been addressed by a number of investigators, despite special challenges inherent in diagnosing comorbidities in this population. In a longitudinal study spanning 30 years (Mouridsen et al. 2008), examined cause of death among 341 Danish ASD patients (median age 43 years) and found that their rate of mortality was twice that which would be expected versus the general population. Several subsequent studies have confirmed the mortality rate in ASD at more than 2X the overall population in the US (Pickett et al. 2006; Shavelle et al. 2001). In the Danish study, epilepsy was associated with one-third of the deaths (8 of 26), whereas clearly identified suicide accounted for two of the 26 deaths. More prominent were accidental drowning and as well as motor vehicle accidents which were seen as more related to patients' difficulties in communications, and these causes of death were also noted in the Shavelle and Pickett studies. While difficult to conclude completed suicide rate from these studies, it remains clear that more work is needed to better understand the subpopulations that may be at highest risk for suicide.

9.3 ADHD

ADHD is characterized as a persistent pattern of inattention and/or hyperactivity-impulsivity that is more frequently displayed and is more severe than is typically observed in individuals at a comparable level of development. There are three subtypes of ADHD, differentiated by (1) inattention as a primary symptom, (2) hyperactivity, or (3) mixed, although systematic study of each as a risk factor has not been conducted. While usually diagnosed in childhood, it is now recognized as a potentially lifelong condition (Wilens et al. 2002; Faraone 2005), and affects roughly 5 % of the population overall (Faraone and Biederman 2005). Response to both stimulant (e.g., D-amphetamine, methylphenidate) and non-stimulant (atomoxetine, guanfacine) medications implicates both dopaminergic and adrenergic systems in the pathophysiology of the disorder. Imaging studies have demonstrated dysregulation in processing of the prefrontal cortex, its inputs, and target areas, although the precise etiology remains elusive (Arnsten 2009).

Several studies have attempted to address whether the incidence of suicide completion or ideation is higher in the ADHD population than in the general population. Most recently (Impey and Heun 2012), have extensively reviewed the literature surrounding the association of ADHD with suicidality. Data were analyzed for completed suicides, attempters, and ideation without attempt, and concluded that despite the variability among populations addressed by various studies, there did appear to be a positive association in the vast majority of studies, but only in males. Attention deficit hyperactivity disorder (ADHD) symptoms occur more frequently in suicidal populations and subjects with ADHD are more likely to have suicidal ideation and to attempt suicide. As in previous discussions, addition of other risk factors, such as substance abuse, anxiety, and depression heighten the risk in this population.

9.4 Chronic Pain/Headache

The chronic pain population is extremely diverse, encompassing neuropathies, MS, migraine, cluster headache, osteoarthritis, fibromyalgia, and low-back pain, to name a few. A number of studies have previously reported higher rates of suicidal behavior in chronic pain populations (Breslau 1992; Magni et al. 1998; Hitchcock et al. 1994; Fishbain 1996; Smith et al. 2004). Depression is highly comorbid in some of these populations, creating ambiguity whether suicidal behavior is secondary to the psychiatric condition or a combination of both the chronic pain and depressive symptoms. Braden and Sullivan (2008) using the National Comorbidity Survey Replication sample found that any increased risk for suicidal behavior in reported chronic pain conditions (arthritic, neck, back, or 'other chronic pain') was largely accounted for by presence of depression or anxiety disorder, with the exception of headache and 'other' pain. However, in a larger sample (Scott et al. 2010), found that many chronic medical conditions, such as hypertension, heart disease, in addition to pain-related conditions such as back and neck pain, in general were associated with higher lifetime rates of suicidal ideation, even after controlling for psychiatric illnesses. Sample and methodological differences likely account for the differing conclusions of these studies, but clearly, chronic pain may present risk, which will be heightened by concomitant depression. Assessment of the relationship between management of chronic pain, pain severity, and suicidal behavior will be crucial in better understanding the risks in these patients.

Besides epilepsy, the neurological condition most clearly associated with suicidal behavior and independent of other factors such as depression is chronic, recurrent headache, such as migraine and cluster headache. Migraine is characterized by moderate to severe headache, usually accompanied by sensory sensitization such as photophobia and phonophobia. There are two main subtypes, delineated by absence or presence of preceding neurologic symptoms referred to as aura. It is clear that irregularity in cerebrovascular and cranial nerve (trigeminal and cervical) function is involved in the disorder, but there is no agreement on initiators or even the exact nature of the irregularity (Cutrer 2010). There are effective acute-phase treatments, however, including the tryptan class of serotonergic 1b/d agonists, and a variety of anticonvulsants and antidepressants have shown some efficacy in phrophylaxis (Pringsheim et al. 2010). The prevalence of migraine in the general population has been recently estimated to be about 11 % (Buse et al. 2012), and migraine is much more prevalent in in and more likely to cause disability in females (Buse et al. 2013a, b). Comorbidity of migraine with risk factors associated with suicidal behavior, such as depression and anxiety disorders, is roughly twice the overall lifetime population averages (Breslau and Davis 1992; Buse et al. 2013a, b). Overall, migraine patients do appear to have a higher risk of suicide attempts than the general population, and the risk may be amplified by comorbid psychiatric illness as well as with increased pain intensity (Breslau et al. 2012). Interestingly, from the standpoint of suicidal ideation, there were few differences among migraine patients with aura and those without. There is no data at present that indicates completed suicide attempts are higher in this population, although previous attempt is a powerful predictor of successive attempts.

Cluster headache is characterized by severe unilateral orbital, supraorbital, or temporal headache lasting between 15 min and up to several hours. Its incidence lower than migraine, recently estimated to be about 0.1–0.2 % of the general population (Fischera et al. 2008). The pathophysiology of cluster headache appears to involve activation of the trigeminal pain pathways, vasodilation of intracranial arteries during attacks, and inflammation of the cavernous sinus, although which of these correlates are primary or secondary is still poorly understood (Leone and Bussone 2009). Involvement of hypothalamic regions is suggested by activation of hypothalamic areas during active headache. Treatments include NSAIDS, calcium channel blockers, such as verapamil, mixed-mechanism anticonvulsant compounds, such as topiramate, lithium and opioids.

While migraine's psychiatric comorbidities have been fairly well studied, perhaps due to the lower population incidence of cluster headache, this linkage appears to have received less attention (Robbins 2013). Rozen and Fishman (2012) surveyed more than 1,000 cluster headache patients and found that depression was observed to be the most frequently comorbid medical condition (nearly 25 %) and the majority (55 %) of patients exhibited suicidal ideation. Among these, 2 % have made suicide attempts. Additionally, half of cluster headache patients have exhibited some form of self-injurious behavior during an episode.

9.5 Parkinson's Disease

Parkinson's disease is the second most common neurodegenerative disease, with a 1 % incidence in the adult population over 60 years of age (de Lau and Breteler 2006). The disease is characterized primarily by motor dysfunction due to loss of dopamine-containing neurons in the midbrain's substantia nigra and hence, loss of their projections to forebrain motor regions. The loss of synaptic input of dopamine can be reflected by a loss of forebrain dopamine transporters or postsynaptic dopamine receptors. Hallmark symptoms are tremor while awake that progresses distally to proximally over the disease course, a shuffling gait, and ultimately progresses to relative immobility. While the motor symptoms are iconic in Parkinson's, it is clear that as importantly the disease results in cognitive, behavioral, and affective symptoms which can be positively or negatively altered by the standard of care-dopamine replacement therapy, as well as by emerging therapies, such as deep brain stimulation. Etiology is multivariate and heterogeneous, and includes factors such as exposure to environmental toxins, coupled to genetic vulnerability and to nutritional history and status. Recently, impulse control disorders which are likely part of the disease and/or treatment (Dagher and Robbins 2009) have been the subject of a number of studies and are characterized by a failure to resist impulses that can lead to harmful outcomes for both themselves and those around them. Examples of these are gambling, which is the most common, but also include hypersexuality, compulsive shopping, and compulsive eating. Impulse control disorders can affect as many as 15 % of patients with Parkinson's disease. It is interesting to consider whether impulsivity, related to the disorder or to its treatment, plays a role in suicidality in the disease. Additionally, given the pivotal role of the dopaminergic system in reward, pleasure, and in cognition, it would certainly be predicted that Parkinson's patients would suffer from depression in much higher proportions than in the general population. This has been demonstrated by Nazem et al. (2008), who estimated that the incidence of depression may be as high as 40 % in the Parkinson's population, accompanied by an alarmingly high level of suicidal ideation of >30 %.

Degeneration of other monoamine neurons could also play a role in depressive symptoms and suicidal behavior in light of evidence that restoration of dopaminergic neural networks by transplantation of dopamine-rich fetal mesencephalic tissue failed to alleviate depressive symptoms despite improving motor symptoms (Politis et al. 2012). Serotonergic neurons and serotonergic terminal fields did not demonstrate recovery with the transplantation and are a reasonable candidate to explain the failure to improve depressive symptoms. This notwithstanding, Parkinson's patients have been shown to have a lower prevalence of completed suicides than age-matched controls (Myslobodsky et al. 2001; Stenager et al. 1994). Depression associated with Parkinson's, however, appears to increase the risk of an attempt, and treatment of the depression therefore becomes quite important (Nazem et al. 2008). Recently, if Parkinson's patients who have undergone DBS treatment are considered, a number of case studies (Burkhard et al. 2004; Soulas et al. 2008), followed by controlled trials (Voon et al. 2008) indicated that DBS patients were indeed at higher risk for suicidal behaviors including completed suicide attempt, especially in the first years following surgery. Interestingly, the increase in suicidal behavior in this population occurs despite otherwise excellent symptomatic outcome (Wolters et al. 2008). There is some retrospective evidence of both affective (Berney et al. 2002) and cognitive (Aybek et al. 2007) changes following DBS surgery, which could potentially play a role in outcome in some patients, although this remains unclear to what degree (if any) the surgery may unmask, induce, or accelerate these symptoms. There does appear to be a clear association with depression in this population, and therefore careful presurgical screening and postoperative monitoring can be useful tools in mitigation.

9.6 Tourette's Syndrome

Tourette's is characterized by involuntary motor tics, sometimes involving vocalizations ranging from grunts to sentences uttered, and commonly involves simple tics, such as jerking of the head or limbs. Tics are often preceded by sensation of impending inevitability. Tourette's affects about 1 % of the population. The pathophysiology involves a loss of inhibitory GABAergic and cholinergic neurons, particularly in the basal ganglia and putamen (Kataoka et al. 2010; Kalanithi et al. 2005). Etiology is complex, where multiple contributing factors including genetics, infection, toxin exposure, and injury can all play a role. The complex etiology is reflected by a high degree of variability in the clinical presentation, but the syndrome appears to consistently appear in childhood, peaks during adolescence, and abates somewhat during adulthood—at least in terms of tic severity. Standard of care are dopamine-blocking drugs—typical and atypical antipsychotics, only two of which, haloperidol and pimozide are FDA-approved for the indication, although a host of other medications have been used, including topiramate, tetrabenazine, SSRIs, and benzodiazepines, all of which, including the antipsychotics, appear to have limited efficacy. DBS and even ECT has been applied to varying degrees of success (Ward et al. 2010; Burdick et al. 2010; Motlagh et al. 2013; Robertson 2006).

Comorbid psychiatric disorders are seen in up to 90 % of Tourette's patients (Kurlan et al. 2002; Freeman and Tourette Syndrome International Database 2007; Zinner and Coffey 2009), especially MDD, Obsessive-Compulsive Disorder (OCD) (Anholt et al. 2006; Kano et al. 2010a, b, 2010). Despite this, there appear to be few studies that specifically address suicide in Tourette's. Comings and Comings (1987) demonstrated a high level of suicidal ideation in this population, with 40–50 % reporting ideation, and up to 15 % reporting actual attempts.

9.7 Epilepsy

Epilepsy is a multifaceted disorder that affects about 3–30 % of a given population over the lifetime, depending upon a number of factors including economic status of the population (Bell et al.2014). While there are many distinct epileptiform disorders, the hallmark characteristic is seizure, with or without loss of consciousness. The seizure, a result of neuronal firing synchrony in a brain region, can have motor involvement that ranges from minimal, as in absence epilepsy up to nearly complete, as in status epilepiticus, depending upon locus, focus, and total amount of tissue involved. Standard of care are a number of classes of antiepileptic drugs, all of which directly or indirectly increase inhibitory tone in brain, usually via enhancement of gabaergic transmission. As in Parkinson's disease, although for different reasons, patients often become refractory to their medications, and an ever-evolving cocktail of medications are sometimes required to maintain the patient. If pharmacotherapy fails, surgical options, including excision of the affected brain region and DBS can provide relief of symptoms. There are clearly congenital forms of epilepsy, although it can develop following acute head trauma, or slowly over the course of neurodegenerative illnesses.

A number of studies have demonstrated a clearly increased risk for suicidal behavior in the epileptic population, even after correcting for socioeconomic status, marital status, and comorbid psychiatric disease (Jones et al. 2003; Rudzinski and Meador 2013; Buljan and Santic 2011). Unlike the general population trend, the length of illness is inversely correlated with risk, in that the risk appears to be highest within the first year of diagnosis (Hesdorffer et al. 2013; Hecimovic et al. 2011). As is almost always the case, concomitant depression is the most prevalent enhancer of risk in this population (Harden and Goldstein 2002). It is of note that some, but certainly not all anti-epileptic drugs appear to have efficacy in bipolar disorder, suggesting some potential overlap between the two types of diseases (Post et al. 1991). Indeed, the suicide rate in bipolar disorder is very high relative to other illnesses (Finseth et al. 2012; Jollant 2010).

9.8 Conclusions and Speculations

The comorbidities of psychiatric and neurologic illness underscores the broad overlap among these disciplines, and by more clearly understanding the relationships among these, further advances in both fields can be made. Among the greatest risk factors for suicidal behavior is presence of depression, which, as we have seen above, is extremely commonly comorbid and can potentially amplify the risk of suicidal behavior if left untreated in any neurological patient population. This may be complicated by the fact that in some patient populations (e.g., Alzheimer's) treatment response to antidepressants is poor. In general, neurological disease results in disrupted cognition (e.g., poor decision-making), which, as described so eloquently by Nazem et al. (this volume) can result in heightened risk for suicidal behavior. Perturbed serotonergic neurotransmission, a common finding in suicidal behavior in general (Mann et al. 1989), is a likely correlate of many neurological diseases, given the widespread distribution and hence influence in brain function. Another pervasive phenomenon in both psychiatric and neurologic diseases in an inflammatory component, that can both result from neurologic insult and maintain a perturbation of circuitry. It is possible than any such disruption can lead to increased risk, exemplified by additional disorders such as fetal alcohol syndrome, multiple sclerosis, ALS, MS, among others. The neurologist should be aware of the complex interplay between symptom severity, chronicity, and concomitant/resultant psychiatric disorders which can lead to fatal outcome. Mitigation can perhaps take the form of making broader use of instruments such as the C-SSRS (Posner et al. This Volume) in assessing risk in individual patients in these populations.

References

Agrawal N, Rickards H (2011) Detection and treatment of depression in neurological disorders. J Neurol Neurosurg Psychiatry 82(8):828–829

Anholt GE et al (2006) Do obsessional beliefs discriminate ocd without tic patients from Ocd with Tic and Tourette's syndrome patients? Behav Res Ther 44(11):1537–1543

Arnsten, AFT (2009) Toward a new understanding of attention-deficit hyperactivity disorder pathophysiology. CNS Drug 23.1:33–41

Aybek S et al (2007) Long-term cognitive profile and incidence of dementia after Stn-Dbs in Parkinson's disease. Mov Disord 22(7):974–981
Bell GS et al (2014) An unknown quantity—The worldwide prevalence of epilepsy. Epilepsia 55 (7):958–962
Berney A et al (2002) Effect on mood of subthalamic Dbs for Parkinson's disease: a consecutive series of 24 patients. Neurology 59(9):1427–1429
Braden JB, Sullivan MD (2008) Suicidal thoughts and behavior among adults with self-reported pain conditions in the national comorbidity survey replication. J Pain 9(12):1106–1115
Brambilla P et al (2003) Brain anatomy and development in autism: review of structural MRI studies. Brain Res Bull 61(6):557–569
Brand S et al (2007) Depression in Parkinson's disease. Assessment and treatment. Nervenarzt 78.6:715–727; quiz 28
Breslau N, Davis GC (1992) Migraine and psychiatric disorders: a prospective epidemiologic study. Clin Neuropharmacol 15(Suppl 1 Pt A): 279A–80A
Breslau N et al (2012) Migraine headaches and suicide attempt. Headache 52(5):723–731
Breslau Naomi (1992) Migraine, suicidal ideation, and suicide attempts. Neurology 42(2):392–392
Buljan R, Santic AM (2011) Suicide attempts in hospital-treated epilepsy patients. Acta Clin Croat 50(4):485–490
Burdick A et al (2010) Lack of benefit of accumbens/capsular deep brain stimulation in a patient with both tics and obsessive-compulsive disorder. Neurocase 16(4):321–330
Burkhard PR et al (2004) Suicide after successful deep brain stimulation for movement disorders. Neurology 63(11):2170–2172
Buse DC et al (2013a) Sex differences in the prevalence, symptoms, and associated features of migraine, probable migraine and other severe headache: results of the American migraine prevalence and prevention (AMPP) study. Headache 53(8):1278–1299
Buse DC et al (2013b) Psychiatric comorbidities of episodic and chronic migraine. J Neurol 260 (8):1960–1969
Buse DC et al (2012) Headache impact of chronic and episodic migraine: results from the American migraine prevalence and prevention study. Headache 52(1):3–17
Carter R et al (2008) Measures matter: the relative contribution of anxiety and depression to suicidal ideation in clinically referred anxious youth using brief versus full length questionnaires. Depress Anxiety 25(8):E27–E35
Center for Disease Control and Prevention (CDC) 2009 Prevalence of autism spectrum disorders—Autism and Developmental Disabilities Monitoring Network, United States, 2006. MMWR Surveill Summ 58(10):1–20
Comings BG, Comings DE (1987) A controlled study of tourette syndrome. V. depression and mania. Am J Hum Genet 41(5):804–821
Cutrer FM (2010) Pathophysiology of migraine. Semin Neurol 30(2):120–130
Dagher A, Robbins TW (2009) Personality, addiction, dopamine: insights from Parkinson's disease. Neuron 61(4):502–510
de Lau LM, Breteler MM (2006) Epidemiology of Parkinson's disease. Lancet Neurol 5 (6):525–535
Faraone SV (2005) The scientific foundation for understanding attention-deficit/hyperactivity disorder as a valid psychiatric disorder. Eur Child Adolesc Psychiatry 14(1):1–10
Faraone SV, Biederman J (2005) What is the prevalence of adult ADHD? results of a population screen of 966 adults. J Atten Disord 9(2):384–391
Finseth PI et al (2012) Risk factors related to lifetime suicide attempts in acutely admitted bipolar disorder inpatients. Bipolar Disord 14(7):727–734
Fischera M et al (2008) The incidence and prevalence of cluster headache: a meta-analysis of population-based studies. Cephalalgia 28(6):614–618
Fishbain DA (1996) Current research on chronic pain and suicide. Am J Public Health 86 (9):1320–1321

Freeman R, Consortium Tourette Syndrome International Database (2007) Tic disorders and ADHD: answers from a world-wide clinical dataset on Tourette syndrome. Eur Child Adolesc Psychiatry 16(Suppl 1):15–23
Harden CL, Goldstein MA (2002) Mood disorders in patients with epilepsy: epidemiology and management. CNS Drugs 16(5):291–302
Hecimovic H et al (2011) Suicidality and epilepsy: a neuropsychobiological perspective. Epilepsy Behav 22(1):77–84
Hesdorffer DC et al (2013) Suicidal ideation and behavior screening in intractable focal epilepsy eligible for drug trials. Epilepsia 54(5):879–887
Hitchcock LS, Ferrell BR, McCaffery M (1994) The experience of chronic nonmalignant pain. J Pain Symptom Manage 9(5):312–318
Impey M, Heun R (2012) Completed suicide, ideation and attempt in attention deficit hyperactivity disorder. Acta Psychiatr Scand 125(2):93–102
Jollant F (2010) Bipolar disorder and suicide risk. Soins Psychiatr 271:17–19
Jones JE et al (2003) Rates and risk factors for suicide, suicidal ideation, and suicide attempts in chronic epilepsy. Epilepsy Behav 4(Suppl 3):S31–S38
Kalanithi PS et al (2005) Altered parvalbumin-positive neuron distribution in basal ganglia of individuals with Tourette syndrome. Proc Natl Acad Sci USA 102(37):13307–13312
Kano Y et al (2010a) Obsessive-compulsive symptom dimensions in japanese tourette syndrome subjects. CNS Spectr 15(5):296–303
Kano Y et al (2010b) Association between Tourette syndrome and comorbidities in Japan. Brain Dev 32(3):201–207
Kano Y et al (2010) Obsessive-compulsive symptom dimensions in Japanese Tourette syndrome subjects. CNS Spectr 15(5):296–303
Kataoka Y et al (2010) Decreased number of parvalbumin and cholinergic interneurons in the striatum of individuals with Tourette syndrome. J Comp Neurol 518(3):277–291
Kim JA et al (2000) The prevalence of anxiety and mood problems among children with autism and asperger syndrome. Autism 4.2:117–132
Kurlan R et al (2002) The behavioral spectrum of Tic disorders: a community-based study. Neurology 59(3):414–420
Leone M, Bussone G (2009) Pathophysiology of trigeminal autonomic cephalalgias. Lancet Neurol 8(8):755–764
Magni G et al (1998) Suicidality in Chronic abdominal pain: an analysis of the hispanic health and nutrition examination survey (hhanes). Pain 76(1-2):137–144
Mann JJ et al (1989) Evidence for the 5-Ht hypothesis of suicide. A review of post-mortem studies. Br J Psychiatry Suppl 8:7–14
Mayes SD et al (2011) Use of Gilliam Asperger's disorder scale in differentiating high and low functioning autism and ADHD. Psychol Rep 108(1):3–13
Mays RM, Janet EG (1993) Autism in young children: an update. J Pediatr Health Care 7.1:17–23
Motlagh MG et al (2013) Lessons learned from open-label deep brain stimulation for tourette syndrome: eight cases over 7 years. Tremor Other Hyperkinet Mov (NY) 3:79
Mouridsen SE et al (2008) Mortality and causes of death in autism spectrum disorders: an update. Autism 12(4):403–414
Muris P et al (1998) Comorbid anxiety symptoms in children with pervasive developmental disorders. J Anxiety Disord 12(4):387–393
Murray MJ, Mayes SD, Smith LA (2011) Brief report: excellent agreement between two brief autism scales (checklist for autism spectrum disorder and social responsiveness scale) completed independently by parents and the autism diagnostic interview-revised. J Autism Dev Disord 41(11):1586–1590
Myslobodsky M, Lalonde FM, Hicks L (2001) Are patients with Parkinson's disease suicidal? J Geriatr Psychiatry Neurol 14(3):120–124
Nazem S et al (2008) Suicidal and death ideation in Parkinson's disease. Mov Disord 23 (11):1573–1579

Pickett JA et al (2006) 1998–2002 update on "causes of death in autism". J Autism Dev Disord 36 (2):287–288

Politis M, Wu K, Loane C, Quinn NP, Brooks DJ, Vertel WH, Bjorkland A, Lindvall O, Piccini P (2012) Serotonin neuron loss and nonmotor symptoms continue in Parkinson's patients treated with dopamine grafts. Sci Transl Med 4:128ra41

Post RM, Findling RL, Kahn RS (1991) Interfaces between seizures and affective disorders: the uses of visually mapping the evolution and longitudinal course of an illness. Mt Sinai J Med 58 (4):310–323

Pringsheim T, Davenport WJ, Becker WJ (2010) Prophylaxis of migraine headache. CMAJ 182 (7):E269–E276

Rickards H (2006) Depression in neurological disorders: an update. Curr Opin Psychiatry 19 (3):294–298

Rickards H (2005) Depression in neurological disorders: Parkinson's disease, multiple sclerosis, and stroke. J Neurol Neurosurg Psychiatry 76(Suppl 1):i48–i52

Robbins MS (2013) The psychiatric comorbidities of cluster headache. Curr Pain Headache Rep 17(2):313

Robertson MM (2006) Mood disorders and gilles de la Tourette's syndrome: an update on prevalence, etiology, comorbidity, clinical associations, and implications. J Psychosom Res 61 (3):349–358

Rozen TD, Fishman RS (2012) Cluster headache in the United States of America: demographics, clinical characteristics, triggers, suicidality, and personal burden. Headache 52(1):99–113

Rudzinski LA, Meador KJ (2013) Epilepsy and neuropsychological comorbidities. Continuum (Minneap Minn) Epilepsy 19.3:682–696

Scott KM et al (2010) Chronic physical conditions and their association with first onset of suicidal behavior in the world mental health surveys. Psychosom Med 72(7):712–719

Shavelle RM, Strauss DJ, Pickett J (2001) Causes of death in autism. J Autism Dev Disord 31 (6):569–576

Smith MT et al (2004) Suicidal ideation, plans, and attempts in chronic pain patients: factors associated with increased risk. Pain 111(1-2):201–208

Soulas T et al (2008) Attempted and completed suicides after subthalamic nucleus stimulation for Parkinson's disease. J Neurol Neurosurg Psychiatry 79(8):952–954

Stanfield AC et al (2008) Towards a neuroanatomy of autism: a systematic review and meta-analysis of structural magnetic resonance imaging studies. Eur Psychiatry 23(4):289–299

Stenager E, Knudsen L, Jensen K (1994) Multiple sclerosis: correlation of anxiety, physical impairment and cognitive dysfunction. Ital J Neurol Sci 15(2):97–101

Storch EA et al (2013) The phenomenology and clinical correlates of suicidal thoughts and behaviors in youth with autism spectrum disorders. J Autism Dev Disord 43(10):2450–2459

Verhoeven JS et al (2010) Neuroimaging of autism. Neuroradiology 52.1:3–14

Voon V et al (2008) A multicentre study on suicide outcomes following subthalamic stimulation for Parkinson's disease. Brain 131(Pt 10):2720–2728

Ward HE, Hwynn N, Okun MS (2010) Update on deep brain stimulation for neuropsychiatric disorders. Neurobiol Dis 38(3):346–353

Wilens, TE, Biederman J, Spencer TJ (2002) Attention deficit/hyperactivity disorder across the lifespan. Annual Rev Med 53.1:113–131

Wolters E et al (2008) Managing Parkinson's disease with continuous dopaminergic stimulation. CNS Spectr 13.4(Suppl 7): 1–14; quiz 15–16

Zinner SH, Coffey BJ (2009) Developmental and behavioral disorders grown up: Tourette's disorder. J Dev Behav Pediatr 30(6):560–573

Chapter 10
Suicide in the Second Half of Life: Cognition and Decision Processes

Katalin Szanto

Abstract The persistent high elderly suicide rates remain an understudied public health problem despite their importance. Suicide, in old age, is often viewed as a rational decision, triggered by loss, illness, disability, and depression. Neither the traditional medical model, which emphasizes the role of psychopathology (especially depression, psychosis, and alcohol and drug abuse), nor the psychosocial models that emphasize the role of social isolation and burdensomeness adequately explains the age-related increase in suicide rates. The importance of different vulnerability factors and certain life-events relative to suicidal behavior may change across the life span. Decision-making deficits due to cognitive decline, and in particular poor cognitive control, are more common in old age. Suicide follows a decision process, and recent studies have shown that suicidal individuals often make disadvantageous decisions in other situations. There is accumulating evidence that impaired cognitive control, deficits in social processing, and impulsivity—expressed in poor decisions both in experimental paradigms and in the context of real-world decision-making—may contribute to the decision to take one's life.

10.1 Introduction

The increase in suicide rates among adolescents in Western countries has drawn much attention in the media and has received research priority, while the persistent high elderly suicide rates remain an understudied public health problem despite their importance (Cardinal 2008). Only recently, the rising suicide rates of the baby-boomer generation (who entered the 50–70 age range) has sparked interest in suicide in the second half of life. In the US, elderly suicide rates decreased from 1991–1999, but the Center for Disease Control reports that suicide rates in individuals aged 45–64 and 65 and older have continued to rise since 2001.

K. Szanto (✉)
Department of Psychiatry, University of Pittsburgh, Pittsburgh, PA 15213, USA
e-mail: szantok@upmc.edu

K.E. Cannon and T.J. Hudzik (eds.), *Suicide: Phenomenology and Neurobiology*,
DOI 10.1007/978-3-319-09964-4_10

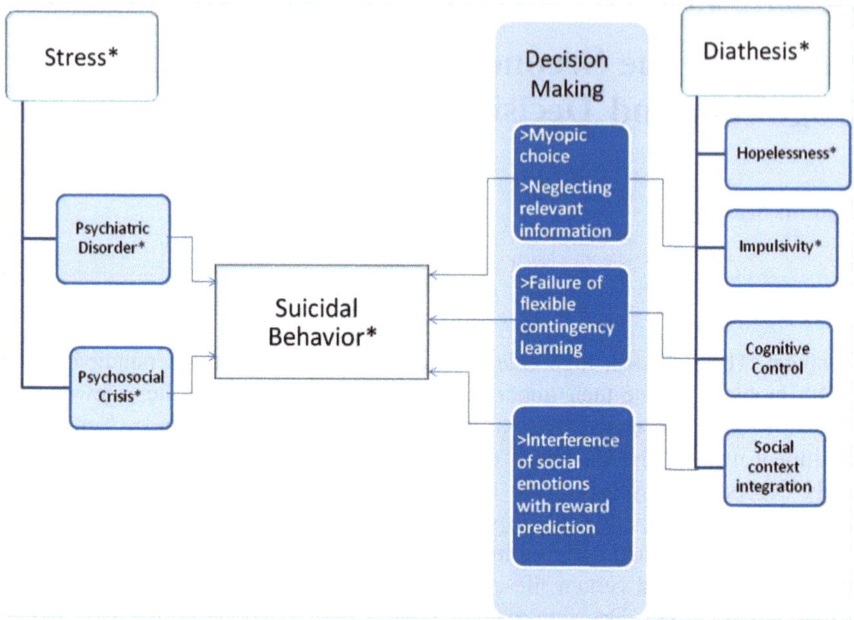

Fig. 10.1 Decision-making in the stress-diathesis model as originally described in Mann (2003)

In particular, suicide rates among men aged 50–59 increased by almost 50 % from 1999 to 2010. Although suicide rates in the United States have decreased over the past two decades, the number of older adults dying by suicide has remained constant, owing to their increased number in the population (Fig. 10.1).

10.2 Epidemiology and Trends

Elderly people have the highest suicide rate in almost all countries in the world where data are available, with the highest suicide rates in persons aged 85 and older (World Health Organization 2005). In many countries such as Hungary, Belarus, and Lithuania, suicide rates increase with age in both genders. However, in other countries, for example in the US and Sri Lanka, the steady increase over the life span is only true for men but not for women. The suicide rates of older men generally surpass that of women with the highest male elderly suicide rates reported in Belarus and Lithuania (approx. 91 per 100,000). In the US, suicide rates among males are highest in the 65+ age group (29.05 suicides per 100,000) and among females, highest in the 45–54 age range (9.34 suicides per 100,000). A different trend exists for Japan, where the highest suicide rate among women is in the 75+

age group (19.4 per 100,000), and the highest rate among men is in the relatively younger 55–64 age range (55.1 per 100,000).

Race and gender are suicide risk modifiers; in the US, African American elders have lower suicide rates than Caucasians, and the suicide rate of elderly men exceeds that of women by 3–1 (Centers for Disease Control and Prevention 2012). Caucasian men over the age of 85 were reported to be at the greatest risk of all age-gender-race groups at 47.3 per 100,000, which is approximately four times the US national suicide rate (11.3 per 100,000). A US study found that men 70 years and older had higher attempt lethality than men 50 years and older (Dombrovski et al. 2008), driven by higher levels of intent. The pattern among women was different, as older women (70+) had lower attempt lethality than those between the ages of 50–69. In the US, firearm suicide rates among males aged 45–64 years were greater than all other suicide methods combined (Centers for Disease Control and Prevention 2012). These trends point to an increasing need to address risk factors that make older adults vulnerable to suicide.

10.2.1 Death by Suicide

A suicide attempt in late life is approximately 25 times more likely to be fatal compared to young adulthood (De Leo et al. 2001). Similar to adolescents and young and middle-aged adults (Mann et al. 1999; Brent et al. 1999), history of suicide attempt is the strongest predictor of death by suicide in old age (Beautrais 2002; Waern et al. 2002a; Conwell et al. 2002). Research experience of recent decades suggests that studies of suicide attempters provide the only practical in vivo window into the biological vulnerability to suicide (Maris et al. 2000). There is, however, considerable skepticism as to how representative suicide attempters are of suicide victims. Indeed, among adolescents and younger adults, the ratio of attempts to completed suicides can be as high as 100:1 (Moscicki 1995). By contrast, this ratio can be as low as 1.2:1 in older men (De Leo et al. 2001), suggesting that elderly suicide attempters may be more similar to those who die of suicide than younger suicide attempters (Pearson and Brown 2000; Frierson 1991). In addition to the fact that the elderly are more likely to be physically frail and live alone than younger adults, the low attempt-to-death ratio is mostly attributed to the fact that older suicide attempters, particularly men over 70, carry out medically serious (high lethality) suicide attempts with a high intent to die (Dombrovski et al. 2008). Thus, it has been proposed that suicidal behavior in old age best approximates lethal suicidal acts. This notion is reinforced by greater clinical and demographic similarity between attempters and suicide victims in older, compared to younger adults (Friedmann and Kohn 2008; De Leo et al. 2001). In summary, attempted suicide in old age is the clinical phenomenon most closely resembling fatal suicidal behavior, thus described as “failed suicide”.

10.2.2 Reattempt, Risk Period

Older adults are more likely to die by suicide within 1 year following a suicide attempt than are younger individuals who made an attempt (Friedmann and Kohn 2008). According to a Finnish study, the first 3 months after hospital discharge represent the highest risk period for reattempts among hospitalized elders (Karvonen et al. 2008). Hawton and Harriss conducted a prospective study investigating repetition of deliberate self-harm and death by suicide in adults aged 60 and older. They followed 730 patients who presented to the hospital after a deliberate self-harm episode for a period of 23 years. Those who had previously attempted suicide were 49 times more likely to die of suicide compared to the demographically similar general population. Nearly three quarters of the sample had high intent during the index episode of self-harm (Hawton and Harriss 2006), which is a greater proportion than found among younger patients.

10.2.3 Age-Specific Diatheses and Stressors

The importance of different vulnerability factors and certain life-events relative to suicidal behavior may change across the life span. Decision-making deficits due to cognitive decline, and in particular poor cognitive control, are more common in old age, while the pathway involving impulsive aggression is more common in young adulthood (McGirr 2008). Bereavement, disability, and pain are often cited as triggering events in old age; in contrast, financial and relationship problems are common motivations in younger age groups.

10.3 Risk Factors Associated with Suicide in the Second Half of Life

10.3.1 Physical Illness

Physical illness and associated disabilities are often cited as motivations for suicide by older suicide attempters, and sometimes mentioned by significant others as a way to rationalize or "understand" the loved ones' suicide. Indeed, research suggests that physical illness is a frequent precipitant to suicidal behavior in older individuals (Waern et al. 2002b; Duberstein et al. 2004b; Harwood et al. 2006). In a sample of 100 suicide victims who were at least 60 years old, Harwood et al. (2006) found that physical illness was one of the three most frequent life problems associated with suicide, along with interpersonal problems and bereavement. This study also noted that pain, breathlessness, and functional limitation were the most frequent physical symptoms associated with death by suicide in late-life. Similarly,

Cattell and Joley found that of the adults aged 65 and older who died by suicide, 43 % used general practitioner services before their death and 23 % had been inpatients in the year preceding their death (Cattell and Jolley 1995). From a prospective study of deliberate self-harm episodes, Hawton and Harriss (2006) identified physical illness as a significant problem in nearly half of the study sample.

Among specific diseases, cancer (Conwell et al. 1990) and diseases associated with breathlessness and pain (Harwood et al. 2006) are the ones most consistently associated with suicide in older adults. Quan et al. (2002) found that cancer, prostate disorders, and chronic pulmonary disease were associated with suicide in the elderly. Waern et al. (2002a) noted that visual impairment, neurological disorders, and malignant disease were associated with increased risk for suicide. Furthermore, using data from 1,354 completed suicides in Ontario, Canada between 1992–2000, Juurlink et al. (2004) found that while many common illnesses—such as congestive heart failure, chronic obstructive lung disease, seizure disorder, urinary incontinence, and moderate to severe pain—were independently associated with an increased risk of suicide in the elderly, the risk was greatest among patients with multiple illnesses.

In contrast to the findings discussed above, an autopsy study conducted by Préville et al. (2005) found no significant difference between health problems reported by suicide victims and controls. However, controls had more functional autonomy than suicide victims had shortly before their deaths.

Physical illness in itself has low predictive value in determining suicide risk, and one should consider other potential vulnerabilities that mediate or accentuate the effect of physical illness on suicidal behavior.

Some studies suggest that gender may play an important role in the extent to which physical illness burden is related to suicidal behavior. Heikkinen and Lonnqvist (1995) found that among victims of suicide aged 60 and older, men had encountered recent somatic illness more often than women. Physical illness may be a stronger risk factor for suicide in men than in women, though it is unclear whether this observation has occurred because studies were underpowered to observe increased suicide risk in women, or because women respond and cope differently to physical illness burden than their male counterparts (Waern et al. 2002b). A psychological autopsy study of late-life suicide victims in which a diagnosis of cancer had played a major role in victims' decisions to end their lives found that all victims were men with a rigid, self-sufficient personality style who had had prior experience with cancer or other debilitating disease (Conwell et al. 1990). Prior to their deaths, victims had expressed fears about cancer-related physical decline, loss of autonomy, stigma of terminal illness, and a fear of becoming a burden to others. They also had diagnosable affective disorders, but had not received mental health care.

Of additional significance in assessing suicide risk is an individual's appraisal of his or her disease burden, including the perceived effect it will have on others and the perceived change on the individual's quality of life. Physical illness could create additional stress for caregivers, reduce functionality, and increase financial strain. Joiner (2002) at al observed that perceived burdensomeness was correlated with suicide attempter status and with the use of more lethal means of suicide, even after controlling for other relevant dimensions such as a desire to control one's own feelings, a desire to control others, emotional pain, and hopelessness. Suicide risk may be particularly amplified among those who perceive their illness to be progressively worsening or terminal, those who previously witnessed loved ones succumb to the disease, and those who put high value on their independence. Receiving the diagnoses of cancer (Conwell et al. 1990) or AIDS increases the risk of suicide. Two time periods appear to be particularly critical to suicide risk in AIDS patients: when the HIV positive diagnosis is communicated and when cognitive complications first appear (McKegney and O'Dowd 1992).

Duberstein's case-control study reported that suicidal elderly were more likely to perceive their illness as incurable and were also more likely to require in-home assistance, according to proxy respondents (victims' next-of-kin). The effect of physical illness remained even after controlling for current psychiatric disorders (Duberstein et al. 2004). Loebel et al. (1991) noted that anticipation of nursing home placement was cited as a precipitating factor in 44 % of persons within their sample who had given reasons for their completed suicides. Research on the hot-cold empathy gap (Loewenstein 2005) suggests that this may be the case because patients are unable to imagine that they will adapt to changing life circumstances and their acute state of fear, anxiety, or pain immediately following an unfavorable diagnosis will not persist. As such, the decision to end one's life may be state-dependent.

10.3.2 Cognition and Decision-Making

Over the last decade there has been an accumulation of evidence that understanding cognitive deficits and decision processes associated with suicidal behavior and their relationship to other risk factors may help to identify people at risk of suicide, and help to develop individualized treatment strategies. This could be particularly true for older suicidal adults, as accelerated age-related cognitive changes may contribute to the inability to solve problems, and to the ultimate decision to take one's life.

Suicide is a heterogeneous behavior resulting from a convergence of individual vulnerability, state, and environmental pressures. Although there is strong evidence for developmental factors, in most countries, suicide rates peak in late adulthood. Although most elderly suicide attempters and those who die by suicide suffer from depression, only a minority of depressed elders attempt suicide, and clinicians still cannot confidently identify depressed elderly who are most likely to attempt or die by suicide. In addition, loss, illness, and disability typical of aging contribute only modestly to suicide risk, leaving an open question of what other factors may account for this pattern.

10.3.2.1 Cognitive Aging, Decision Processes, and Suicidal Behavior

It remains unclear to what extent accelerated cognitive aging explains higher suicide rates in older adults (Haw et al. 2009). There may be a certain phase of cognitive decline or a particular cognitive profile that predisposes one to suicidal behavior. For example, a Danish population study found a marked increase in suicide rates in dementia patients after an inpatient admission (Erlangsen et al. 2008). It is likely that age-related neurodegenerative and vascular changes (Alexopoulos et al. 1997; Chan et al. 2007) modify older adults' vulnerability to suicide. The ability to make cognitively demanding decisions declines in old age even in non-demented elderly (Denburg et al. 2007). Older adults are more likely to be the victims of misleading advertising or other scams, and also make less advantageous decisions in the laboratory than younger individuals (Fein et al. 2007; Brown and Ridderinkhof 2009). This is partly explained by an age-related decline in cognitive control (MacPherson et al. 2002), related to the disproportionate effect of aging on the prefrontal cortex (Raz et al. 2005).

Originally described by Mann (2003), the stress-diathesis model differentiates temporary stressors such as psychosocial strain and mood states from a stable diathesis encompassing heritable impulsive-aggressive traits and hopelessness. An emerging literature suggests that the tendency to make disadvantageous decisions is the link between some aspects of the diathesis and suicidal behavior. Early studies described suicide attempters as poor problem solvers and the suicidal crisis as a state with low-level, concrete thinking, increased impulsivity, and a focus on immediate goals, where consequences of the attempt are not considered. There is increasing evidence to support the view that the suicide diathesis involves cognitive deficits and maladaptive decision-making. Extending the stress-diathesis model, we propose that the trait-like diatheses—impaired cognitive control, deficits in social processing, and impulsivity—are expressed in poor decisions.

10.3.2.2 Decision-Making Biases as a Link Between the Stable Diathesis and the Suicidal Crisis

Providing initial evidence, Jollant and colleagues found impaired decision-making on the Iowa Gambling Task in euthymic younger suicide attempters with mood disorders: suicide attempters failed to switch from high-initial payoff, high-loss options to low-initial payoff, long-term winning options (Jollant et al. 2005). Studies replicated these findings in younger (Bridge et al. 2006) and bipolar (Malloy-Diniz et al. 2009) patients; however, there was a negative report as well (Oldershaw et al. 2009). A similar decision-making task without working memory demands (Cambridge Gambling Task), (Clark et al. 2011) showed decision-making impairment in older suicide attempters compared to depressed non-suicidal and healthy controls. While these findings support the notion of altered decision-making in suicide attempters, the mechanisms of impairment on such a complex task remain unclear.

10.3.2.3 Cognitive Control Deficits and High-Lethality Suicide Attempts

Population studies have linked poor cognitive abilities (Andersson et al. 2008; Gunnell et al. 2011) to suicidal behavior. Deficits in cognitive control represent the most consistent finding in both middle-aged (Keilp et al. 2008, 2001; Marzuk et al. 2005; Raust et al. 2007; Nock et al. 2010) and older (Gujral et al. 2012; McGirr et al. 2012a; Richard-Devantoy et al. 2012) suicide attempters, as well as in euthymic first-degree relatives of suicide victims (McGirr et al. 2012a). Cognitive control is the active maintenance of patterns of activity that represent goals and the means to achieve them (Miller and Cohen 2001). This construct is related to the older term *executive function*. In the domain of decision-making, cognitive control is required to represent goals and to organize information about rewards, punishments, and available actions. Interference control; measured by the Stroop, appears to be a particularly sensitive index (Richard-Devantoy 2011; Keilp et al. 2013), related to higher lethality of suicide attempts (Keilp et al. 2001, 2013, 2008). One study found a relationship between high-lethality suicide attempts and poor cognitive control, as assessed by the Wisconsin Card Sort (McGirr et al. 2012; Dombrovski et al. 2011, 2013), independent of medication exposure, substance use disorders, and possible brain injury from suicide attempts. It is unclear, however, if these deficits are selective, and whether attention and working memory are also affected (Dougherty et al. 2004; Keilp et al. 2008). Our studies show that a basic deficit in cognitive control, which undermines decision-making in complex environments, is linked to high-lethality suicide attempts. Poor decision-making can result from several distinct decision-making biases, suggesting the existence of different pathways or subgroups en route to suicidal decisions. One of the pathways has been linked to impulsivity.

10.3.2.4 Decision-Making Deficits Related to Impulsivity in Late-Life Suicide

Impulsivity is a complex, multidimensional construct (Klonsky and May 2010; Kirby and Finch 2010; Dougherty et al. 2004). Dougherty and colleagues proposed that impulsivity includes at least three testable components: response initiation prior to complete processing, response inhibition, and myopic choice (Dougherty et al. 2009, 2010). Risk-taking impulsivity is also often considered as a separate component. It is possible that the importance of these components vary across the life-cycle in suicidal individuals, given the larger cooccurrence of substance abuse and conduct disorder in younger compared to older suicide attempters. Using Kirby's Monetary Choice Questionnaire (Kirby 1997), Dombrovski and colleagues (Dombrovski et al. 2011) found that the preference for immediate reward over larger delayed reward, i.e., myopic choice, differentiated between low lethality (mostly impulsive) and high lethality (mostly premeditated) suicidal acts. The same group also reported that older suicide attempters neglected key information when making decisions (Dombrovski et al. 2013), linking specific decision-making patterns to low-medical lethality, poorly planned attempts (Dombrovski et al. 2011, 2013).

10.3.2.5 Social Cognition and Social Decision-Making

Lack of feeling connected (Duberstein et al. 2004b) and poor social problem solving (Gibbs et al. 2009) have been described in older suicide attempters. However, cognitive substrates of this apparent social impairment in suicide attempters remain unknown. Social cognition (i.e., the encoding, storage, retrieval, and application of social information) is a prerequisite of social understanding and empathy. One possible deficit, the inability to recognize others' complex emotional states has been observed not only in disorders characterized by prominent social deficits (autism-spectrum disorders and frontotemporal dementia), but also in depression, alcohol dependence, and in normal aging. Szanto and colleagues reported that older suicide attempters committed significantly more errors in social emotion recognition and showed poorer global cognitive performance than elders with no psychiatric history (Szanto et al. 2012). Attempters had restricted social networks: they were less likely to talk to their children, had fewer close friends, and did not engage in volunteer activities, compared to nonsuicidal depressed elders and those with no psychiatric history.

Suicide is often a solution to mounting conflicts, albeit at a catastrophic personal cost. Economic bargaining games can model social influences on decision-making. These tasks are beginning to shed light on social decision processes in psychiatric illness (King-Casas and Chiu 2012; Kishida et al. 2010), such as distrust in borderline personality disorder; however, so far there has been only one study that investigated social decision-making in suicidal individuals. Using an economic bargaining game that involves unfairness (the Ultimatum Game), Szanto and colleagues found that suicidal elderly, in particular high medical lethality suicide attempters, had disadvantageous tendencies in resolving conflicts on this game (Szanto et al. 2013a). In contrast to the control groups and low-medical lethality suicide attempters, they did not adjust their responses to unfairness based on the money at stake. One of the deficits that may contribute to these patterns of suboptimal social decision-making is social interference of emotions with reward prediction. Indeed, maladaptive interference of social emotions in striatal reward responses during an economic exchange have been described (Delgado et al. 2005).

10.3.3 Social Connectedness

Research has shown that poor social connectedness, or the lack of enduring, stable interpersonal relationships, can amplify the risk for suicide in older adults. Suicidal behavior and social connectedness have been linked through several subjective indicators such as social isolation and perceived sense of loneliness, and objective indicators such as living alone and the loss of loved ones.

Subjective indicators of social connectedness include the individual's own perception of social supports and interactions. Using the Interpersonal Theory of Suicide proposed by Joiner et al. (2009), Van Orden (Van Orden et al. 2010) suggests that a thwarted sense of belongingness is one of the subjective constructs that contribute significantly to suicide risk. Prolonged loneliness and the absence of reciprocally caring relationships can induce negative emotional and interpersonal states, which may result in suicidal ideation or behavior. Kissane and McLaren note that adults who report a higher sense of belonging cite a greater number of reasons for living, which may be linked to reduced risk for suicide. (Kissane and McLaren 2006). Harrison et al. (2010) found that suicidal elderly report lower levels of perceived support and prolonged interpersonal difficulties. This is consistent with the idea that depressed elderly are typically characterized as dealing with rejection or criticism poorly/incompetently. Perceived weak social supports and deteriorating relationships could result in guilt and feelings of worthlessness, which in turn could increase their likelihood of considering suicide. The findings also suggest a persistent pattern of hostility, sensitivity, and ambivalence in interpersonal relationships, which could be associated with high rigidity and inflexibility common in elderly people who may be at high risk for suicide. Poor social integration and perceived lack of community support were also found by Dennis and his colleagues (Dennis et al. 2005) to be important in predicting suicidal behavior. In somewhat similar findings, Awata et al. (2005) showed that lack of perceived 'instrumental support' related to inability to function independently could lead to increased suicidal thinking.

Adults in this phase of life typically experience a range of stressful events such as loss of a spouse or loved ones, retirement, change in living arrangements, and physical illness that serve as objective indicators of social connectedness. Support from family and friends during such events is important in order to cope effectively with these stressors and to serve as a "buffer" against their negative impact. Harwood et al. (2006) suggest that suicidal individuals experience more problems related to bereavement. Chronic distress due to loss of a spouse or loved one can pose as a risk factor for suicide. Our study found that complicated grief resulting from bereavement is an important indicator of suicidal ideation in the elderly (Szanto 1997). Vanderhorst and McLaren (2010) explored states of relatedness in adults 65 or older and found that limited availability of social support was associated with higher levels of depression and suicidal ideation. Duberstein et al. (2004b) found that those who died from suicide were more likely to be unemployed, widowed or single/divorced, and less likely to have had siblings or children. They were also less likely to have been engaged in community activities or social networks. Our findings found associations between suicide risk and subjective as well as objective indicators of social connectedness. Even after accounting for other factors such as depression and physical illness burden, suicidal elderly were found to have more disruptive interpersonal relationships and restricted social networks than non-suicidal elderly. They reported lower levels of belonging, tangible support, and were less likely to maintain regular contact with their children (Szanto et al. 2012).

There is some evidence that making resources available can improve these subjective and objective indicators that affect social connectedness among the elderly. De Leo et al. (2002) and Oyama et al. (2005) show that intervention methods and community programs that bolster social connectedness may have a positive impact on the elderly and prevention of suicide.

10.3.4 Socioeconomic Status and Suicidal Behavior

Low socioeconomic status may be a risk factor for suicide, both as a chronic stressor in itself and as a potential barrier to accessing treatment (Cohen et al. 2009). Some research also suggests that individuals of lower socioeconomic status may be more likely to report suicidal ideation at the beginning and throughout the treatment of late-life depression (Cohen et al. 2006).

Interestingly, some evidence suggests that employment status may be more relevant to suicidal behavior than pure socioeconomic status. Cubbin et al. (2000) noted that in a noninstitutionalized civilian US sample, no significant difference was found in the risk of suicide by income or education after adjustment for other relevant characteristics (e.g., age, race, sex, ethnicity). However, those not in the labor force were more than twice as likely to die from suicide compared to white-collar workers (adults?). Lewis and Sloggett (1998) similarly noted that the association between suicide and unemployment was stronger than the association with other socioeconomic measures in a representative 1 % sample of the population in England and Wales in which census variables were linked to mortality data. Blakely et al. (2003) found that among 2 million respondents to the New Zealand 1991 census aged 25–64, being unemployed was associated with a two- to three-fold increased relative risk of death by suicide compared to being employed. The authors note that about half of the association might be confounded by mental illness.

Research by Link et al. (1993) goes further, suggesting that the relationship between socioeconomic status and depression/distress (but not explicitly suicide) is linked to the social causation model, which states that increased education, occupational prestige, and the degree to which one is able to exercise direction, control, and planning (i.e., autonomy) in one's occupation is protective against depression.

Indeed, while some studies have tried to parse out the cause/effect bi-directional relationship between lower socioeconomic status and mental illness, our search suggested no studies have examined suicide in this context specifically.

10.3.5 Personality Pathology and Late-Life Suicide

Personality disorders (PDs)—especially borderline personality disorder—are associated with high impulsivity (Wilson et al. 2007), emotion regulation difficulties (Bornovalova et al. 2008), and suicidal behavior (Wilson et al. 2006). The prevalence rate of PDs and severe personality pathology among older adults who attempt or complete suicide is reported to be lower (Henriksson et al. 1995; Harwood et al. 2001; Blasco-Fontecilla et al. 2009) than the prevalence rate of PDs among younger suicide attempters or completers (Henriksson et al. 1995), and the rate of cluster B PDs is relatively low as well (Abrams and Horowitz 1999, 1996). Nonetheless, the presence of a PD confers increased risk for suicide attempt and completion among older adults (Harwood et al. 2001). In psychological autopsy studies, low openness to experience (Duberstein et al. 2004) and anxious and obsessional (anankastic) personality accentuation (Harwood et al. 2001) have been associated with death by suicide in late life. Personality features may alter or attenuate with age. The lack of agreement regarding the role of PDs in late-life suicide may indicate heterogeneity: it is possible that both emotionally inflexible and emotionally labile elderly are at risk. There is also some evidence for an association between suicide attempts and impulsivity; these data were collected primarily from self-report measures (McGirr et al. 2008) and are primarily from young adult groups (Horesh 2001). A study by Wilson and colleagues (Wilson et al. 2007) using the Barratt Impulsiveness Scale reported greater non-planning impulsiveness in patients with borderline PD than in patients without borderline PD, independent of Axis I diagnoses. Among people with PDs, more "impulsive" individuals are not necessarily at higher risk for suicide (Soloff et al. 2005). Some studies even find lower impulsivity in people who commit the most serious suicidal acts and demonstrate the greatest degree of 5HT vmPFC abnormalities (Oquendo et al. 2003; Soloff et al. 2005). Trait impulsivity may decline with age (Stepp and Pilkonis 2008): studies of late-life attempters report lower impulsivity (McGirr et al. 2008) and higher degrees of premeditation compared to younger suicide attempters. In summary, personality factors seem to play a smaller role in late-life suicide than in mid-life suicide, and specific personality profiles that predispose individuals to suicidal behavior in old age remain poorly understood.

10.4 Treatment and Prevention

10.4.1 Intervention and Prevention

There are a number of both promising and already proven treatment strategies that focus on reducing depression and suicidal behavior in the elderly (While et al. 2012). Similar to other age groups, evidence supports approaches that focus on high suicide risk groups, such as the early detection and effective treatment of those with mental health problems, increased outreach to depressed and homebound older adults (especially those with a history of suicidal behavior), education of treatment providers, and restriction of lethal means (Mann et al. 2005; Szanto et al. 2007; Lapierre et al. 2011). In addition, the elderly in particular would greatly benefit from resilience training, improved coping mechanisms, and positive aging schemas

(Szanto et al. 2013). However, research on suicide prevention and treatment in this age group is limited due to the underrepresentation of elderly in suicide studies. A systematic review conducted by Lapierre and colleagues observed that, out of 149 publications on suicide prevention or intervention programs, only 19 focused on older adults (Lapierre et al. 2011). The lack of research in suicide prevention in old age contrasts sharply with the fact that, in most countries worldwide, elderly people have the highest suicide rates (World Health Organization) and many suicidal depressed older adults have difficult-to-treat depression (Szanto et al. 2003).

Five main categories emerged among the programs in Lapierre's review: primary care interventions, community-based outreach, telephone counseling, clinical treatment, and resilience training. Older adults who die by suicide are more likely to have been seen by primary care providers than by mental health professionals; therefore, practitioners require training and support in the assessment and management of suicidal patients. Promising primary care interventions trials include the PROSPECT (Prevention of Suicide in Primary Care Elderly: Collaborative Trial) (Bruce et al. 2004) and IMPACT (Improving Mood: Promoting Access to Collaborative Treatment) (Unutzer et al. 2002) studies. The PROSPECT study tested the effectiveness of elderly-focused care management intervention strategies, and found that the intervention group had a greater reduction in depressive symptoms, as well as a faster decline in suicidal ideation than the standard control care group (Bruce et al. 2004). Patients of the IMPACT intervention received access to a depression care manager who offered treatments including antidepressant management and psychotherapy. Compared to patients receiving standard care, those enrolled in IMPACT's intervention arm had significantly fewer depressive symptoms, exhibited less functional impairment, and reported a higher quality of life (Unutzer et al. 2002). The successes of PROSPECT and IMPACT indicate that there are more beneficial means of treatment than standard care for elderly patients afflicted with depressive disorders. However, the effectiveness of these trials was limited to the improvement of suicidal ideation and both trials were underpowered to show differences in suicidal behavior in the treatment arms vs. standard care. Of the clinical treatments, the Lapierre review mentions only the study by Szanto et al. (2003). This study found that suicidal ideation improved in both the antidepressant only and in the combined intervention arms (medication plus interpersonal psychotherapy). However, those who had high suicide risk (evidenced by current suicidal ideation or a history of suicide attempt), or recurrent thoughts of death (moderate suicide risk), were less likely to respond to treatment and they needed significantly longer time to remit from depression (median time to response, 6 and 5 vs 3 weeks) than low-suicide risk elders.

Of the community-based outreach programs, Lapierre et al. found that mental-health workshops run by municipal public health organizations that focused on strengthening social support showed a decrease in the suicide rate of older women (Chiu et al. 2003; Oyama et al. 2005). In men, there was no statistically significant difference at follow-up, suggesting that community-based suicide prevention programs still are not efficient for older men, who have much higher suicide rates than older women.

Telephone counseling, in the form of both a 24-h emergency number and a twice-weekly support call offered to elderly users, resulted in a significant decrease in the number of completed suicides among the elderly relative to the region's expected suicide rate (De Leo et al. 1995, 2002; Fiske and Arbore 2001; Morrow-Howell et al. 1998). Participants also reported less severe depression, improved psychosocial functioning, and required less home visits by GPs. However, like the community-based programs, these results held only for women.

Two studies of resilience training (Lapierre et al. 2007; Heisel et al. 2009) were included in the review. Lapierre et al. (2007) focused on increasing the meaningfulness of life among the patients, and the Heisel et al. (2009) study provided interpersonal psychotherapy to improve social functioning skills. Both studies reported that the experimental group had a decrease in depressive symptoms, and in the Lapierre study, a significant portion of the participants reported a complete absence of suicidal ideation by the end of the intervention.

There is lack of studies on substance abuse and suicidal behavior in this age group. It is unclear whether alcohol and drugs (including prescription opioids) contribute to an increased risk of suicide in the baby-boomer generation in the US. The underlying difficulty of developing tailored and personalized treatment options may also be linked to a lack of treatment access and stigma surrounding mental disorders in general and suicidality in particular. These factors may explain why a large portion of the old age population in need of psychiatric interventions does not seek out mental health facilities. By providing additional settings for suicide assessment that stray from traditional locations, e.g., integrated clinics for physical and mental diseases, elderly may be increasingly able to receive treatment. Potential approaches for this age group may also include online resources, which could be especially advantageous for those adults who are very isolated or frail. These new technologies would offer baby-boomer generations a more accessible and private means of independent initiation into a treatment plan. With the development of these online resources, attempts are being made to provide more effective self-testing, crisis-intervention, safety planning, and other means of support to those suffering from suicidality (Mishara and Côté 2013). In summary, long-term programs that integrate preventive interventions at multiple levels will be the most effective.

10.4.2 Psychotropic Medications and Suicidal Behavior

Although the oldest age groups have the highest suicide rate and the majority of older suicide attempters and completers suffer from depression (Conwell and Brent 1995; Waern et al. 2003) they have the lowest percentage of antidepressant use (Abrams et al. 2009) in the US and elsewhere. In addition, there is some indication that older depressed suicidal adults may benefit the most from adequate antidepressant treatment compared to younger adults (Kalmar et al. 2008). The FDA meta-analyses (Stone et al. 2009) also highlighted the beneficial effects of antidepressants in the elderly population and concluded that there is no indication of antidepressant-related increased suicide risk in older age groups.

In contrast, sedatives and hypnotics should be used with more caution in suicidal elderly. A case-control study performed by Carlsten and Waern 2009) found a significant increase in suicide risk among elderly users of sedatives and/or hypnotics, and no increase of risk in elderly users of SSRIs. Possible causes of the increased risk include the triggering of uncharacteristic aggressive behavior, adverse reactions between the medication and alcohol, and the possibility that the medication was used as a means to commit suicide. Carlsten and Waern stress that the increased suicide risk among elderly calls for an evaluation of suicide risk prior to prescribing hypnotics or sedatives.

References

Abrams RC, Horowitz SV (1996) Personality disorders after age 50: a meta-analysis. J Personality Disord 10:271–281

Abrams RC, Horowitz SV (1999) Personality disorders after age 50: a meta-analytic review of the literature. In: Rosowsky E, Abrams RC, Zweig RA (eds) Personality disorders in older adults: emerging issues in diagnosis and treatment. Psychology Press

Abrams RC et al (2009) Antidepressant use in elderly suicide victims in New York City: an analysis of 255 Cases. J Clin Psychiatry Print

Alexopoulos GS et al (1997) Vascular depression' hypothesis. Arch Gen Psychiatry 54.10:915–922 (Print)

Abrams RC, Sandra V (1996) Personality disorders after age 50: a meta-analysis. J Pers Disord 10.3:271–281 (Print)

Andersson L et al (2008) Association of Iq scores and school achievement with suicide in a 40-year follow-up of a Swedish Cohort. Acta Psychiatrica Scandinavica 118.2:99–105 (Print)

Awata S et al (2005) Factors associated with suicidal ideation in an elderly Urban Japanese population: a community-based, cross-sectional study. Psychiatry Clinic Neurosci 59.3:327–36 (Print)

Beautrais AL (2002) A case control study of suicide and attempted suicide in Older Adults. Suicide Life-Threatening Behav 32.1:1–9 (Print)

Blakely TA, Sunny CDC, June A (2003) Unemployment and suicide. evidence for a causal association? J Epidemiol Commun Health 57.8:594–600 (Print)

Blasco□Fontecilla H et al (2009) Severity of personality disorders and suicide attempt. Acta Psychiatrica Scandinavica 119.2:149–55 (Print)

Bornovalova MA et al (2008) A multimodal assessment of the relationship between emotion dysregulation and borderline personality disorder among inner-city substance users in residential treatment. J Psychiatric Res 42.9:717–726 (Print)

Brent DA et al (1999) Age- and sex-related risk factors for adolescent suicide. J Am Acad Child Adolesc Psychiatry 38.12:1497–505 (Print)

Bridge JA, Goldstein TR, Brent DA (2006) Adolescent suicide and suicidal behavior. J Child Psychol Psychiatry 47.3–4:372–394 (Print)

Brown SBRE, Ridderinkhof KR (2009) Aging and the neuroeconomics of decision making: a review. Cogn Affect Behav Neurosci 9.4:365–379 (Print)

Bruce ML et al (2004) Reducing suicidal ideation and depressive symptoms in depressed older primary care patients: a randomized controlled trial (See Comment). JAMA 291.9:1081–1091 (Print)

Cardinal C (2008) Three decades of suicide and life-threatening behavior: a bibliometric study. Suicide Life-Threat Behav 38.3:260–273 (Print)
Carlsten A, Margda W (2009) Are sedatives and hypnotics associated with increased suicide risk of suicide in the elderly? BMC Geriatr 9.1:20(Print)
Cattell, H, David JJ (1995) One hundred cases of suicide in elderly people. British J Psychiatry 166.4:451–457 (Print)
Centers for Disease Control and Prevention, National Center for Injury Prevention and Control (2012) National suicide statistics at a glance. May 11, 2012. Web. August 9, 2013
Chan SS, Lyness JM, Conwell Y (2007) Do cerebrovascular risk factors confer risk for suicide in later life? a case-control study. Am J Geriatr Psychiatry 15.6:541–544 (Print)
Clark L et al (2011) Impairment in risk-sensitive decision-making in older suicide attempters with depression. Psychol Aging 26.2:321–330 (Print)
Cohen A et al (2006) Social inequalities in response to antidepressant treatment in older adults. Arch Gen Psychiatry 63.1:50–56 (Print)
Cohen A et al (2009) Socioeconomic status and anxiety as predictors of antidepressant treatment response and suicidal ideation in older adults. Soc Psychiatry Psychiatr Epidemiol 44.4:272–277 (Print)
Conwell Y, David B (1995) Suicide and aging i: patterns of psychiatric diagnosis. Int Psychogeriatr 7.2:149–164 (Print)
Conwell Y, Duberstein PR, Caine ED (2002) Risk factors for suicide in later life. Biol Psychiatry 52.3:193–204 (Print)
Conwell Y, Eric DC, Kurt O (1990) Suicide and cancer in late life. Hosp. Commun Psychiatry 41.12:1334–1338 (Print)
Cubbin C, Felicia BL, Gordon SS (2000) Socioeconomic status and the occurrence of fatal and nonfatal injury in the United States. Am J Public Health 90.1:70 (Print)
De Leo D, Carollo G, Dello Buono M (1995) Lower suicide rates associated with a tele-help/tele-check service for the elderly at home. Am J Psychiatry 152.4:632–634 (Print)
De Leo D, Dello Buono M, Dwyer J (2002) Suicide among the elderly: the long-term impact of a telephone support and assessment intervention in Northern Italy. British J Psychiatry 181:226–229 (Print)
De Leo D et al (2001) Attempted and completed suicide in older subjects: results from the who/euro multicentre study of suicidal behaviour. Int J Geriatr Psychiatry 16.3:300–310 (Print)
Delgado MR, Frank RH, Phelps EA (2005) Perceptions of moral character modulate the neural systems of reward during the trust game. Nature Neurosci 8.11: 1611–1618 (Print)
Denburg NL et al (2007) The orbitofrontal cortex, real-world decision making, and normal aging. Ann New York Acad Sci 1121:480–498 (Print)
Dennis M et al (2005) Self-harm in older people with depression. British J Psychiatry 186:538–539 (Print)
Dombrovski AY et al (2008) Sex differences in correlates of suicide attempt lethality in late life. Am J Geriatr Psychiatry 16.11:905–913 (Print)
Dombrovski AY et al (2011) Lethal forethought: delayed reward discounting differentiates high- and low-lethality suicide attempts in old age. Biol Psychiatry 70.2:138–44 (Print)
Dombrovski AY et al (2013) Reward signals, attempted suicide, and impulsivity in late-life depression. JAMA Psychiatry (Print)
Dougherty DM et al (2004) Laboratory measured behavioral impulsivity relates to suicide attempt history. Suicide Life Threatening Behav 34.4:374–385 (Print)
Dougherty DM et al (2009) Distinctions in behavioral impulsivity: implications for substance abuse research. Addict Dis Treat 8.2:61–73 (Print)
Dougherty DM et al (2010) Effects of acute tryptophan depletion on three different types of behavioral impulsivity. Int J Tryptophan Res 3:99–111 (Print)
Duberstein PR, Conwell Y, Caine ED (2004) Age differences in the personality characteristics of suicide completers: preliminary findings from a psychological autopsy study. Psychiatry 57.3:213–224 (Print)

Duberstein PR et al (2004a) Suicide at 50 years of age and older: perceived physical illness, family discord and financial strain. Psychol Med 34.1:137–146 (Print)
Duberstein PR et al (2004b) Poor social integration and suicide: fact or artifact? a case-control study. Psychol Med 34.7:1331–1337 (Print)
Erlangsen A, Zarit SH, Conwell Y (2008) Hospital-diagnosed dementia and suicide: a longitudinal study using prospective, nationwide register data. Am J Geriatr Psychiatry 16.3:220–228 (Print)
Fein G, McGillivray S, Finn P (2007) Older adults make less advantageous decisions than younger adults: cognitive and psychological correlates. J Int Neuropsychol Soc 13.3:480–489 (Print)
Fiske A, Patrick A (2001) Future directions in late life suicide prevention. Omega-Detroit New York 42.1:37–54 (Print)
Friedmann H, Kohn R (2008) Mortality, or probability of death, from a suicidal act in the United States. Suicide Life Threat Behav 38.3:287–301 (Print)
Frierson RL (1991) Suicide attempts by the old and the very old. Archiv Intern Med 151.1:141 (Print)
Gibbs LM et al (2009) When the solution is part of the problem: problem solving in elderly suicide attempters. Int J Geriatric Psychiatry 24.12:1396–404 (Print)
Gujral S et al (2012) Impaired executive function in contemplated and attempted suicide in late life. Am J Geriatric Psychiatry (Print)
Gunnell D et al (2011) School performance and risk of suicide in early adulthood: follow-up of two national cohorts of swedish schoolchildren. J Affect Dis 131.1–3:104–112 (Print)
Harrison KE et al (2010) Alone? perceived social support and chronic interpersonal difficulties in suicidal elders. Int Psychogeriatr 22.3:445–454 (Print)
Harwood D et al (2001) Psychiatric disorder and personality factors associated with suicide in older people: a descriptive and case-control study. Int J Geriatric Psychiatry 16.2:155–165 (Print)
Harwood D et al (2006) Life problems and physical illness as risk factors for suicide in older people: a descriptive and case control study. Psychol Med 36.9:1265–1274 (Print)
Haw C, Harwood D, Hawton K (2009) Dementia and suicidal behavior: a review of the literature. Int Psychogeriatr 21.3:440–453 (Print)
Hawton K, Harriss L (2006) Deliberate self-harm in people aged 60 years and over: characteristics and outcome of a 20-year cohort. Int J Geriatr Psychiatry 21.6:572–581 (Print)
Heikkinen ME, Jouko K (1995) Recent life events in elderly suicide: a nationwide study in Finland. Int Psychogeriatr 7.2:287–300 (Print)
Heisel MJ et al (2009) Adapting interpersonal psychotherapy for older adults at risk for suicide: preliminary findings. Prof Psychol: Res Pract 40.2:156 (Print)
Henriksson MM et al (1995) Mental disorders in elderly suicide. Int Psychogeriatr 7.2:275–286 (Print)
Horesh N (2001) Self-report versus computerized measures of impulsivity as a correlate of suicidal behavior. Crisis 22.1:27–31 (Print)
Joiner TE et al (2002) Perceived burdensomeness and suicidality: two studies on the suicide notes of those attempting and those completing suicide. J Soc Clin Psychol 21.5:531–545 (Print)
Joiner TE Jr et al (2009) The interpersonal theory of suicide: guidance for working with suicidal clients. American Psychological Association (Print)
Jollant F et al (2005) Impaired decision making in suicide attempters. Am J Psychiatry 162.2:304–310 (Print)
Juurlink DN et al (2004) Medical illness and the risk of suicide in the elderly. Arch Intern Med 164.11:1179–1184 (Print)
Kalmar S et al (2008) Antidepressant prescription and suicide rates: effect of age and gender. Suicide Life Threat Behav 38.4:363–74 (Print)
Karvonen K et al (2008) Suicide after hospitalization in the elderly: a population based study of suicides in Northern Finland between 1988–2003. Int J Geriatric Psychiatry 23.2:135–141 (Print)

Keilp JG et al (2001) Neuropsychological dysfunction in depressed suicide attempters. Am J Psychiatry 158.5:735–741 (Print)
Keilp JG et al (2008) Attention deficit in depressed suicide attempters. Psychiatry Res 159.1–2:7–17 (Print)
Keilp JG et al (2013) Neuropsychological function and suicidal behavior: attention control, memory and executive dysfunction in suicide attempt. Psycholog Med 43.3:539–551 (Print)
King-Casas B, Chiu PH Understanding interpersonal function in psychiatric illness through multiplayer economic games. Biol Psychiatry 72.2:119–25 (Print)
Kirby KN (1997) Bidding on the future: evidence against normative discounting of delayed rewards. J Exp Psychology-General 126.1:54–70 (Print)
Kirby KN, Finch JC (2010) The hierarchical structure of self-reported impulsivity. Person Individual Differ 48.6:704–713 (Print)
Kishida KT, King-Casas B, Montague PR (2010) Neuroeconomic approaches to mental disorders. Neuron 67.4:543–554 (Print)
Kissane M, McLaren S (2006) Sense of belonging as a predictor of reasons for living in older adults. Death Stud 30.3:243–258 (Print)
Klonsky ED, May A (2010) Rethinking impulsivity in suicide. Suicide Life Threat Behav 40.6:612–619 (Print)
Lapierre S et al (2007) Addressing suicidal ideations through the realization of meaningful personal goals. Crisis: J Crisis Intervent Suicide Prevent 28.1:16–25 (Print)
Lapierre S et al (2011) A systematic review of elderly suicide prevention programs. Crisis: J Crisis Interv Suicide Prev 32.2:88–98 (Print)
Lewis G, Andy S (1998) Suicide, deprivation, and unemployment: record linkage study. Bmj 317.7168:1283–1286 (Print)
Link BG, Mary Clare L, Bruce PD (1993) Socioeconomic status and depression: the role of occupations involving direction, control, and planning. Am J Sociol 98.6:1351–1387 (Print)
Loebel JP et al (1991) Anticipation of nursing home placement may be a precipitant of suicide among the elderly. J Am Geriatrics Soc (Print)
Loewenstein G (2005) Hot-cold empathy gaps and medical decision making. Health Psychol 24.4S:S49 (Print)
MacPherson SE, Phillips LH, Della Sala S (2002) Age, executive function and social decision making: a dorsolateral prefrontal theory of cognitive aging. Psychol Aging 17.4:598–609 (Print)
Malloy-Diniz LF et al (2009) Suicide behavior and neuropsychological assessment of type i bipolar patients. J Affect Dis 112.1–3:231–236 (Print)
Mann JJ (2003) Neurobiology of suicidal behaviour. Nature Rev Neurosci 4.10:819–828 (Print)
Mann JJ et al (1999) Toward a clinical model of suicidal behavior in psychiatric patients. Am J Psychiatry 156.2:181–189 (Print)
Mann JJ et al (2005) Suicide prevention strategies: a systemic review. JAMA 294.16:2064–2074 (Print)
Maris RW et al (2000) Comprehensive textbook of suicidology, 1st edn. Guilford Press (Print)
Marzuk PM et al (2005) Executive functioning in depressed patients with suicidal ideation. Acta Psychiatrica Scandinavica 112.4:294–301 (Print)
McGirr A et al (2008) Impulsive-aggressive behaviours and completed suicide across the life cycle: a predisposition for younger age of suicide. Psychol Med 38.3:407–417 (Print)
McGirr A et al (2012) Deterministic learning and attempted suicide among older depressed individuals: cognitive assessment using the wisconsin card sorting task. J Psychiatric Res 46.2:226–32 (Print)
McGirr AFJ, Turecki G (2012) Neurocognitive alterations in first degree relatives of suicide completers. J Affect Dis (Print)
McKegney F, Mary AO (1992) Suicidality and hiv status. Am J Psychiatry 149.3:396–398 (Print)
Miller EK, Cohen JD (2001) An integrative theory of prefrontal cortex function. Ann Rev Neurosci 24:167–202 (Print)

Mishara BL, Côté L-P (2013) Suicide prevention and new technologies: towards evidence based practice. Suicide Prevent New Technol 1 (Print)
Morrow-Howell N, Susan B-K, Lee J (1998) Evaluating an intervention for the elderly at increased risk of suicide. Res Soc Work Pract 8.1:28–46 (Print)
Moscicki EK (1995) Epidemiology of suicide. Int Psychogeriatr 7.2:137–48 (Print)
Nock MK et al (2010) Measuring the suicidal mind: implicit cognition predicts suicidal behavior. Psycholog Sci 21.4:511–517 (Print)
Oldershaw A et al (2003) Decision making and problem solving in adolescents who deliberately self-harm. Psychol Med 39.1:95–104 (Print)
Oquendo MA et al (2003) Positron emission tomography of regional brain metabolic responses to a serotonergic challenge and lethality of suicide attempts in major depression. Archiv Gen Psychiatry 60.1:14–22 (Print)
Oyama H et al (2005) Community-based suicide prevention through group activity for the elderly successfully reduced the high suicide rate for females. Psychiatry Clin Neurosci 59:337–355 (Print)
Pearson JL, Brown GK (2000) Suicide prevention in late life: directions for science and practice. Clin Psychol Rev 20.6:685–705 (Print)
Préville M et al (2005) Physical health and mental disorder in elderly suicide: a case-control study. Aging Mental Health 9.6:576–584 (Print)
Quan H et al (2002) Association between physical illness and suicide among the elderly. Soc Psychiatry Psychiatr Epidemiol 37.4:190–197 (Print)
Raust A et al. (2007) Prefrontal cortex dysfunction in patients with suicidal behavior. Psychol Med 37.3:411–4199 (Print)
Raz N et al (2005) Regional brain changes in aging healthy adults: general trends, individual differences and modifiers. Cereb Cortex 15.11: 676–689 (Print)
Richard-Devantoy S et al (2011) P03-470—cognitive inhibition in suicidal depressed elderly. Eur Psychiatry 26.1:1640 (Print)
Richard-Devantoy S et al (2012) Deficit of cognitive inhibition in depressed elderly: a neurocognitive marker of suicidal risk. J Affect Dis140.2:193–99 (Print)
Soloff PH et al (2005) High-lethality status in patients with borderline personality disorder. J Per Dis 19.4:386–399 (Print)
Stepp, SD, Paul AP (2008) Age-related differences in individual dsm criteria for borderline personality disorder. J Pers Dis 22.4:427 (Print)
Stone M et al (2009) Risk of suicidality in clinical trials of antidepressants in adults: analysis of proprietary data submitted to us food and drug administration. BMJ: British Medical J 339 (Print)
Szanto K et al (1997) Suicidal ideation in elderly bereaved: the role of complicated grief. Suicide Life-Threatening Behav 27.2:194–207 (Print)
Szanto K et al (2003) Occurrence and course of suicidality during short-term treatment of late-life depression. Archiv Gen Psychiatry 60.6:610–617 (Print)
Szanto K et al (2007) A suicide prevention program in a region with a very high suicide rate. Arch Gen Psychiatry 64.8:914–920 (Print)
Szanto K et al (2012) Social emotion recognition, social functioning, and attempted suicide in late-life depression. Am JGeriatric Psychiatry 20.3:257–265 (Print)
Szanto K et al (2013a) The cost of social punishment and high-lethality suicide attempts. Psychol Aging (in press) (Print)
Szanto K et al (2013b) Research to reduce the suicide rate among older adults: methodology roadblocks and promising paradigms. Psychiatric Serv 64.6:586–589 (Print)
Takahashi CHFY, Suh GH (2003) Elderly suicide prevention in east asia. Int J Geriatr Psychiatry 18.11:973–976 (Print)
Unutzer J et al (2002) Collaborative care management of late-life depression in the primary care setting: a randomized controlled trial (See Comment). JAMA 288.22:2836–2845 (Print)
Van Orden KA et al (2010) The interpersonal theory of suicide. Psychol Rev 117.2:575–600 (Print)

Vanderhorst RK, McLaren S (2010) Social relationships as predictors of depression and suicidal ideation in older adults. Aging Mental Health 9.6:517–525 (Print)

Waern M, Rubenowitz E, Wilhelmson K (2003) Predictors of suicide in the old elderly. Gerontology 49.5:328–334 (Print)

Waern M et al (2002a) Mental disorder in elderly suicides: a case-control study. Am J Psychiatry 159.3:450–455 (Print)

Waern M et al (2002b) Burden of illness and suicide in elderly people: case-control study. Bmj 324.7350:1355 (Print)

While D et al (2012) Implementation of mental health service recommendations in england and wales and suicide rates, 1997–2006: a cross-sectional and before-and-after observational study. Lancet 379.9820:1005–1012 (Print)

Wilson ST et al (2006) Impulsivity, suicidality and alcohol use disorders in adolescents and young adults with borderline personality disorder. Int J Adolesc Med Health 18.1:189–196 (Print)

Wilson ST et al (2007) Comparing impulsiveness, hostility, and depression in borderline personality disorder and bipolar ii disorder. J Clin Psychiatry 68.10:1533–1539 (Print)

World Health Organization (2005) Suicide prevention. Web

Chapter 11
Early Life Trauma and Suicide

Aaron T.O. Short and Charles B. Nemeroff

Abstract Abuse, neglect, trauma, and other adversities experienced as a child or young adolescent have repeatedly and conclusively been shown to increase one's risk of developing major psychiatric disorders later in life. A growing body of literature supports the view that child abuse and neglect lead to a multitude of poor health outcomes including increased rates of post-traumatic stress disorder (PTSD), attention deficit—hyperactivity disorder, bipolar disorder, schizophrenia, major depression, as well as other major medical disorders including cardiovascular disease, diabetes, asthma, and obesity (Felitti et al. 1998; Heim and Nemeroff 2001). Early life trauma (ELT) is associated with alterations in emotional, behavioral, and cognitive arenas. There is considerable evidence to support ELT as an independent risk factor for suicidal ideation and behaviors in adulthood (Gunter et al. 2013; Friestad et al. 2014; Daigle and Cote 2006; Sarchiapone et al. 2009) whereas traumatic exposure in adulthood does not share a similar magnitude of suicidal risk as compared to childhood trauma. Impulsivity is one risk factor for suicidal behaviors, and is associated with early, prolonged, and severe trauma exposure (Braquehais et al. 2010; Kendall-Tackett 2002; Roy 2005). Indeed, suicides characterized by impulsivity are more likely in those with a history of ELT (Zouk et al. 2006). In this chapter, we review ELT origens, and how these can produce or interact with other risk factors contributing to suicide.

A.T.O. Short · C.B. Nemeroff (✉)
Department of Psychiatry and Behavioral Sciences, University of Miami,
Miami, FL, USA
e-mail: CNemeroff@med.miami.edu

C.B. Nemeroff
Center on Aging, Jackson Memorial Hospital, University of Miami Hospital,
1120 Northwest 14 Street, Suite 1455, Miami, FL 33136, USA

K.E. Cannon and T.J. Hudzik (eds.), *Suicide: Phenomenology and Neurobiology*,
DOI 10.1007/978-3-319-09964-4_11

11.1 Introduction

The increasing prevalence of suicidal ideation and behaviors in childhood populations has become recognized as a serious public health concern (Herba et al. 2008; O'Leary et al. 2006; Gould et al. 1998a). A recent CDC publication reported that approximately 13 % of child and young adult deaths are attributable to suicide each year in the United States (2012). It is the second leading cause of death amongst 7–12th grade students in the United States, and fourth amongst ages 1–17 (CDC WISQARS 2013). The identification of leading risk factors is crucial as awareness of this phenomenon grows. There is now ample data to support the view that suicidal behaviors arise from an assortment of factors: psychological, biological, societal, and cultural (US Department of Health and Human Services 2012). Individual factors such as ELT, depression, substance use disorder, bipolar disorder, schizophrenia, PTSD, access to lethal means, anxiety, male gender, age, and barriers to treatment are all important risk contributors (US Public Health Service 1999). In order to better understand suicidal behaviors, it is important to define and differentiate these acts. Recently, there has been increased focus on the incidence of suicide among young children and adolescents who have been bullied. This emerging area of research is described in detail below. In this monograph, we focus on recent studies that have sought to determine the relationship between child abuse and neglect and risk for suicide. We review the consequences of early life trauma (ELT) on both childhood and adulthood risk for suicide and its associated psychiatric disorders.

Approximately, one in 12 high-school students report that they have engaged in suicidal behavior, and one in six reports having seriously considered it (Eaton et al. 2006). Suicidal behavior can encompass passive ideation, planning, and/or attempting the act. "The world would be better if I weren't here, I wish that I was dead," are examples of passive ideation whereas, "I'm thinking about ways to end my life" is an example of planning. A suicide attempt includes self-directed harmful behavior that could result in potential injury or loss of life.

Pre-adolescent suicidal ideation is a risk factor for suicidal behavior later in adolescence (Jackson and Nuttall 2001; Lewinsohn et al. 1994; Beautrais Beautrais 1999). Data, compiled from 16 states, published on the CDC website illustrate the most common mechanisms of injury in childhood suicide attempts, namely hanging, suffocation, and firearms, in that order. Approximately 30 % of completed cases were apparently premeditated. Roughly 35 % were diagnosed with a syndromed psychiatric disorder at the time of death, 26 % were involved in active treatment, and 21 % had a history of previous suicide attempt (CDC Mental 2013). In a mixed study of adolescents and young adults, the nonfatal rate of suicidal behavior was the highest in younger cohorts (Goldsmith et al. 2002). However, adults have the highest rate of completed suicide. Individuals with a history of suicidal behaviors are significantly more likely to engage in these behaviors later in life (Groleger et al. 2003). In Sweden, suicide was reported to be the most common cause of death for 15–24-year-olds, irrespective of gender (Jiang et al. 2010).

Gender and race impact the risk of suicidal behaviors. A large CDC surveillance study, with a median cohort age of 16, reported that suicidal ideation was highest in girls (19.3 %) compared to boys (12.5 %), with an increased incidence in Hispanics (16.7 %) followed by whites (15.5 %) and blacks (13.2 %). Girls more commonly made plans as to how the act might be carried out (15.0 %) relative to boys (10.8 %), and planning is highest in the Hispanic community (14.3 %), followed by white (12.1 %) and black (11.1 %). Over the study's 6-year span, 89 % of completed suicides were males, 86 % were white, 11 % were black, and 3 % Hispanic. The majority of completed suicides (82 %) involved the use of firearms (CDC Surveillance 2012).

Substance use is a strong risk factor for the emergence of suicidal thoughts and behaviors in American high school students. The risk dramatically increases with particular illicit drugs and with the total number of substances historically abused. By engaging nearly 75,000 high school students in a survey, Wong et al. (2013) found that a lifetime history of substance abuse was a strong independent risk factor associated with suicidal behaviors and serious attempts within the previous year. Heroin was the most closely linked with these risks (OR = 5–23.6), followed by methamphetamines (OR = 4.3–13.1), steroids (OR = 3.7–11.8), cocaine, ecstasy, hallucinogens, and inhalants (OR = 3.1–10.8). After controlling for socio-demographic variables, interpersonal violence, symptoms of depression, and eating disorders, the findings remained significant.

Although the number of substances used had a graded relationship to suicidal behaviors, it remains unclear whether there is a propensity for those with these behaviors to abuse substances, or whether the substances themselves promote these behaviors or a combination of the two. MacDonald et al. (2009) have shown that early age suicidal ideation is a predictor of later substance dependence, and Friestad et al. (2014) note that ELT increases the risk of substance abuse as well as suicide attempts in adulthood.

11.2 Early Life Trauma

There is a strong correlation between ELT and the subsequent development of psychiatric disorders, inclusive of major depression, generalized anxiety disorder, panic disorder, bipolar disorder, schizophrenia, and post-traumatic stress disorder (PTSD) (Heim et al. 2010; Agid et al. 1999; Famularo et al. 1992; Heim and Nemeroff 2001; Katerndahl et al. 2005; Kendler et al. 1992, 2000, 2004; McCauley et al. 1997; Molnar et al. 2001; Mullen et al. 1996; Nemeroff and Vale 2005; Saunders et al. 1992; Stein et al. 1996; Hill et al. 2000). Early life traumatic experiences are also linked to increased rates of personality disorders, as well as attachment and eating disorders (Heim et al. 2010; Agid et al. 1999; Famularo et al. 1992; Felitti et al. 1998; Romans et al. 1995; Saunders et al. 1992; Zeanah et al. 2004). Several links between child abuse, neglect, and later substance use have also been published (Goldman-Mellor et al. 2013; Briere and Woo 1989; Burnam et al. 1988; Kendler et al. 2000; Wilsnack and Beckman 1984).

Data from the National Center of Child Abuse and Neglect reveal that roughly one million cases of child maltreatment are confirmed in the United States each year, from nearly three million reported. Of the confirmed cases, approximately 60 % are due to neglect, 20 % to physical abuse, and 10 % to sexual abuse (Heim et al. 2010; Children's Bureau, Administration of Children, Youth, and Families. U.S. Department of Health and Human Services 2006). It is important to note that many, if not most, maltreatment cases are never reported.

Self-reported prevalence rates of childhood abuse vary from 25 to 40 % in structured interviews (McCloskey and Walker 2000; Costello and Angold 2000), with one group publishing higher rates for men (41 %) compared to women (30 %) based on phone interviews (Scher et al. 2004). Others found childhood sexual abuse (before the age of 18) to range from 20 to 25 % in women and 8–9 % in men (McCauley et al. 1997; Holmes and Slap 1998; Gorey and Leslie 1997). In a cohort of 16-year-old females with a history of sexual abuse, 28 % also reported a history of physical abuse (Horowitz et al. 1997). In this group, those with a history of sexual abuse were at increased risk of having experienced physical abuse as well.

Throughout maturation, we are naturally subjected to increased rates of potential trauma exposure (PTE); this might, for example, include dog bites, car accidents, or exposure to violence from within the family or in the community. One group followed 213 2–4-year-old northeastern US children through development. After 12 months, there were notable increases in PTE experiences, with a greater than 50 % increase in reports throughout the cohort, implying that a substantial number of children who had not experienced a PTE by the first assessment, were exposed to ELT within a 12-month period. Girls were more susceptible to developing internalizing symptoms when affected by the combination of PTEs and stressors. The risk for externalizing problems was comparable in boys and girls (Grasso et al. 2012). Those with a history of PTE were more vulnerable to behavioral and emotional dysregulation when faced with nontraumatic stressors later in life. Repeated stress exposure adversely affects the manner in which one handles later life stressors, with more PTEs over the course of one's life increasing the likelihood of a syndrome psychiatric disorder. This study was limited in that it relied on parents' reports in a retrospective fashion.

Concordant with these findings are those of Hammen et al. (2000) who reported that children with a history of abuse and neglect are at greater risk of developing exaggerated stressful responses to later life events. Some authors posited a cumulative effect of trauma exposure that increases the rate of mood symptoms (Briggs-Gowan et al. 2010).

11.3 Adverse Childhood Experiences

The adverse childhood experience (ACE) scale has been used to evaluate and monitor the presence of ELT over time. An ACE might include physical, sexual, or psychological abuse, physical or emotional neglect, exposure to substance use, divorce, mental illness, criminal behavior, or a battered parent. In the ACE study funded by the CDC, Dube et al. (2001) demonstrated increased rates of suicide attempts in adults with a history of ACEs. The cohort was comprised of 17,337 adults followed in the San Diego, 1995–1997. They reported that 3.8 % of those with a suicide attempt history reported one or more ACEs, compared to 1.1 % without an ACE history. This data also positively correlated attempted suicide in childhood and adolescence with the number of ACEs. In those with seven or more self-reported ACEs, approximately one-third of the subjects reported a suicide attempt, an OR of 31.1 (Dube et al. 2001).

This correlation was replicated in New Zealand population, which revealed that participants 16 years of age and younger with a history of sexual trauma exposure were at an 18-fold increased risk of suicide behavior. Exposure to physical abuse in childhood resulted in a fourfold increase in adult suicidal behavior (Mullen et al. 1996). In self-reports, US adolescents with three ACEs had an eightfold increased risk of developing pre adulthood suicidal behavior, with a threefold risk persisting throughout adulthood (Dube et al. 2001).

In a community based study of nearly 2,000 women, those with a history of sexual or physical abuse in childhood had more symptoms of depression, anxiety and frequent suicide attempts, as well as substance abuse and inpatient psychiatric hospitalization (McCauley et al. 1997). Isohookana et al. (2013) identified sexual abuse as an independent risk factor for suicidal behaviors amongst young women. Those with a history of sexual abuse had twice the risk of suicide attempts. This connection was confirmed in a Chinese study of 16 and younger females with a history of sexual victimization; they noted a 2.7-fold increased risk of suicide (Lin et al. 2011).

A Taiwanese group showed that although young females were 3.5 times more likely to exhibit self-mutilating behaviors, an additional fourfold risk was observed when there was also a history of sexual abuse (Tsai et al. 2011). Other forms of adolescent or childhood trauma, such as sexual abuse, life-threatening accidents/conditions, or natural disasters similarly increased suicidal behaviors (Isohookana et al. 2013). Women are clearly more susceptible than men to PTSD, which increases lifetime suicide risk (Pagura et al. 2010). Breslau et al. (1997) reported that those females that experienced traumatic events at 15 years of age or younger were even more vulnerable to developing PTSD compared to older women. In a New York-based study of 12–18 year-olds with a history of psychiatric inpatient treatment, one-third reported having practiced self-mutilating behaviors; half reported at least one previous suicide attempt. In this population, 43 % reported a history of abuse and 3 % sexual victimization. Each form of abuse significantly heightened the risk for attempted suicide later in life (Lipschitz et al. 1999).

Apart from increasing one's risk for developing psychiatric syndromes, ELT may also predict longer mood episodes. A 5-year prospective study assessing anxiety and depression which controlled for trauma history found that those with a positive history of ELT were less likely to remit from symptoms (Zlotnick et al. 1997). In another study of 235 patients, Zlotnick et al. (2001) found that those with history of anxiety and/or depression with comorbid ELT were found to exhibit symptomatology for extended intervals.

In a longitudinal follow-up of 676 children, Widom et al. (2007) reported that those with a history of physical abuse or multiple types of abuse were at increased risk of developing depression (OR = 1.59 and 1.75, respectively). Heim et al. (2010) affirmed that ELT victims showed a trend toward early onset of major depression, adding that increased severity, frequency, and duration of abuse result in an increased risk for psychological sequelae. In a primary care-based cross-sectional study, McQuaid et al. (2001) found that ELT was positively associated with a greater lifelong risk of developing major depressive disorder. These associations have also been consistent in other population-based studies (Tanskanen et al. 2004).

Dube et al. (2003) investigated various consequences of childhood abuse. As the number of ACEs increased, a 30 % increase in depressed affect, a 50–75 % increased rate of suicide attempts, 20–30 % increased likelihood of contracting a sexually-transmitted disease, 20–30 % increased risk for smoking, and 40–50 % increased risk for self-reported alcoholism (Dube et al. 2003). A recent study (Etain et al. 2013) demonstrated a marked effect of ELT on the course of bipolar disorder including an earlier age of onset, more depressive episodes and increased suicide attempts.

11.4 Bullying

Bullying in youth is a problem of international concern (Carney and Merrell 2001). It is pervasive and well documented throughout several Western societies (Nansel et al. 2004; Karatzias et al. 2002; Kaltiala-Heino et al. 2000; Forero et al. 1999; Wolke et al. 2001), and across continents. A person is bullied when he or she is repeatedly exposed to negative actions on the part of one or more persons (Olweus 1991). Despite the setting, bullying can be classified into four major categories: direct/physical (violence, robbery), direct/verbal (taunting, intimidation), indirect/relational (ostracization, deprecation), and cyberbullying. Rivers and Noret (2010) add bystanders as a separate classification. The pervasiveness of bullying is increasingly recognized as a public health hazard of considerable magnitude. Peer relationships have been identified as a predictor of psychopathology for at risk adolescents (Bearman and Moody 2004). Kim et al. (2005) described how the effects of this relationship appear to be independent of race, culture, or varying settings. Both bully and victim experience emotional challenges, poorer social relationships, and report poorer subjective health. Childhood bullying has long-lasting effects that may persist throughout adolescence (Bond et al. 2001; Kumpulainen and Rasanen 2000) and even into adulthood (Nansel et al. 2004; Olweus 1992, 1994).

Prevalence rates range from region to region with one recent UK self-report investigation revealing a 25 % rate (Radford et al. 2011), and another group finding that 8 % of children were victimized over the course of 1 month and 18 % in their lifetime (Hinduja and Patchin 2009). A 2007 publication revealed that 28 % of students in the 12–18 age group were bullied over a 6-month course, 25 % were bullied once or twice a month, 11 % twice a week, and 8 % reported daily victimization (Dinkes et al. 2007). In a cohort of 4th through 12 grade US students, slightly less than half reported abstaining from bullying practices, and/or having not been a victim of bullying over the past school year; 15 % reported having been frequently or severely antagonized by their peers (Hoover and Olsen 2001).

Bullying is pervasive and is not exclusively related to societal values but rather associated with adolescent development (Smith et al. 1999). In one study of 113,000 11–15-year-olds students from 25 countries, reports of bullying behaviors ranged from 9 to 54 %. Although the prevalence varies across the globe, there is remarkable consistency in the long-term consequences (Nansel et al. 2004). Bully and victimization practices are related to poor family functioning and inter-parental violence or maltreatment (Rigby et al. 1997; Baldry 2003; Shields and Cicchetti 2001).

Bullies have been known to have higher likelihoods for developing depression, engaging in antisocial behaviors, and having legal problems later in life (Salmon et al. 1996; Olweus 1994). In self-report studies, being bullied and fighting with peers are associated with an increased risk of suicidal ideation (Kim et al. 2005; Klomek et al. 2007). Moreover, being a victim and bullying coupled with a preexistent mental health diagnosis further increases the risk of suicidal behavior. Clearly, school bullying should no longer be considered a “normal” process where “kids are just being kids.”

Investigations into bullying practices can be traced back to the 1960s and have been associated with links to adverse physical health, behavioral, psychotic, depressive, emotional, as well as academically detrimental outcomes. The most commonly noted methods used to assess childhood bullying behavior are through self-reporting (Klomek et al. 2007), parent reporting (Arseneault et al. 2006), peer reporting (Kim et al. 2006), teacher reporting (Olweus 1993), or a combination of the above (Kumpulainen and Rasanen 2000). Bullying truly became the forefront of public attention in 1982 following three separate suicides in Norway, where all three of the victims left suicide notes alluding to the fact that they had been “whipping boys” (Stassen 2007; Olweus 1993).

As noted above, bullies and victims report greater health problems, difficulties adjusting emotionally at school, and even a higher likelihood of weapon carrying. Victims are more likely to relate difficulties in relating to peers while there is a strong probability for bullies to abuse alcohol (Nansel et al. 2004). It is important to note that because not all children who are involved in bullying behaviors harm themselves or have suicidal behavior, identifying at risk children and adolescents who are most endangered should be a major public health goal. Historically, this has largely focused on identifying victims of bullying, with bullies overlooked.

Although earlier studies suggested that bullies reported higher self-esteem (Salmivalli et al. 1999; Rigby and Slee 1991), or no significant difference in self-esteem in comparison to peers (Seals and Young 2003), more recent data suggest that bullies also exhibit an increased risk for suicidal behaviors. Middle school self-reported studies show that those who were exposed to bullying practices, or were bullies themselves, had significantly lower self-worth relative to peers (Patchin and Hinduja 2010; Jankauskiene et al. 2008; Frisen et al., 2007; Yang et al. 2006). Both bullies and victims of bullies are at higher risk of exhibiting suicidal behaviors. There is growing support that the mixed bully victim group, those who are both bullies and victims, is the most vulnerable for development of depression later in life (Klomek et al. 2007).

11.5 Cyber Bullying

Bullying is not only limited to the schoolyard or playground. Patchin and Hinduja (2006) point out that cyberbullying is a relatively new concept, and as such, there is confusion as to its characterization. There is agreement that cyber bullying can result in severe distress for the victim (Ybarra et al. 2006) and might be better defined as a deliberate act or behavior carried out repeatedly over time. This assumes that the target experiences real and disruptive pain, which is associated with emotional, psychological, or relational problems with peers. By definition, cyber bullying must be performed by use of an electronic device. Common examples include text messages, malicious messages posted on social networking sites, or defaming photos or videos uploaded on the Internet without the consent of the victim (Patchin and Hinduja 2010).

Cyberbullying extends to the home, "following" the victim beyond the traditional locale of school, outside the observation of teachers (Patchin and Hinduja 2006). It is increasingly difficult for the victim to escape the reaches of the bully's exploits (Slonje and Smith 2008). It is suggested that it is easier for the bully to attack his/her victims in cyberspace, because there are a lack of physical and or social cues that would prevent him/her from otherwise relenting (Dehue et al. 2008). Cyberbullies are not always aware of the nonverbal/expressive reactions of their victims, and may be more assaultive in the absence of these signs.

Suzuki et al. (2012) maintain that there are seven different types of cyberbullying. The first three types are conducted via mobile phones.

1. Mobile phone call bullying (e.g., abusive or silent call)
2. Text message bullying (via abusive text message)
3. Picture/video clip bullying (includes taking a picture or clip of someone else to use it in an abusive manner, e.g., sending it to others or uploading it onto a website to embarrass a target)

The other four types of cyberbullying are conducted via the Internet.

4. Email bullying (sending or receiving abusive emails)
5. Chat room bullying (being abusive or being abused in chat room features)
6. Bullying through instant messaging (e.g., a bully can interact with online communities to see whether a target is logged on and proceed to send vicious instant messages)
7. Bullying via websites (e.g., create a website that is abusive toward a specific person)

As the frequency of Internet use rises, so does the risk of cyberbullying (Ybarra et al. 2006; Li 2008). Instant messaging is the most common method of cyberbullying in the United States (Raskauskas and Stoltz 2007; Kowalski and Limber 2007; Ybarra and Mitchell 2007), and United Kingdom (Smith et al. 2008; Dehue et al. 2008). Email attacks are more common in other regions (Slonje and Smith 2008). In terms of age groups, 13–14-year-olds have been reported to be at the highest risk for experiencing cyber-attacks (Kowalski and Limber 2007; Ybarra et al. 2006), though other studies failed to yield similar results, with little difference in age of cyber victims (Patchin and Hinduja 2006; Smith et al. 2008; Beran and Li 2007).

In order to assess the prevalence of bullying, data were collected from 3,767 students in six middle schools in the United States. Eleven percent of students reported they had been cyberbullied within 2 months, 4.1 % claimed to be cyber bully antagonizers, and 6.8 % said they assumed both role of victim and bully (Kowalski and Limber 2007). Another investigation revealed that 10 % of middle school students had been cyber bullied over the course of 1 month and closer to 20 % had been cyber bullied over the course of their life. In a review of surveys distributed to 13–18-year-old students in the USA, 49 % reported they had been a cyber-victim and 21 % served as a cyber-bully over the past school year (Raskauskas and Stoltz 2007).

Victims in the cyber world are more likely to exhibit the role of victim in the real world, suggesting that a victim's status remains consistent in the real world and online. Cyber victims are also likely to act as cyber bullies (Ybarra et al. 2006; Li 2008; Patchin and Hinduja 2006, Hinduja and Patchin 2008; Sourander et al. 2010; Schultze-Krumbholz and Scheithauer 2009; Raskauskas and Stoltz 2007). Increased severity and frequency of bullying has been linked with a heightened risk of self-harm. There is evidence that bully victims are at an increased risk for suicidal behaviors and adverse long-term mental-health sequelae (Kim et al. 2009; Klomek et al. 2011). Patterns of self-harm not only persist into adulthood but that these behaviors engender mental health problems later in life (Skegg 2005; Fergusson et al. 2005; Harrington et al. 2006; Steinhausen et al. 2006).

Klomek et al. (2009) reported that girls have a greater likelihood of suicide attempts/completions, which is correlated with the severity and frequency of victimization experienced (Klomek et al. 2009). These findings were not confirmed in boys. In a NY State High School self-report study where 9 % of the children reported being victimized frequently and 13 % bullied others frequently, there was a strong correlation (OR = 3.6–4.5) between being bullied/bullying others and suicide attempts across both sexes. Recurrent victimization or bullying was related to high risks of depression, suicidal ideation and attempts compared to peers.

A Swedish study that sought influences of self-mutilation, suicide attempts, and bullying behaviors found that after adjusting for age, family factors, school factors, and psychiatric history, there was an increased risk of suicide attempts in girls but not boys, who were victims of bullying (OR = 2.07) or assumed the role of bully (3.27). Although girls were less commonly bullied, the consequences were more severe in terms of long-term sequelae. The boys were less likely to report bullying behaviors, however the lack of response might partly be explained by a smaller representation within the sample (208 males: 300 females). This study was limited by a small sample size and was exclusively comprised of adolescents in an inpatient psychiatric setting (Luukkonen et al. 2009).

Several investigators have suggested that bully victims have a tendency toward heightened emotional arousal/dysregulation, poor impulse control (Sterzer et al. 2005; Woods and White 2005; Arseneault et al. 2006; Wolke et al. 2001) and are more ready to engage in verbal and physical aggression (Kumpulainen and Rasanen 2000; Kim et al. 2006; Sourander et al. 2007). Bully victims also suffer from low self-worth, impaired social acceptance, and poor academic standing (Kumpulainen et al. 1998; Austin and Joseph 1996; Woods and White 2005).

In order to assess the enduring effects of early life bullying/victimization, previous studies have followed the cohort for a few months or at most a few years into adolescence, without assessing the long-lasting effects into adulthood. In a recent population-based study, Copeland et al. (2013) assessed 1,420 participants, aged 9–16-year-olds from North Carolina, to predict whether childhood bullying would lead to psychiatric problems and suicidality in adulthood. This investigation accounted for pre-existing psychiatric comorbidities as well as family hardships, where four different types of family hardships were evaluated, inclusive of low socioeconomic status, unstable family structure, family dysfunction, and maltreatment at home. Their data support a direct, pleiotropic, and long-lasting effect for victims, bullies, and bully victims, alike. Specifically, victims of childhood bullying were more susceptible to the development of anxiety disorders (agoraphobia, generalized anxiety disorder, and panic disorder) in adulthood, bully victims have an increased risk of adult depression as well as panic disorder and agoraphobia, and pure-bullies exhibited an increased risk for antisocial personality disorder in adulthood. Of note, only female bully victims exhibit an increased risk of agoraphobia, while male counterparts were at increased risk for suicidality.

11.6 Developmental Cognitive Considerations

Trauma experienced by the developing brain has repeatedly been shown to have persistent and widespread neurobiological consequences contributing to lasting cognitive effects. Home, family environments, and ELT have strong influences on cognitive, emotional, social, and physiological functioning later in life (Gould et al. 2012; DeBellis et al. 1999a, b; Perry and Pollard 1998; Baram et al. 2012). Childhood trauma (abusive, physical, sexual, or emotional) surely predisposes to borderline personality disorder later in life (Herman et al. 1989; Zanarini and Frankenburg 1997). One investigation notably observed that those with a history of sexual abuse exhibited a fourfold increased risk of borderline personality in adulthood (Zelkowitz et al. 2001).

An 18-year prospective study (Noll et al. 2010) followed 84 women with a history of sexual abuse and 108 controls. A history of sexual abuse was negatively associated with acquired receptive language proficiency, as well as lower baseline levels of intellectual functioning. Notably, this difference was largely apparent by mid-adolescence, was associated with depression, anxiety, dissociative tendencies, behavioral problems, and negative affect (Trickett et al. 1994). Those with a history of sexual abuse had lower rates of high-school graduation and other higher educational attainments. It remains unclear as to the direct cause and effect of historical abuse and subsequent cognitive deficits, though we do know that these events can disrupt critical neuropsychological development during childhood (Watts-English et al. 2006). Family dysfunction, low parental education, and economic disadvantages could all possibly add to these deficits; further studies are necessary to gain a better understanding (Noll et al. 2010).

Brown et al. (1986) identified the lengthy separation of a child from his mother, inclusive of death before a child's 11th birthday, as a risk factor for depression later in life. Hill et al. (2000) showed that low maternal care and a history of early-life sexual abuse are independent contributors to the risk of developing a depressive disorder in adulthood. Agid et al. (1999) compared the loss of a parent figure, before the age of 17, in controls and those with mental illness. There is a significantly higher likelihood of developing adulthood depression later in life in the parent-loss group (OR = 3.8, p: 0.001), whereas early separation (before 9-year-olds) predicates a stronger risk (OR = 11, p: 0.03) as compared to later separation. Early loss of a parent has been correlated with increased rates of bipolar disorder, and the loss of a sibling has been associated with increased susceptibility for depression in adulthood (Brent et al. 1993).

11.7 Neurobiological Alterations

Maltreatment in childhood has been linked with increased catecholamine and cortisol activity, suggesting a dysregulation of the neuroendocrine system (Carrion et al. 2002; DeBellis et al. 1994). As levels of glucocorticoids (cortisol) rise and act on the hippocampus and amygdala, memory, and learning are impaired (Lupien et al. 1998). Some authors postulate that early trauma results in an accelerated loss of neurons (Sapolsky et al. 2000), delay or slowing of myelin formation (Dunlop et al. 1997), impairments of neuronal pruning associated with normal development (Todd 1992), inhibition of neurogenesis (Gould et al. 1998a, b), and even inhibitions of brain growth factors (Smith et al. 1995). Magnetic resonance imaging investigations have demonstrated that women with a history of severe sexual abuse have reduced intracranial and cerebral volumes as well as decreased hippocampal volumes compared to individuals without a shared history of abuse (Heim et al. 2013; Stein et al. 1997; DeBellis et al. 1999a, b; Fleglar et al. 2011).

Several studies revealed a relationship between ELT and the subsequent cascade of neurobiological and inflammatory changes in the central nervous system that persist throughout adulthood (Neigh et al. 2009; Gould et al. 2012; Goldman-Mellor et al. 2013, O'Donovan et al. 2013). Elevated levels of inflammation have been associated with the pathophysiology of suicidality (Lindqvist et al. 2009), with specific elevations of interleukin-2 (IL-2) having been observed in depressed, nonsuicidal individuals, with increased levels of interleukin-6 (IL-6) in those with suicidal behaviors and depressive symptoms (Janlidze et al. 2011; Kim et al. 2008). Moreover, increased inflammatory markers, including C-reactive protein (CRP) and tumor necrosis factor (TNF) are observed in individuals with depressive pathology (Currier and Nemeroff 2010) as well as in those with a history of ELT exposure (Nemeroff and Seligman 2013; Danese et al. 2007; Pace et al. 2006).

It is clear that child abuse and neglect, including bullying, is a significant contributor to an increased risk for several major psychiatric disorders, suicide attempts as well as completed suicide. The precise neurobiological consequences of ELT are becoming more evident. Because victims of child abuse represent a clear at risk group, preventative measures should be developed in this population. Additional suicide prevention efforts in coordination with long-term surveillance are needed.

References

Agid O, Shapira B, Zislin J, Ritsner M, Hanin B, Murad H et al (1999) Environment and vulnerability to major psychiatric illness: a case control study of early parental loss in major depression, bipolar disorder and schizophrenia. Molecular Psychiatry 4:163–172

Austin S, Joseph S (1996) Assessment of bully/victim problems in 8 to 11-year-olds. Br J Educ Psychol 66:447–456

Arseneault LE, Walsh E, Trzesniewski K, Newcombe R, Caspi A, Moffitt TE (2006) Bullying victimization uniquely contributes to adjustment problems in young children: a nationally representative cohort study. Pediatrics 118:130–138

Baldry AC (2003) Bullying in schools and exposure to domestic violence. Child Abuse Negl 27:713–732

Baram T, Davis E, Obenaus A, Sandman C, Small S, Solodnkin A, Stern H (2012) Fragmentation and unpredictability of early-life experience in mental disorders. Am J Psychiatry 169 (9):907–915

Beautrais AL (1999) Further suicidal behavior among medically serious suicide attempters. Suicide Life Threat Behav 34:1–11

Bearman PS, Moody J (2004) Suicide and friendships among American adolescents. Am J Public Health 94:89–95

Beran T, Li Q (2007) The relationship between cyberbullying and school bullying. J Stud Wellbeing 1:15–33

Bond L, Carlin JB, Thomas L, Rubin K, Patton G (2001) Does bullying cause emotional problems? A prospective study of young teenagers. BMJ 323:480–484
Braquehais MD, Oquendo MA, Baca-Garcia E, Sher L (2010) Is impulsivity a link between childhood abuse and suicide? Compr Psychiatry 51:121–129
Brent DA, Perper JA, Moritz G, Liotus L, Schweers J, Roth C et al (1993) Psychiatric impact of the loss of an adolescent sibling to suicide. J Affect Disord 28:249–256
Breslau N, Davis GC, Andreski P, Peterson EL, Schultz LR (1997) Sex differences in posttraumatic stress disorder. Arch Gen Psychiatry 54(11):1044–1048
Briere J, Woo R (1989) Child abuse sequelae in adult psychiatric emergency room patients. Am J Psychiatry 146(12):1602–1606 (Print)
Briggs-Gowan MJ, Ford JD, Fraleigh L, McCarthy K, Carter AS (2010) Prevalence of exposure to potentially traumatic events in a healthy birth cohort of very young children in the northeastern United States. J Trauma Stress 23:725–733. doi:10.1002/jts.20593
Brown GW, Harris TO, Bifulco A (1986) Long-term effects of early loss of parent. In: Rutter M, Izard CE, Read PB (eds) Depression in young people: developmental and clinical perspective. Guilford Press, New York, pp 251–296
Burnam MA, JA Stein, JM Golding, JM Siegel, SB Sorenson, AB Forsythe, Telles CA (1988) Sexual assault and mental disorders in a community population. J Consult Clin Psychol 56 (6):843–850 (Print)
Carney AG, Merrell KW (2001) Bullying in schools: perspectives on understanding and preventing an international problem. School Psychol Int 22:364–382
Carrion VG, Weems CF, Ray RD, Glaser B, Hessl D, Reiss AL (2002) Diurnal salivary cortisol in pediatric post-traumatic stress disorder. Biol Psychiatry 51(7):575–582
Centers for Disease Control and Prevention (2013) Mental Health Surveillance Among Children—United States, 2005–2011. Morb Mortal Wkly Rep 62(2):1–35 (Print)
Centers for Disease Control and Prevention (2012) Youth Risk Behavior Surveillance—United States, 2011. Morb Mortal Wkly Rep 61(4):1–162 (print)
Centers for Disease Control and Prevention (2013) Web-based injury statistics query and reporting system (WISQARS). http://www.cdc.gov/ncipc/wisqars/default.htm. Accessed 17 August 2013
Children's Bureau, Administration of Children, Youth, and Families. U.S. Department of Health and Human Services (2006) Child maltreatment 2004. U.S. Government Printing Office, Washington, DC
Copeland W, Wolke D, Angold A, Costello J (2013) Adult psychiatric outcomes of bullying and being bullied by peers in childhood and adolescence. JAMA Psychiatry 70(4):419–426
Costello E, Angold A (2000) Developmental psychopathology and public health: past, present, and future. Dev Psychopathol 12:599–618
Currier MB, Nemeroff CB (2010) Inflammation and mood disorders: proinflammatory cytokines and the pathogenesis of depression. AntiInflamm Antiallergy Agents Med Chem 9:212–220
Daigle DM, Cote G (2006) Nonfatal suicide-related behavior among inmates: testing for gender and type differences. Suicide Life Threat Behav 36:670–681
Danese A, Pariante CM, Caspi A, Taylor A, Poulton R (2007) Childhood maltreatment predicts adult inflammation in a life-course study. Proc Natl Acad Sci USA. 104(4):1319–1324
DeBellis MD, Baum AS, Birmaher B, Keshavan MS, Eccard CH, Boring AM, Jenkins FJ, Ryan ND (1999a) A.E. Bennett Research Award. Developmental traumatology. Part I. Biological stress systems. Biol Psychiatry 45:1259–1270
DeBellis MD, Keshavan MS, Clark DB, Casey BJ, Giedd JN, Boring AM, Frustaci K, Ryan ND (1999b) A.E. Bennett Research Award. Developmental traumatology. Part II. Brain development. Biol Psychiatry 45:1271–1284
DeBellis MD, Lefter L, Trickett PK, Putnam FW (1994) Urinary catecholamine excretion in sexually abuse girls. J Am Acad Child Adolesc Psychiatry 33(3):320–327
Dehue F, Bolman C, Völlink T (2008) Cyberbullying: youngsters' experiences and parental perception. Cyberpsychol Behav 11:217–223

Dinkes R, Cataldi EF, Lin-Kelly W, Snyder TD (2007) Indicators of school crime and safety: 2007. US Department of Education, US Department of Justice, Office of Justice Programs, Washington, DC

Dube SR, Anda RF, Felitti VJ (2001) Childhood abuse, household dysfunction, and the risk of attempted suicide throughout the life span: findings from the adverse childhood experiences study. JAMA 286(24):3089–3096

Dube S, Vincent J, Dong M, Giles W, Anda R (2003) The impact of adverse childhood experiences on health problems. Prev Med 37:268–277. doi:10.1016/S0091-7435(03)0123-3

Dunlop SA, Archer MA, Quinlivan JA, Beazley LD, Newnham JP (1997) Repeated prenatal corticosteroids delay myelination in the ovine central nervous system. J Matern Fetal Med 6 (6):309–313

Etain B, Aas M, Andreassen O, Lorentzen S, Dieset I, Gard S, Kahn J, Bellivier F, Leboyer M, Melle I, Henry C (2013) Childhood trauma is associated with severe clinical characteristics of bipolar disorders. J Clin Psychiatry 74(10):991–998. doi:10.4088/JCP.13m08353

Eaton DK, Kann L, Kinchen SA, Ross J, Hawkins J, Harris WA et al (2006) Youth risk behavior surveillance—United States. MMWR Surveill Summ 55(SS-5):1–108

Famularo R, Kinscherff R, Fenton T (1992) Psychiatric diagnoses of maltreated children: preliminary findings. J Am Acad Child Adolesc Psychiatry 31:863–867

Felitti VJ, Anda RF, Nordenberg D, Williamson DF, Spitz AM, Edwards V et al (1998) Relationship of childhood abuse and household dysfunction to many of the leading causes of death in adults. The adverse childhood experiences (ACE) study. Am J Prev Med 14:245–258

Fergusson DM, Horwood LJ, Ridder EM, Beautrais AL (2005) Suicidal behaviour in adolescence and subsequent mental health outcomes in young adulthood. Psychol Med 35:983–993

Fleglar SJ, Fouche JP, Jordaan E, Marais S, Spottiswoode B, Stein DJ, Vythilingum B (2011) The neural correlates of intimate partner violence in women. Afr J Psychiatry (Johannesberg) 14 (4):310–314

Forero R, McLellan L, Rissel C, Bauman A (1999) "Bullying behaviour and psychosocial health among school students in New South Wales, Australia". Cross sectional survey. BMJ 319:344–348

Friestad C, Ase-Bente R, Kjelsberg E (2014) Adverse childhood experiences among women prisoners: relationships to suicide attempts and drug abuse. Int J Soc Psychiatry 60(1):40–46. doi:10.1177/0020764012461235

Frisen A, Jonsson AK, Persson C (2007) Adolescents' perception of bullying: who is the victim? Who is the bully? What can be done to stop bullying. Adolescence 42(168):749–761

Goldman-Mellor S, Caspi A, Harrington H, Hogan S, Nada-Raja S, Poulton R, Moffitt T (2013) Suicide attempt in young people: a signal for long-term health care and social needs. JAMA Psychiatry. doi:10.10001/jamapsychiatry.2013.2803

Goldsmith SK, Pellmar TC, Kleinman AM, Bunney WE (2002) Reducing suicide: a national imperative. National Academy Press, Washington, DC

Gorey KM, Leslie DR (1997) The prevalence of child sexual abuse: integrative review adjustment for potential response and measurement biases. Child Abuse Negl 21:391–398

Gould F, Clarke J, Heim C, Harvey PD, Majer M, Nemeroff CB (2012) The effects of child abuse and neglect on cognitive functioning in adulthood. J Psychiatry Res 45(4):500–506

Gould MS, King R, Greenwald S et al (1998a) Psychopathology associated with suicidal ideation and attempts among children and adolescents. J Am Acad Child Adolesc Psychiatry 37:915–923

Gould E, Tanapat P, McEwen BS, Fluggae G, Fuchs E (1998b) Proliferation of granule cell precursors in the dentate gyrus of adult monkeys is diminished by stress. Proc Natl Acad Sci USA 95(6):3168–3171

Grasso D, Ford J, Briggs-Gowan M (2012) Early life trauma exposure and stress sensitivity in young children. J Pediatr Psychol 38(1):94–103. doi:10.1093/jpepsy/jss101

Groleger U, Tomori M, Kocmur M (2003) Suicidal ideation in adolescence—an indicator of actual risk. Isr J Psychiatry Relat Sci 40:202–208

Gunter TD, Chibnall JT, Antoniak SK, Philibert RA, Black DW (2013) Childhood trauma, traumatic brain injury, and mental health disorders associated with suicidal ideation and suicide-related behavior in a community corrections sample. J Am Acad Psychiatry Law 41:245–255
Hammen C, Henry R, Daley SE (2000) Depression and sensitization to stressors among young women as a function of childhood adversity. J Consult Clin Psychol 68:782–787
Harrington R, Pickles A, Aglan A, Harrington V, Burroughs H, Kerfoot M (2006) Early adult outcomes of adolescents who deliberately poisoned themselves. J Am Acad Child Adolesc Psychiatry 45:337–345
Heim C, Mayberg H, Mletzko T, Nemeroff C, Pruessner J (2013) Decreased cortical representation of genital somatosensory field after childhood sexual abuse. Am J Psychiatry 170(6):616–623 (print)
Heim C, Nemeroff C (2001) The role of childhood trauma in the neurobiology. Soc Biol Psychiatry 49:1023–1039
Heim C, Shugart M, Craighead WE, Nemeroff CB (2010) Neurobiological and psychiatric consequences of child abuse and neglect. Dev Psychobiol 52(7):671–690
Herba CM, Ferdinand RF, Stijnen T et al (2008) Victimization and suicide ideation in the TRAILS study: specific vulnerabilities of victims. J Child Psychol Psychiatry 49:867–876
Herman JL, Perry J, Van der Kolk BA (1989) Childhood trauma in borderline personality disorder. Am J Psychiatry 46:490–495
Hill J, Davis R, Byatt M, Burnside E, Rollinson L, Fear S (2000) Childhood sexual abuse and affective symptoms in women. Psychol Med 30:1283–1291
Hinduja S, Patchin JW (2009) Bullying beyond the schoolyard: preventing and responding to cyberbullying. Sage Publications, Thousand Oaks (Corwin Press)
Hinduja S, Patchin JW (2008) Cyberbullying: an exploratory analysis of factors related to offending and victimization. Deviant Behav 29:129–156
Holmes WC, Slap GB (1998) Sexual abuse of boys: definition, prevalence, correlates, sequelae, and management. J Am Med Assoc 280:1855–1862
Hoover J, Olsen G (2001) Teasing and harassment: the frames and scripts approach for teachers and parents. National Educational Service, Bloomington
Horowitz LA, Putman FW, Noll JG, Trickett PK (1997) Factors affecting utilization of treatment services by sexually abused girls. Child Abuse and Neglect 21:35–48
Isohookana R, Riala K, Hakko H, Rasanen P (2013) Adverse childhood experiences and suicidal behavior of adolescent. Eur Child Adolesc Psychiatry 22:13–22. doi:10.1007/s00787-012-0311-8
Jackson H, Nuttall RL (2001) Risk for preadolescent suicidal behavior: an ecological model. Child Adolesc Social Work J 18:189–203
Jankauskiene R, Kardelis K, Sukys S, Kardeliene L (2008) Associations between school bullying and psychosocial factors. Soc Behav Pers 2:145–162
Janlidze S, Mattei D, Westrin A, Traskman-Bendz L, Brundin L (2011) Cytokine levels in the blood may distinguish suicide attempters from. Brain Behav Immun 25(2):335–339
Jiang G-X, Floderus B, Wasserman D (2010) Sja¨lvmord i Stockholms la¨n och Sverige 1980–2008. Karolinska Institutets folkha¨lsoakademi" Pa uppdrag av Stockholm la¨ns landsting. Karolinska Institutet 30
Kaltiala-Heino R, Rimpela M, Rantanen P, Rimpela A (2000) Bullying at school: an indicator of adolescents at risk for mental disorders. J Adolesc 23:661–674
Karatzias A, Power KG, Swanson V (2002) Bullying and victimisation in Scottish secondary schools: same or separate entities? Aggress Behav 28:45–61
Katerndahl D, Burge S, Kellogg N (2005) Predictors of development of adult psychopathology in female victims of childhood sexual abuse. J Nerv Mental Dis 193:258–264
Kendall-Tackett K (2002) The health effects of childhood abuse: four pathways by which abuse can influence health. Child Abuse Neglect 26(6–7):715–729
Kendler KS, Bulik CM, Silberg J, Hettema JM, Myers JMS, Prescott CA (2000) Childhood sexual abuse and adult psychiatric and substance use disorders in women: an epidemiological and cotwin control analysis. Arch Gen Psychiatry 57:953–959

Kendler KS, Kuhn JW, Prescott CA (2004) Childhood sexual abuse, stressful life events and risk for major depression in women. Psychol Med 34:1475–1482
Kendler KS, Neale MC, Kessler RC, Heath AC, Eaves LJ (1992) A population-based twin study of major depression in women: the impact of varying definitions of illness. Arch Gen Psychiatry 49:257–266
Kim YS, Koh Y-J, Leventhal B (2005) School bullying and suicidal risk in Korean middle school students. Pediatric 115:357–363
Kim YK, Lee SW, Kim SH, Han SW, Choi SH, Lee BH (2008) Differences in cytokines between non-suicidal patients and suicidal patients in major depression. Prog Neuropsychopharmacol Biol Psychiatry 15(32):356–361
Kim YS, Leventhal BL, Koh YJ, Hubbard A, Boyce AT (2006) School bullying and youth violence: causes or consequences of psychopathology? Arch Gen Psychiatry 63:1035–1041
Kim YS, Leventhal BL, Yun-Joo K, Boyce WT (2009) Bullying increased suicide risk: prospective study of Korean adolescents. ArchSuicide Res 13:15–30
Klomek AB, Kleinman M, Altschuler E, Marrocoo F, Amakawa L, Gould MS (2011) High school bullying as a risk for later depression and suicidality. Suicide Life Threat Behav 41:501–516
Klomek AB, Marrocco F, Kleinman M, Schonfeld IS, Gould M (2007) Bullying, depression, and suicidality in adolescents. J Am Acad Child Adolesc Psychiatry 1:40–49
Klomek AB, Sourander A, Niemela S et al (2009) Childhood bullying behaviors as a risk for suicide attempts and completed suicides: a population-based birth cohort study. J Am Acad Child Adolesc Psychiatry 48:2540–2561
Kowalski RM, Limber SP (2007) Electronic bullying among middle school students. J Adolesc Health 41:S22–S30
Kumpulainen K, Rasanen E (2000) Children involved in bullying at elementary school age: their psychiatric symptoms and deviance in adolescence: an epidemiological sample. Child Abuse Negl 24:1567–1577
Kumpulainen K, Rasanen E, Henttonen I et al (1998) Bullying and psychiatric symptoms among elementary school-age children. Child Abuse Negl 22:705–717
Lewinsohn PM, Rohde P, Seeley JR (1994) Psychosocial risk factors for future adolescent suicide attempts. J Consult Clin Psychol 62:297–305
Li Q (2008) A cross-cultural comparison of adolescents' experience related to cyberbullying. Educ Res 50:223–234
Lin D, Li X, Fan X, Fang X (2011) Child sexual abuse and its relationship with health risk behaviors among rural children and adolescents in Hunan, China. Child Abuse Negl 35 (9):680–687
Lindqvist D, Janelidze S, Hagell P, Erhardt S, Samuelsson M, Minthon L, Hansson O, Bjorkqvist M, Traskman-Bendz L, Brundin L (2009) Interleukin-6 is elevated in the cerebrospinal fluid of suicide attempters and related to symptom severity. Biol Psychiatry 1(66):287–292
Lipschitz DS, Winegar RK, Nicolaou AL, Hartnick EW, Michele BA, Southwick SM (1999) Perceived abuse and neglect as risk factors for suicidal behavior in adolescent inpatients. J Nerv Ment Dis 187(1):32–39
Lupien S, Sharma S, Nair NP et al (1998) Glucocorticoids and human brain aging. Nat Neurosci 1 (1):69–73 (published correction appears in Nat Neurosci 1(4):329 (1998))
Luukkonen A, Rasanen P, Helina H, Riala K (2009) Bullying behavior is related to suicide attempts but not to self-mutilation among psychiatric inpatient adolescents. Psychopathology, 42:131–138. doi:10.1159/000204764
MacDonald R, Taylor J, Clarke D (2009) The relationship between early suicide behaviors and mental health: results from a nine-year panel study. J Adolesc 32(5):1159–1172
McCauley J, Kern DE, Kolodner K, Dill L, Schroeder AF, DeChant et al (1997) Clinical characteristics of women with a history of childhood abuse. JAMA 277:1362–1368
McCloskey LA, Walker M (2000) Posttraumatic stress in children exposed to family violence and single-event trauma. J Am Acad Child Adolesc Psychiatry 39:108–115
McQuaid JR, Pedrelli P, McCahill ME, Stein MB (2001) Reported trauma, post-traumatic stress disorder and major depression among primary care patients. Psychol Med 31:1249–1257

Molnar BE, Buka SL, Kessler RC (2001) Child sexual abuse and subsequent psychopathology: results from the national comorbidity survey. Am J Public Health 91:753–760
Mullen PE, Martin JL, Anderson JC, Romans SE, Herbison GP (1996) The long-term impact of the physical, emotional, and sexual abuse of children: a community study. Child Abuse Negl 20(1):7–21
Nansel TR, Craig W, Overpeck MD, Saluja G, Ruan WJ (2004) Health behaviour in school-aged children bullying analyses working group. Cross-national consistency in the relationship between bullying behaviors and psychosocial adjustment. Arch Pediatr Adolesc Med 158:730–736
Neigh GN, Gillespie CF, Nemeroff CB (2009) The neurobiological toll of child abuse and neglect. Trauma Violence Abuse 10(4):389–410
Nemeroff CB, Seligman F (2013) Commentary: the pervasive and persistent neurobiological and clinical aftermath of child abuse and neglect. J Clin Psychiatry 74(10):999–1001 (print)
Nemeroff CB, Vale W (2005) The neurobiology of depression: inroads to treatment and new drug discovery. J Clin Psychiatry 66(supp 7):5–13. Pubmed:16124836
Noll J, Shenk C, Yeh M, Ji J, Putnam F, Trickett P (2010) Receptive language and educational attainment for sexually abused females. Pediatrics 126:e615–e622. doi:10.1542/peds.2010-0496
O'Donovan A, Rush G, Hoatam G, Hughes BM, McCrohan A, Kelleher C, O'Farrelly C, Malone KM (2013) Suicidal ideation is associated with elevated inflammation in patients with major depressive disorder. Depress Anxiety 30(4):307–314
O'Leary CC, Frank DA, Grant-Knight W et al (2006) Suicidal ideation among urban nine and ten year olds. J Dev Behav Pediatr 27:33–39
Olweus D (1992) Bullying among schoolchildren: intervention and prevention. In: Peters RD, McMahon RJ, Quinsey VL (eds) Aggression and violence throughout the life span. Sage Publications, Newbury Park, pp 100–125
Olweus D (1991) Bully/victim problems among school children: basic facts and effects of a school based intervention program. In: Pepler D, Rubin K (eds) The development and treatment of childhood aggression. Erlbaum, Hilsdale, pp 411–448
Olweus D (1994) Bullying at school: long-term outcomes for the victims and an effective school-based intervention program. In: Huesmann LR (ed) Aggressive behavior: current perspectives. Plenum Press, New York, pp 97–130
Olweus D (1993) Bullying at school: what we know and what we can do. Blackwells, Oxford
Pace TW, Mletzko TC, Alagbe O, Musselman DL, Nemeroff CB, Miller AH, Heim CM (2006) Increased stress-induced inflammatory responses in male patients with major depression and increased early life stress. Am J Psychiatry 163(9):1630–1633
Patchin JW, Hinduja S (2006) Bullies move beyond the schoolyard: a preliminary look at cyberbullying. Youth Violence Juv Justice 4:148–169
Patchin JW, Hinduja S (2010) Cyberbullying and self-esteem. J School Health 80:614–621
Pagura J, Stein MB, Bolton JM, Cox BJ, Grant B, Sareen J (2010) Comorbidity of borderline personality disorder and posttraumatic stress disorder in the U.S. population. J Psychiatry Res 44(16):1190–1198
Perry BD, Pollard R (1998) Homeostasis, stress, trauma, and adaptation—a neurodevelopmental view of childhood trauma. Child Adolesc Psychiatry Clin North Am 7:33–51
Radford L, Corral S, Bradley C, Fisher H, Bassett C, Howat N et al (2011) Child abuse and neglect in the UK today. National Society for the Prevention of Cruelty to Children, London
Raskauskas J, Stoltz AD (2007) Involvement in traditional and electronic bullying among adolescents. Dev Psychol 43:564–575
Rigby K, Cox I, Black G (1997) Cooperativeness and bully/victim problems among Australian school children. J Soc Psychol 137:357–368
Rigby K, Slee PT (1991) Bullying among Australian school children: reported behavior and attitudes toward victims. J Soc Psychol 131:615–627
Rivers I, Noret N (2010) Participant roles in bullying behavior and their association with thoughts of ending one's life. Crisis 31(3):143–148

Romans S, Douglass H, Martin J (1995) Child sexual abuse. Curr Opin Pediatr 7(4):405–409 (print)
Roy A (2005) Childhood trauma and impulsivity. Possible relevance to suicidal behavior. Arch Suicide Res 9(2):147–151
Salmivalli C, Kaukiainen A, Kaistaniemi L, Lagerspetz KM (1999) Self-evaluated self-esteem, peer-evaluated self-esteem, and defensive egotism as predictors of adolescents' participation in bullying situations. Pers Soc Psychol Bull 25:1268–1278
Salmon G, James A, Smith DM (1996) Bullying in schools: self reported anxiety, depression, and self esteem in secondary school children. BMJ 317:924–925
Sapolsky RM, Romero LM, Munck AU (2000) How do glucocorticoids influence stress responses? Integrating permissive, suppressive, stimulatory, and preparative actions. Endocr Rev 21(1):55–89
Sarchiapone M, Carli V, Giannantonio M et al (2009) Risk factors for attempting suicide in prisoners. Suicide Life Threat Behav 39:343–350
Schultze-Krumbholz A, Scheithauer H (2009) Social-behavioral correlates of cyberbullying in a German student sample. Z Psychol/J Psychol 217:224–226
Scher CD, Forde DR, McQuaid JR, Stein MB (2004) Prevalence and demographic correlates of childhood maltreatment in an adult community sample. Child Abuse Negl 28:167–180
Seals D, Young J (2003) Bullying and victimization: prevalence and relationship to gender, grade level, ethnicity, self-esteem and depression. Adolescence 38:735–747
Shields A, Cicchetti D (2001) Parental maltreatment and emotion dysregulation as risk factors for bullying and victimization in middle childhood. J Clin Child Psychol 30:349–363
Skegg K (2005) Self-harm. Lancet 366:1471–1483
Slonje R, Smith PK (2008) Cyberbullying: another main type of bullying? Scand J Psychol 49:147–154
Smith MA, Makino S, Kvetnansky R, Post RM (1995) Effects of stress on neurotrophic factor expression in the rat brain. Ann NY Acad Sci 771:234–239
Smith PK, Mahdavi J, Carvalho M, Fisher S, Russell S et al (2008) Cyberbullying: its nature and impact in secondary school pupils. J Child Psychol Psychiatry 49:376–385
Smith PK, Morita Y, Junger-Tas J, Olweus D, Catalano R, Slee P (1999) The nature of school bullying: a cross-national perspective. Routledge, London, New York
Stassen BK (2007) Update on bullying at school: science forgotten? Dev Rev 27:90–126
Stein MB, Koverola C, Hanna C, Torchia MG, McClarty B (1997) Hippocampal volume in women victimized by childhood sexual abuse. Psychol Med 27(4):951–959
Stein MB, Walker JR, Anderson G et al (1996) Childhood physical and sexual abuse in patients with anxiety disorders and in a community sample. Am J Psychiatry 153:275–277
Steinhausen HC, Bösiger R, Metzke CW (2006) Stability, correlates, and outcome of adolescent suicidal risk. J Child Psychol Psychiatry 47:713–722
Saunders BE, Villoponteaux LA, Lipovsky JA (1992) Child sexual assault as a risk factor for mental disorders among women: A community survey. J Interpers Violence 7:189–204
Sterzer P, Stadler C, Krebs A, Kleinschmidt A, Poustka F (2005) Abnormal neural responses to emotional visual stimuli in adolescents with conduct disorder. Biol Psychiatry 57:7–15
Sourander A, Jensen P, Ronning JA et al (2007) Childhood bullies and victims and their risk of criminality in late adolescence. Arch Pediatr Adolesc Med 161:546–552
Sourander A, Klomek AB, Ikonen M, Lindroos J, Luntamo T et al (2010) Psychosocial risk factors associated with cyberbullying among adolescents: a population-based study. Arch Gen Psychiatry 67:720–728
Suzuki K, Asaga R, Sourander A, Mandell D (2012) Cyberbullying and adolescent mental health. Int J Adolesc Med Health 24(1):27–35 (print)
Tanskanen A, Hintikka J, Honkalampi K, Haatainen K, Koivumaa-Honkanen H, Viinamäki H (2004) Impact of multiple traumatic experiences on the persistence of depressive symptoms—a population-based study. Nord J Psychiatry 58:459–464
Todd RD (1992) Neural development is regulated by classical neuro-transmitters: dopamine D2 receptor stimulation enhances neurite outgrowth. Biol Psychiatry 31(8):794–807

Trickett PK, McBride-Chang C, Putnam FW (1994) The classroom performance and behavior of sexually-abused females. Dev Psychopathol 6:183–194
Tsai MH, Chen YH, Chen CD, Hsiao CY, Chien CH (2011) Deliberate self-harm by Taiwanese adolescents. Acta Pediatr 100(11):223–226
US Department of Health and Human Services (2012) National strategy for suicide prevention: goals and objectives for action. Office of the Surgeon General and National Action Alliance for Suicide Prevention, Washington, DC
US Public Health Service (1999) The surgeon general's call to action to prevent suicide. US Department of Health and Human Services, Washington, DC
Watts-English T, Fortson BL, Gibler N, Hooper SR, De Bellis MD (2006) The psychobiology of maltreatment in childhood. J Soc Issues 63(4):717–736
Widom CS, DuMont K, Czaja SJ (2007) A prospective investigation of major depressive disorder and comorbidity in abused and neglected children grown up. Arch Gen Psychiatry 64:49–56
Wilsnack SC, Beckman LJ (1984) Alcohol problems in women: antecedents, consequences, and intervention. Guilford, New York
Wolke D, Woods S, Schulz H (2001) Bullying and victimization of primary school children in England and Germany: prevalence and school factors. Br Psychiatry 92:673–696
Wong SS, Zhou B, Goebert D, Hishinuma ES (2013) The risk of adolescent suicide across patterns of drug use: a nationally representative study of high school students in the United States from 1999 to 2009. Soc Psychiatry Psychiatr Epidemiol 48(10):1611–1620 (print)
Woods S, White E (2005) The association between bullying behaviour, arousal levels and behavior problems. J Adolesc 28:381–395
Yang SJ, Kim JM, Kim SW, Shin IS, Yoon JS (2006) Bullying and victimization behaviors in boys and girls at South Korean Primary Schools. J Am Acad Child Adolesc Psychiatry 45 (1):69–77
Ybarra ML, Mitchell KJ, Wolak J, Finkelhor D (2006) Examining characteristics and associated distress related to internet harassment: findings from the second youth internet safety survey. Pediatrics 118:1169–1677
Ybarra ML, Mitchell KJ (2007) Prevalence and frequency of internet harassment instigation: implications for adolescent health. J Adolesc Health 41:189–195
Zanarini MC, Frankenburg FR (1997) Pathways to the development of borderline personality disorder. J Pers Disord 11:93–104
Zeanah CH, Scheeringa M, Boris NW, Heller SS, Smyke AT, Trapani J (2004) Reactive attachment disorder in maltreated toddlers. Child Abuse Negl 28(8):877–888 (print)
Zelkowitz P, Paris J, Guzder J, Feldman R (2001) Diatheses and stressors in borderline pathology of childhood: the role of neuropsychological risk and trauma. J Am Acad Child Adolesc Psychiatry 40:100–105
Zlotnick C, Mattia J, Zimmerman M (2001) Clinical features of survivors of sexual abuse with major depression. Child Abuse Negl 25:357–367
Zlotnick C, Warshaw M, Shea MT, Keller MB (1997) Trauma and chronic depression among patients with anxiety disorders. J Consult Clin Psychol 65:333–336
Zouk H, Tousingnant M, Seguin M, Lesage A, Turecki G (2006) Characterization of impulsivity in suicide completers: clinical, behavioral and psychosocial dimensions. J Affect Disord 92(2-3):195–204

Part III
Treatment Approaches

Chapter 12
Experimental Pharmacologic Approaches for the Reduction of Suicidal Ideation and Behavior

Elizabeth D. Ballard, Erica M. Richards, Dawn F. Ionescu, Mark J. Niciu, Jennifer Vande Voort and Carlos A. Zarate Jr

Abstract Treatment of the suicidal patient is limited by existing antidepressant medications, which can take weeks for an adequate response. New treatment approaches associated with rapid reduction of acute suicide risk are greatly needed. Experimental therapeutics—including intravenous ketamine and scopolamine—have rapid, robust, and relatively sustained reductions in suicidal thoughts within minutes to hours of administration. These findings have the potential to transform emergent treatment of the acutely suicidal patient and implicate the glutamatergic and muscarinic system in the development of suicidal thoughts and behaviors. Other putative targets for antisuicidal intervention include the thyroid and purinergic system, the latter involving the impulsive/aggressive suicide endophenotype. Benefits of research involving rapid-acting therapeutics include smaller sample sizes, short length of clinical trials, and assured compliance with study interventions. This approach also permits the evaluation of possible biomarkers of response and relapse to be incorporated into clinical trial design to more rapidly identify neurobiological correlates of suicide risk.

Each year, an estimated 1,000,000 individuals worldwide, and 30,000 in America alone, die by suicide (Centers for Disease Control and Prevention 2013). Clinically, over 420,000 individuals seek treatment for suicidal thoughts or behavior in U.S. emergency departments each year (Ting et al. 2012). Consequently, suicidal ideation is a common presentation in psychiatric practice with potentially fatal consequences; 50 % of psychiatrists have had a patient die by suicide (Ruskin et al. 2004). Unfortunately, few psychopharmacologic approaches have been consistently associated with a reduction in suicidal behavior (Mathews et al. 2013) and only one psychiatric medication, clozapine, has Food and Drug Administration (FDA) approval for suicidal behavior in patients with schizophrenia. Existing antidepressant mediations, which also may be used to treat depressed suicidal individuals, can take weeks to take effect. This delay in improvement of suicidal ideation places

E.D. Ballard · E.M. Richards · D.F. Ionescu · M.J. Niciu · J.V. Voort · C.A. Zarate Jr (✉)
Experimental Therapeutics and Pathophysiology Branch, Intramural Research Program, National Institute of Mental Health, National Institutes of Health, Bethesda, MD 20892, USA
e-mail: zaratec@mail.nih.gov

K.E. Cannon and T.J. Hudzik (eds.), *Suicide: Phenomenology and Neurobiology*,
DOI 10.1007/978-3-319-09964-4_12

individuals at risk for suicidal behavior (Jick et al. 2004). Therefore, in addition to the FDA approved psychopharmacologic medications, there is a great need for new approaches that are associated with rapid reduction of acute suicide risk.

12.1 Obstacles to Suicide Research

There are a number of obstacles to suicide research, which can become even more intransigent in the development and evaluation of novel compounds. First, death by suicide is a low base rate phenomenon even among patients with major psychiatric disorders like major depressive disorder, bipolar disorder, and schizophrenia. Since extremely large sample sizes would be required to detect changes in death by suicide, most clinical trials use suicide ideation or attempts as primary outcomes. Patients who contemplate and attempt suicide—but live—may be clinically different from those individuals who die by suicide (DeJong et al. 2010), which creates a significant limitation in suicide research and again attests to the need for large sample sizes. Second, the timing of a clinical trial in relation to the suicidal thoughts or behavior can be problematic, as attempts may be impulsive with little contemplation beforehand. By the time a researcher is able to identify, contact, and fully consent a participant, the "suicidal crisis" may be over or already treated in an emergency setting. Lastly, ethical concerns inherent in clinical treatment research with suicidal individuals are numerous, including the capacity to consent while a patient is suicidal, the potential to do harm if treatment is withheld in a placebo-controlled study, safety monitoring throughout the trial (including emergency coverage) and criteria for study withdrawal (Pearson et al. 2001). As a result, most of the neurobiological literature on suicide risk is conducted with participants who have attempted suicide in their lifetime and rarely proximal to the event itself. Nonetheless, considering the impact of suicidal behavior on patients, clinicians and communities, clinical trials with patients at acute risk are essential. The following chapter details potential neurobiological targets in suicidal patients and describes new progress in experimental therapeutics with the hope that faster, more efficacious interventions can be developed.

12.2 A New Research Model to Develop and Evaluate Rapid-Acting Treatments for Depression and Suicidal Ideation

The evaluation of treatments for suicidal patients and identification of biomarkers of treatment response have been limited by existing pharmacologic interventions. Treatment response may take weeks-to-months with standard antidepressants, which is inadequate for the urgent need to treat suicidal thoughts and behavior immediately in emergency settings. Furthermore, to detect a treatment effect on suicidal behaviors, follow-up observation would need to last well beyond the duration of most clinical trials in order to capture sufficient events. Consequently, ascertaining treatment effects and potential response biomarkers for conventional antidepressants (often cited as the primary treatments for suicidal behavior) is lengthy, costly, and requires many participants. In contrast, new experimental therapeutics—including intravenous infusions with ketamine and scopolamine—have rapid, robust, and relatively sustained antidepressant effects in major depression (Zarate et al. 2012, 2013b; Murrough et al. 2013). The benefits of this research model or paradigm include smaller sample sizes, decreased costs from longer trials, and assured compliance unlike with daily oral medications, which addresses some of the ethical obstacles to research with suicidal individuals. Furthermore, this paradigm allows evaluation of possible biomarkers of response and relapse to be incorporated into clinical trial design. Specifically, exploratory biomarkers of treatment response, such as neuroimaging, peripheral blood markers, genomics, and proteomics can be assessed before, during and after the administration of the experimental compound; the post-administration evaluation then occurs on a time scale of hours-to-days instead of weeks-to-months. Treatment response biomarkers may then be validated in larger trials and, in an iterative process, lead to enrichment strategies for future drug screening and development (for a full discussion of this process, please see Zarate et al. (2013a); Niciu (2014)).

Within this paradigm, the treatment of the suicidal patient warrants specific consideration, as the primary outcome of interest shifts away from suicidal behavior to suicidal thoughts. If an intravenous antidepressant compound has effects within an hour, it is improbable to see an observable effect on suicidal behavior(s) in a highly supervised research setting. In other words, since suicide attempts are relatively rare, it is not possible to demonstrate a short-term impact on suicidal behavior in the research environment. Further, while suicidal ideation is associated with later suicide attempt and death (Baca-Garcia et al. 2011), it is not an appropriate proxy for suicidal behavior, due to the clinical differences between ideators and attempters (DeJong et al. 2010; Smith et al. 2010; Borges et al. 2010). Instead, in evaluating rapid-acting antidepressants, trajectories of suicidal ideation are assessed using such measures as the Scale for Suicidal Ideation (SSI) (Beck et al. 1979), Montgomery-Asberg Depression Rating Scale (MADRS) (Montgomery and Asberg 1979), and Columbia-Suicide Severity Rating Scale (C-SSRS) (Posner et al. 2011) which are sensitive to change over short periods of time. While individuals who contemplate suicide may differ from those who attempt (DeJong et al. 2010), a robust antisuicidal effect of rapid-acting antidepressants on these standardized measures entails fewer participants and/or more rapid throughput in a controlled (typically inpatient) milieu. Such a research model may minimize risk associated with participation with experimental trials, including less time off of mediations or traditional clinical treatment and closer observation during the experimental phase.

12.3 Potential Targets for Suicidal Behavior

Putative targets in the development of pharmacologic approaches to the treatment of suicidal thoughts and behavior are displayed in Fig. 12.1. There are several other in-depth analyses of the neurobiology of suicide (Ernst et al. 2009; Mann and Currier 2010), including a recent review from our group (Mathews et al. 2013). The most researched potential targets include: (1) the serotonergic system as lower serotonergic functioning and lower 5-hydroxyindoleacetic acid (HIAAA) levels have been found in the cerebrospinal fluid (CSF) of individuals who die by suicide (Asberg et al. 1976; Nordstrom et al. 1994; Mann et al. 1995); (2) the hypothalamic-pituitary-adrenal (HPA) axis, which may be affected by epigenetic influences related to early life stress (Turecki et al. 2012) and; (3) other hormonal systems, including low cholesterol and high testosterone, which are associated with increased suicide attempts (Kunugi et al. 1997; Sher 2012).

While historically understudied in the suicide research literature, the glutamatergic system has received great attention in the past two decades in the etiology, pathogenesis, pathophysiology, and treatment of major mood disorders (Sanacora et al. 2008; Zarate et al. 2006). In the large real-world major depressive disorder effectiveness trial, Sequenced Treatment Alternatives to Relieve Depression (STAR*D), treatment-emergent suicidal ideation, was associated with single nucleotide polymorphisms for GRIA3 and GRIK2, whose genes encode ionotropic glutamate receptors (Laje et al. 2007). Similar associations were found in the Munich Antidepressant Response Signature (MARS) trial (Menke et al. 2008). Alterations in N-methyl-D-aspartate (NMDA) receptor function have also been found in individuals who died by suicide (Nowak et al. 1995). Such findings have led to the investigation of glutamate-based compounds such as ketamine in the treatment of depression and suicidal ideation. Table 12.1 depicts clinical compounds implicated in the treatment of suicidal thoughts and behaviors.

12.3.1 Endophenotypes of Suicidal Behavior

Due to the heterogeneity in molecular pathways and clinical presentations associated with suicide, an endophenotypic approach may be beneficial for identifying treatment targets. An endophenotype represents an intermediary step from genes-to-clinical phenotype, which can simplify intermediate players in multifactorial disorders and identify mediators/moderators underpinning complex clinical presentations (Gottesman and Gould 2003). Several proposed suicide-salient endophenotypes, using criteria set forward by Gottesman and Gould (2003), include impulsive and aggressive traits, early onset of major depression, neurocognitive dysfunction (including executive functioning and impaired decision-making), and cortisol response to psychosocial stress (Mann et al. 2009; Courtet et al. 2011). Other proposed candidate endophenotypes for suicidal behavior with relatively less

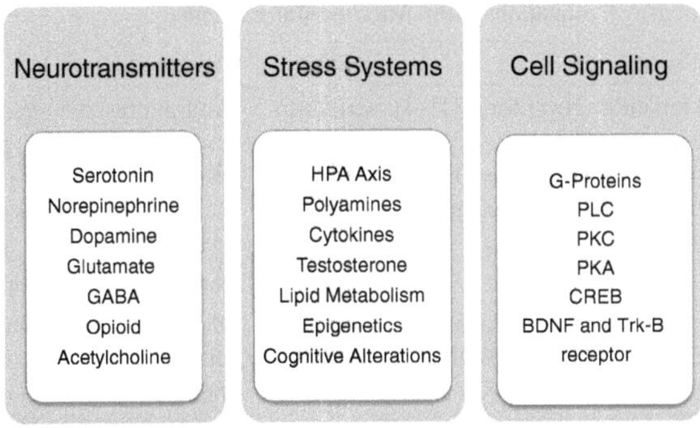

Fig. 12.1 Putative targets in the neurobiology of suicide. Adapted from:(Mathews et al. 2013). *BDNF* brain-derived neurotrophic factor; *CREB* cyclic AMP-response element binding protein; *GABA* gamma-aminobutyric acid; *HPA* hypothalamic-pituitary-adrenal; *PLC* Phospholipase C; *PKC* Protein Kinase C; *PKA* Protein Kinase A; *Trk* tyrosine kinase receptor

research evidence are dysfunctional serotonergic neurotransmission, second-messenger systems aberrations, and traits consistent with borderline personality disorder, including affective dysregulation and difficulties in interpersonal relationships. Each of these constructs could be used to identify treatment targets for experimental therapeutics for suicidal behavior, with allopurinol as a case example discussed in the following section.

12.3.2 Purinergic System and Allopurinol

The purinergic system has been implicated in the impulsive and aggressive behavior associated with mania (Machado-Vieira 2012) and has therefore been targeted in drug development. Purinergic metabolism is involved in the regulation of neurotransmitters (ATP and adenosine) and affects sleep, motor activity, appetite, cognition, and social interaction (Machado-Vieira 2012). An adenosine antagonist, caffeine is also a GABA receptor antagonist and phosphodiesterase inhibitor; excessive consumption is associated with irritability, anxiety, tachycardia, and increased blood pressure (presumably via its effects on GABA). In contrast, increased caffeine consumption has been linked with a lower risk of death by suicide (Lucas et al. 2014). The end product of purinergic metabolism is uric acid, which has been positively associated with increased drive/motivation, disinhibition, hyperthymia, and irritable temperament (Lorenzi et al. 2010). As a syndrome model, Lesch-Nyhan Disease is a congenital disorder associated with the overproduction of uric acid associated with increased de novo purine synthesis and deficient salvage of purine bases. Among the characteristics associated with this disorder is intense self-injurious behavior, including self-biting and self-hitting

Table 12.1 Psychiatric Medications with AntiSuicidal Evidence

Drug	Target	Findings
Clozapine	Dopamine receptors (D1-4), serotonin receptors (1A, 2A, 2C), adrenergic receptors, histamine (H1) receptors, muscarinic (M2) receptors	Anti-aggressive effects, antipsychotic and mood stabilizing effects, close clinical monitoring (Hennen and Baldessarini 2005; Frogley et al. 2012)
		FDA approved for suicidal behavior in patients with schizophrenia
Lithium	cAMP mediated signal transduction; CREB activation; BDNF; PI cascade; PKC inhibition; GSK-3 inhibition; Bcl-2 expression	Mood stabilizing and anti-depressant effects; thought to also target impulsivity and aggression (oral formulation) (Quiroz et al. 2010; McCarthy et al. 2010)
Ketamine	NMDA receptor antagonist; mTOR activation; eEF2 de-suppression; BDNF production/release; Arc; GSK-3 inhibition	Rapid antidepressant and antisuicidal effects (0.1–0.5 mg/kg IV) (Kavalali 2012)
TRH	HPT axis	Rapid antidepressant effect (IV) and antisuicidal effects (IT) (Callahan et al. 1997; Bonnin et al. 2010)
Scopolamine	Muscarinic receptor antagonist; NMDA receptor expression; mTOR activation	Rapid antidepressant effects (IV); decreased suicidal ideation (Furey and Drevets 2006; Drevets and Furey 2010)
Allopurinol	Xanthine oxidase inhibitor: decreased purines and free radicals	Efficacy in bipolar mania; may reduce impulsivity associated with suicidal behavior (Machado-Vieira et al. 2002; Sperlagh et al. 2012)

Adapted from: (Mathews et al. 2013)
Arc activity-regulated cytoskeletal associated protein; *Bcl-2* B-cell lymphoma 2; *BDNF* brain-derived neurotrophic factor; *cAMP* cyclic adenosine monophosphate; *CREB* cAMP response element binding protein; *eEF* eukaryotic elongation factor; *GSK-3* glycogen synthase kinase 3; *HPT* hypothalamic-pituitary-thyroid; *IV* intravenous; *IT* intrathecal; *mTOR* mammalian target of rapamycin; *NMDA* N-methyl-D-aspartate; *PI* phosphatidylinositide; *PKC* protein kinase C; *TRH* thyrotropin releasing hormone

(Torres et al. 2012). Therefore, the purinergic system may be a potential target for suicidal/self-injurious behaviors and a model for the study of impulsivity.

Allopurinol is a xanthine oxidase inhibitor, which decreases production of uric acid, superoxide, and hydrogen peroxide and is widely used as a treatment for gout. Because of its role in the purinergic system, it has been proposed as a possible treatment for acute mania. In a randomized placebo-controlled trial of 180 bipolar I patients in a current manic episode, adjunctive allopurinol to lithium was associated with greater Young Mania Rating Scale (YMRS) (Young et al. 1978) score reductions when compared to adjunctive dipyridamole, another agent that regulates purine metabolism, plus lithium, or lithium plus placebo (Machado-Vieira et al. 2008). Similar results were found in a randomized clinical trial of lithium, haloperidol, and allopurinol compared to lithium, haloperidol, and placebo (Akhondzadeh et al. 2006). While the relationship of allopurinol to suicidal behavior has yet to be evaluated, it has a theoretical therapeutic role for patients with high impulsivity and aggression.

12.3.3 Ketamine

The recent interest in glutamatergic pathways in depression has been led by promising results with subanesthetic doses of the non-competitive N-methyl-D-aspartate receptor antagonist ketamine. Originally used clinically as a dissociative anesthetic and analgesic, recent research on ketamine's rapid and potent antidepressant properties has opened promising avenues for future development of treatments for acutely suicidal patients (Zarate et al. 2006, 2013b; Murrough et al. 2013). After initial reports as an antidepressant, an open-label single subanesthetic infusion of ketamine (0.5 mg/kg given intravenously over 40 min) in 33 major depressive disorder (MDD) patients decreased suicidal ideation (as assessed by the decreased mean SSI) immediately following infusion, which continued over the next 4 h. Suicide items from the MADRS, Hamilton Depression Rating Scale (HDRS) (Hamilton 1960), and Beck Depression Inventory (BDI) (Beck and Beamesderfer 1974), as well as indicators of anxiety and hopelessness also significantly decreased over the same time period (DiazGranados et al. 2010). Analogous reductions in suicidal ideation were further demonstrated in a double-blind, placebo-controlled study of the glutamatergic modulator riluzole or placebo following a single open-label ketamine infusion in treatment-resistant unipolar depression (Ibrahim et al. 2012). Similarly, in a double-blind, randomized, crossover study of 15 participants with bipolar I or II depression, suicidal ideation (assessed by the MADRS) significantly improved within 40 min after a single infusion of ketamine (Zarate et al. 2006). A comparable decrease in suicidal ideation was demonstrated 24 h after ketamine infusion in 25 participants with treatment-resistant depression (Price et al. 2009), a finding which has been replicated in a trial of ketamine compared to midazolam (Price et al. 2014). A subset of the participants ($n = 9$) received multiple infusions over 12 days, and the antisuicidal effects were maintained. Similar results have been found in a study involving patients in India with treatment-resistant depression (Thakurta et al. 2012). When collapsing across multiple ketamine clinical trials, the effect of ketamine on suicidal ideation is independent of its effect on depression and anxiety (Ballard et al. In Press).

Several case reports and naturalistic studies have also hinted how ketamine could be used with suicidal patients in clinical practice. In a naturalistic study, 14 depressed patients in the emergency department with active suicidal ideation received low-dose ketamine (0.2 mg/kg intravenous push) and were followed for up to 10 days (Larkin and Beautrais 2011). Improvements in suicidal ideation were demonstrated over the 10 days of follow-up. A case report in an urgent outpatient psychiatric clinic described the use of ketamine in a patient with depression and suicidal ideation, intent, and plan (Zigman and Blier 2013). The patient was offered the option of ketamine or psychiatric hospitalization/electroconvulsive therapy (ECT). After opting for ketamine, suicidal ideation resolved within 30 min and improvements in depressive symptoms were maintained at 8 days post-infusion. Suicidal thoughts had not returned after a month post-infusion. Lastly, in a letter to the editor, a palliative care team advocated the clinical use of ketamine for terminally ill patients with suicidal ideation, depression, and anxiety, reporting a 20 year track record of using a combination of ketamine and narcotics at acceptable/tolerable doses (Thangathurai and Mogos 2011).

These antidepressant effects of ketamine are likely mediated by enhanced synaptic plasticity in key brain circuits, e.g. prefrontal cortex and hippocampus (Duman and Aghajanian 2012). Potential cellular and molecular mechanisms for these effects include presynaptic glutamate release increasing α-amino-3-hydroxy-5-methylisoxazole-4-propionate (AMPA)/NMDA receptor throughput, the activation/phosphorylation of mammalian target of rapamycin (mTOR), and GSK-3 inhibition. Eukaryotic elongation factor (eEF2), a translation repressor, may be deactivated through ketamine-mediated blockade of NMDA receptors, which then leads to reductions in eEF2 phosphorylation and de-suppression of rapid dendritic protein translation such as increased brain-derived neurotrophic factor (BDNF) release in the hippocampus (Kavalali and Monteggia 2012). Cytoskeleton-associated proteins (Arc) may also be activated by ketamine, leading to dynamic changes in the actin cytoskeleton and remodeling of dendritic spines. Therefore, the antisuicidal effects of ketamine may be related to any or all of these cellular and molecular targets.

While the antisuicidal effects of ketamine appear promising, there remain several cautionary tales. First, in an open-label trial of subanesthetic intravenous ketamine in 10 patients with treatment-refractory obsessive-compulsive disorder (OCD), two patients reported passive suicidal ideation, worsening anxiety, and dysphoria at 1 day post-infusion in previously non-syndromal depression at the time of infusion (Niciu et al. 2013). The authors hypothesize that the delayed-onset suicidal ideation may be related to: (1) worsening obsessional and free-floating anxiety and psychomotor agitation post-infusion, (2) the interaction of ketamine-related acute dysphoria with existing psychiatric comorbidities, or (3) ketamine-induced derealization/depersonalization, activating past vulnerabilities (both patients had extensive trauma histories). Consequently, off-label use of ketamine is not indicated at this time for individuals with substantial psychiatric comorbidities and past trauma. If ketamine is used in a non-research setting, close follow-up in the peri-infusion period is mandatory.

Another concern with ketamine administration is psychotomimetic or dissociative adverse effects. Consequently, different opportunities for NMDA receptor modulation have been explored. AZD6765/lanicemine, a proprietary low-trapping NMDA receptor antagonist, was administered to inpatients with treatment-resistant depression in a double-blind, placebo-controlled, proof-of-concept study, and demonstrated a brief (80–110 min) antidepressant effect (Zarate et al. 2013a; Mathews et al. 2013). Albeit less potent, this compound was not associated with dissociative, psychotomimetic, or other effects seen with ketamine; in fact, neither clinicians nor patients could correctly guess whether the patient had been administered the study drug or placebo. A placebo-controlled trial has demonstrated that repeated infusions of AZD6765 is associated with maintained mood improvements (Sanacora et al. 2013; Smith et al. 2010). Compounds such as AZD6765, which are able to replicate the rapid antidepressant and anxiolytic effects of ketamine without psychogenic experiences would be exceptionally useful in clinical practice.

12.3.4 Scopolamine

Scopolamine hydrobromide is a muscarinic cholinergic receptor antagonist, which may also have antisuicidal effects via its effects of multifarious pathways: muscarinic neurotransmission and glutamatergic neurotransmission (leading to downstream mTOR phosphorylation/activation) (Voleti et al. 2013). Scopolamine has been shown to have rapid antidepressant effects in recurrent MDD and bipolar depression when administered intravenously (4 mcg/kg) (Furey and Drevets 2006). Antidepressant response to scopolamine has been associated with activation in the bilateral middle occipital cortex during emotional visual stimuli processing (Furey et al. 2013), potentially identifying a biomarker for treatment response. In a double blind, placebo-controlled, crossover trial, scopolamine was associated with a reduction on the suicidal ideation item on the MADRS (Drevets and Furey 2010). Further prospective investigation of scopolamine's putative antisuicidal properties is critically needed.

12.3.5 Thyrotropin-Releasing Hormone

Thyrotropin-releasing hormone (TRH) is a hypothalamic tripeptide that regulates the hypothalamic-pituitary-thyroid axis by stimulating the production and release of thyroid stimulating hormone (TSH) from the pituitary. The greatest concentration of TRH receptors is in the amygdala and hippocampus with lower densities in the cortex, diencephalon, and basal ganglia (Manaker et al. 1986). Results on the efficacy of oral and intravenous TRH in major mood disorders have been mixed (Callahan et al. 1997) and may be limited by inadequate blood-brain barrier penetration and extremely short half-life (Marangell et al. 1997). In a pilot study of lumbar intrathecal TRH injection in eight patients with treatment-resistant depression, there was a reduction of depression and suicidal ideation within 1 day of administration (Marangell et al. 1997). Similar results were demonstrated after intravenous and intrathecal administration of TRH to two patients with treatment-resistant bipolar II disorder (Callahan et al. 1997). These findings in small cohorts have not been replicated, but novel delivery routes with increased CNS penetrance, e.g. intranasal administration, may revitalize TRH research in depressive illnesses.

12.4 Future Directions

With the rise of rapid-acting antidepressant research, psychiatry is poised for novel, mechanistically distinct treatments for depression and suicidal ideation. While much of the suicide research literature has focused on alterations in serotonergic and HPA functioning, new findings implicate the glutamatergic, muscarinic, and thyroid hormonal systems. In addition, the impulsive/aggressive endophenotype may also be a potential target for experimental intervention development, especially with high-risk suicidal patients with substance use disorders and borderline personality disorder. Current research on ketamine and scopolamine may further our understanding of underlying neurobiological processes as an enrichment strategy to develop more targeted treatments. Consistent with the NIMH's Research Domain Criteria (RDoC) initiative, which will emphasize constructs/dimensions of observable behavior and neurobiological measures, further research must also evaluate these compounds outside the context of traditional diagnostic categories and in real-world settings to evaluate how they perform with community samples. Furthermore, since the literature on the impulsive/aggressive endophenotype is robust, the evaluation of substances such as ketamine in individuals with impulsive and/or aggressive tendencies is warranted to determine possible antisuicidal and self-injurious efficacy.

As stated in the introduction to this chapter, our work with rapid-acting antidepressants has necessitated a focus on suicidal ideation, rather than suicidal behavior, as our primary outcome. This focus could significantly impact the clinical care of emergent suicidal ideation, e.g. emergency departments. The ability to reduce suicidal thoughts *within hours* instead of days-to-weeks could facilitate a short-term reduction in suicide risk and preclude recidivism and frequent psychiatric hospitalizations (thereby cutting long-term health costs). Such treatment provides time to both connect the patient with more comprehensive long-term resources, such as regular psychopharmacological follow-up and therapeutic resources (such as Cognitive Behavioral Therapy or Dialectical Behavioral Therapy) to allow such interventions to take effect. Albeit difficult to assess prospectively due to its low incidence, future studies will need to evaluate the relationship between suicide-related biomarkers and subsequent suicide attempt(s) and/or death to truly impact public health.

References

Akhondzadeh S et al (2006) Allopurinol as an adjunct to lithium and haloperidol for treatment of patients with acute mania: a double-blind, randomized, placebo-controlled trial. Bipolar Disord 8(5) Part 1:485–489 (print)

Asberg M, Traskman L, Thoren P (1976) 5-HIAA in the cerebrospinal fluid. A biochemical suicide predictor? Arch Gen Psychiatry 33(10):1193–1197 (print)

Baca-Garcia E et al (2011) Estimating risk for suicide attempt: are we asking the right questions? Passive suicidal ideation as a marker for suicidal behavior. J Affect Disord 134(1–3):327–332 (print)
Ballard ED et al (In Press) Improvement in suicidal ideation after ketamine infusion: relationship to reductions in depression and anxiety. J Psychiat Res
Beck AT, Beamesderfer A (1974) Assessment of depression: the depression inventory. Mod Probl Pharmacopsychiatry 7:151–169 (print)
Beck AT, Kovacs M, Weissman A (1979) Assessment of suicidal intention: the scale for suicide ideation. J Consult Clin Psychol 47(2):343–252 (print)
Bonnin CM et al (2010) Bipolar disorder, cognitive functioning and hypothalamic-pituitary-thyroid axis. Actas Esp Psiquiatr 38:223–228 (print)
Borges G et al (2010) Twelve-month prevalence of and risk factors for suicide attempts in the World Health Organization world mental health surveys. J Clin Psychiatry 71(12):1617–1628 (print)
Callahan AM et al (1997) Comparative antidepressant effects of intravenous and intrathecal thyrotropin-releasing hormone: confounding effects of tolerance and implications for therapeutics. Biol Psychiatry 41(3):264–272 (print)
Centers for Disease Control and Prevention, National Center for Injury Prevention and Control (2013) Web-based injury statistics query and reporting system (WISQARS), 5 Dec 2013
Courtet P et al (2011) The neuroscience of suicidal behaviors: what can we expect from endophenotype strategies? Transl Psychiatry 1(pii):e7 (print)
DeJong TM, Overholser JC, Stockmeier CA (2010) Apples to oranges?: a direct comparison between suicide attempters and suicide completers. J Affect Disord 124(1–2):90–97 (print)
DiazGranados N et al (2010) Rapid resolution of suicidal ideation after a single infusion of an N-methyl-D-aspartate Antagonist in patients with treatment-resistant major depressive disorder. J Clin Psychiatry 71(12):1605–1611. Epub 13 Jul 2010 (print)
Drevets WC, Furey ML (2010) Replication of scopolamine's antidepressant efficacy in major depressive disorder: a randomized, placebo-controlled clinical trial. Biol Psychiatry 67 (5):432–438. Epub 15 Jan 2010 (print)
Duman RS, Aghajanian GK (2012) Synaptic dysfunction in depression: potential therapeutic targets. Science 338(6103):68–72. doi:10.1126/science.1222939 print
Ernst C, Mechawar N, Turecki G (2009) Suicide neurobiology. Prog Neurobiol 89(4):315–333 (print)
Frogley C et al (2012) A systematic review of the evidence of Clozapine's anti-aggressive effects. Int J Neuropsychopharmacol 15(9):1351–1371 (print)
Furey ML, Drevets WC (2006) Antidepressant efficacy of the antimuscarinic drug scopolamine: a randomized, placebo-controlled clinical trial. Arch Gen Psychiatry 63(10):1121–1129 (print)
Furey ML et al (2013) Potential of pretreatment neural activity in the visual cortex during emotional processing to predict treatment response to scopolamine in major depressive disorder. JAMA Psychiatry 70(3):280–290 (print)
Gottesman II, Gould TD (2003) The endophenotype concept in psychiatry: etymology and strategic intentions. Am J Psychiatry 160(4):636–645 (print)
Hamilton M (1960) A rating scale for depression. J Neurol Neurosurg Psychiatry 23:56–62 (print)
Hennen J, Baldessarini RJ (2005) Suicidal risk during treatment with clozapine: a meta-analysis. Schizophr Res 73(2–3):139–145 (print)
Ibrahim L et al (2012) Course of improvement in depressive symptoms to a single intravenous infusion of ketamine versus add-on Riluzole: results from a 4-Week, double-blind, placebo-controlled study. Neuropsychopharmacology 37(6):1526–1533 (print)
Jick H, Kaye JA, Jick SS (2004) Antidepressants and the risk of suicidal behaviors. JAMA 292 (3):338–343 (print)
Kavalali ET, Monteggia LM (2012) Synaptic mechanisms underlying rapid antidepressant action of ketamine. Am J Psychiatry 3(10):12040531 (print)
Kunugi H et al (1997) Low serum cholesterol in suicide attempters. Biol Psychiatry 41(2):196–200 (print)

Laje G et al (2007) Genetic markers of suicidal ideation emerging during citalopram treatment of major depression. Am J Psychiatry 164(10):1530–1538 (print)
Larkin GL, Beautrais AL (2011) A preliminary naturalistic study of low-dose ketamine for depression and suicide ideation in the emergency department. Int J Neuropsychopharmacol 14 (8):1127–1131 (print)
Lorenzi TM et al (2010) Association of serum uric acid levels with emotional and affective temperaments. J Affect Disord 121(1–2):161–164 (print)
Lucas M et al (2014) Coffee, caffeine, and risk of completed suicide: results from three prospective cohorts of american adults. World J Biol Psychiatry 15(5):377–386 (print)
Machado-Vieira R (2012) Purinergic system in the treatment of bipolar disorder: uric acid levels as a screening test in mania. J Clin Psychopharmacol 32(5):735–736 (print)
Machado-Vieira R et al (2002) Purinergic dysfunction in mania: an integrative model. Med Hypotheses 58(4):297–304 (print)
Machado-Vieira R et al (2008) A double-blind, randomized, placebo-controlled 4-week study on the efficacy and safety of the purinergic agents allopurinol and dipyridamole adjunctive to lithium in acute bipolar mania. J Clin Psychiatry 69(8):1237–1245 (print)
Manaker S et al (1986) Autoradiographic localization of thyrotropin releasing hormone receptors in human brain. Neurology 36(5):641–646 (print)
Mann JJ et al (2009) Candidate endophenotypes for genetic studies of suicidal behavior. Biol Psychiatry 65(7):556–563 (print)
Mann JJ, Currier DM (2010) Stress, genetics and epigenetic effects on the neurobiology of suicidal behavior and depression. Eur Psychiatry 25(5):268–271 (print)
Mann JJ et al (1995) Blunted serotonergic responsivity in depressed inpatients. Neuropsychopharmacology 13(1):53–64 (print)
Marangell LB et al (1997) Effects of intrathecal thyrotropin-releasing hormone (protirelin) in refractory depressed patients. Arch Gen Psychiatry 54(3):214–222 (print)
Mathews DC et al (2013) Neurobiological aspects of suicide and suicide attempts in bipolar disorder. Transl Neurosci 4(2):121–124 (print)
McCarthy MJ, Leckband SG, Kelsoe JR (2010) Pharmacogenetics of lithium response in bipolar disorder. Pharmacogenomics 11:1439–1465 (print)
Menke A et al (2008) Genetic markers within glutamate receptors associated with antidepressant treatment-emergent suicidal ideation. Am J Psychiatry 165(7):917–918 (print)
Montgomery SA, Asberg M (1979) A new depression scale designed to be sensitive to change. Br J Psychiatry 134:382–389 (print)
Murrough JW et al (2013) Antidepressant efficacy of ketamine in treatment-resistant major depression: a two-site randomized controlled trial. Am J Psychiatry 170(10):1134–1142 (print)
Niciu MJ et al (2013) Two cases of delayed-onset suicidal ideation, dysphoria and anxiety after ketamine infusion in patients with obsessive-compulsive disorder and a history of major depressive disorder. J Psychopharmacol 27(7):651–654 (print)
Niciu MJ, Mathews DC, Nugent AC, Ionescu DF, Furey ML, Richards EM, Machado-Viera R, Zarate CA (2014) Developing biomarkers in mood disorders research thourgh the use of rapid-acting antidepressants. Depress Anxiety 31(4):297–307 (print)
Nordstrom P et al (1994) CSF 5-HIAA predicts suicide risk after attempted suicide. Suicide Life Threat Behav 24(1):1–9 (print)
Nowak G, Ordway GA, Paul IA (1995) Alterations in the N-methyl-D-aspartate (NMDA) receptor complex in the frontal cortex of suicide victims. Brain Res 675(1–2):157–164 (print)
Pearson JL et al (2001) Intervention research with persons at high risk for suicidality: safety and ethical considerations. J Clin Psychiatry 62(Suppl 25):17–26 (print)
Posner K et al (2011) The Columbia-Suicide Severity Rating Scale: initial validity and internal consistency findings from three multisite studies with adolescents and adults. Am J Psychiatry 168(12):1266–1277 (print)
Price RB et al (2009) Effects of intravenous ketamine on explicit and implicit measures of suicidality in treatment-resistant depression. Biol Psychiatry 66(5):522–526

Price RB et al (2014) Effects of ketamine on explicit and implicit suicidal cognition: a randomized controlled trial in treatment-resistant depression. Depress Anxiety 31(4):335–343

Quiroz JA et al (2010) Novel insights into lithium's mechanism of action: neurotrophic and neuroprotective effects. Neuropsychobiology 62(1):50–60. Epub 7 May 2010 (print)

Ruskin R et al (2004) Impact of patient suicide on psychiatrists and psychiatric trainees. Acad Psychiatry 28(2):104–110 (print)

Sanacora G et al (2013) Lanicemine: a low-trapping NMDA channel blocker produces sustained antidepressant efficacy with minimal psychotomimetic adverse effects. Mol Psychiatry. Epub ahead of print (print)

Sanacora G et al. (2008) Targeting the glutamatergic system to develop novel, improved therapeutics for mood disorders. Nat Rev Drug Discov 7(5):426–437 (print)

Sher L (2012) Testosterone and suicidal behavior. Expert Rev Neurother 12(3):257–259 (print)

Smith PN et al. (2010) The acquired capability for suicide: a comparison of suicide attempters, suicide ideators, and non-suicidal controls. Depress Anxiety 27(9):871–877 (print)

Sperlagh B et al (2012) The role of purinergic signaling in depressive disorders. Neuropsychopharmacol Hung 14:231–238 (print)

Thakurta RG et al (2012) Rapid response with ketamine on suicidal cognition in resistant depression. Indian J Psychol Med 34(2):170–175 (print)

Thangathurai D, Mogos M (2011) Ketamine alleviates fear, depression, and suicidal ideation in terminally Ill patients. J Palliat Med 14(4):389 (print)

Ting SA et al (2012) Trends in us emergency department visits for attempted suicide and self-inflicted injury, 1993–2008. Gen Hosp Psychiatry 34(5):557–565

Torres RJ, Puig JG, Jinnah HA (2012) Update on the phenotypic spectrum of Lesch-Nyhan disease and its attenuated variants. Curr Rheumatol Rep 14(2):189–194 (print)

Turecki G et al (2012) The neurodevelopmental origins of suicidal behavior. Trends Neurosci 35 (1):14–23. Epub 15 Dec 2011 (print)

Voleti B et al (2013) Scopolamine rapidly increases mammalian target of rapamycin complex 1 signaling, synaptogenesis, and antidepressant behavioral responses. Biol Psychiatry 74 (10):742–749 (print)

Young RC et al (1978) A rating scale for mania: reliability, validity and sensitivity. Br J Psychiatry 133:429–435 (print)

Zarate CA Jr et al (2012) Replication of ketamine's antidepressant efficacy in bipolar depression: a randomized controlled add-on trial. Biol Psychiatry 71(11):939–946 (print)

Zarate CA Jr, Mathews DC, Furey ML (2013a) Human biomarkers of rapid antidepressant effects. Biol Psychiatry 73(12):1142–1155 (print)

Zarate CA Jr et al (2013b) A randomized trial of a low-trapping nonselective N-methyl-D-aspartate channel blocker in major depression. Biol Psychiatry 74(4):257–264 (print)

Zarate CA Jr et al (2006) A randomized trial of an N-methyl-D-aspartate antagonist in treatment-resistant major depression. Arch Gen Psychiatry 63(8):856–864 (print)

Zigman D, Blier P (2013) Urgent ketamine infusion rapidly eliminated suicidal ideation for a patient with major depressive disorder: a case report. J Clin Psychopharmacol 33(2):270–272 (print)

Chapter 13
Psychotherapeutic Treatment Approaches for Suicidal Individuals

Megan S. Chesin, Sadia Chaudhury and Barbara Stanley

Abstract In the past 20 years, rigorous empirical study has shown that Dialectical Behavior Therapy (DBT) and Cognitive-Behavioral Therapy (CBT) treatment approaches for suicide prevention work to reduce recurrent suicidal behavior among high suicide-risk groups. In addition, very brief psychotherapeutic approaches comprised of supportive contact post-discharge and/or CBT techniques have been developed and tested. These interventions aim to increase safety among the many acutely suicidal individuals who present to acute care settings but will not engage in follow-up mental healthcare. This chapter outlines both long-term and very brief psychotherapeutic interventions to prevent suicide, as well as the evidence base for these treatments. Additionally, one promising mindfulness-based approach to suicide prevention (MBCT-S) is also detailed. Proposed directions for future research include more rigorous testing of MBCT-S and the proposal and testing of treatment targets so existing treatments may be refined and new treatments can be efficiently developed.

13.1 Introduction

Suicide is a leading cause of death. In the U.S., more than 38,000 individuals died by suicide in 2010 (National Center for Injury Prevention and Control 2012). Worldwide, almost one million people die by suicide each year (World Health Organization 2012). Suicide attempts in the U.S. occur at rates up to 25 times higher than suicides (Goldsmith et al. 2002). Given the incidence and prevalence of suicide and

M.S. Chesin (✉) · B. Stanley
Department of Psychiatry, Columbia University College of Physicians and Surgeons, 1051 Riverside Drive, Unit 42, New York, NY 10032, USA
e-mail: mchesin@nyspi.columbia.edu

M.S. Chesin · S. Chaudhury · B. Stanley
Molecular Imaging and Neuropathology Division, New York State Psychiatric Institute, 1051 Riverside Drive, Unit 42, New York, NY 10032, USA

K.E. Cannon and T.J. Hudzik (eds.), *Suicide: Phenomenology and Neurobiology*,
DOI 10.1007/978-3-319-09964-4_13

suicide attempt, identifying interventions to prevent suicidal behavior in individuals identified as at risk is imperative. However, designing and testing such interventions is challenging for several reasons: (1) There are ethical concerns to consider when offering novel treatment to some but not all individuals at acute risk for suicidal behavior, e.g., when randomizing high suicide-risk patients to enhanced treatment or treatment as usual (TAU). (2) Pinpointing efficacious treatments is difficult given the nature of the primary outcomes in suicide intervention research. That is, when suicidal ideation and suicide attempts are the primary outcomes of interest, natural regression to the mean and the low incidence of suicide-related events, limit power to detect pre- to postôtreatment gains. (3) Suicidal patients are a heterogeneous group (Carballo et al. 2008), posing a challenge to identifying what works and what works for whom among the different types of suicide attempters and completers.

Despite such difficulties, several psychotherapeutic treatments to prevent suicide and suicide-related behavior are available and empirically supported. In this chapter, we provide a comprehensive review of multi-session psychotherapeutic treatments to prevent suicidal behavior among high suicide-risk groups, and we summarize the most promising very brief (i.e., one session) interventions for suicidal patients that are begun or even completed at the time and place where suicidal individuals present for help (e.g., emergency departments). Our review is focused on describing treatments for suicidal adults and adolescents and the evidence base. We also suggest directions for future research, highlighting the need for research that could lead to the refinement of available psychotherapeutic treatments for suicidal behavior and the development of additional brief interventions.

13.2 Longer-Term Treatments for Suicidal Behavior

13.2.1 Dialectical Behavioral Therapy

Dialectical Behavioral Therapy (DBT) (Linehan 1993) combines change strategies and techniques from behavioral treatments with acceptance-based strategies and techniques. DBT was originally designed as a treatment for individuals who chronically engage in suicidal and self-injurious behaviors (Linehan 1987). Because chronic non-suicidal self-injury, defined as the intentional, direct destruction of one's own body tissue without any conscious intent to die (Favazza 1998; Linehan 1987), and repetitive suicidal behavior occur frequently in Borderline Personality Disorder (BPD) (Association 2000; Jacobson and Gould 2007), DBT was quickly considered and tested as a treatment for BPD. Thus, most of the evidence for using DBT to treat suicidal behavior comes from studies testing DBT to treat self-inflicted injury with and/or without suicidal intent, among BPD patients, and DBT is manualized as a treatment for individuals with BPD (Linehan 1987).

Findings from eight randomized controlled trials (RCTs) conducted by six different groups (Carter et al. 2010; Clarkin et al. 2007; Koons et al. 2001; Linehan et al. 1991, 1999, 2006; McMain et al. 2009; Pistorello et al. 2012; Verheul et al. 2003) consistently show that DBT is an effective and efficacious treatment for self-injury and suicidal behavior among individuals with BPD. When compared to TAU, patients who have received DBT show greater reductions in suicidal ideation (Koons et al. 2001; Pistorello et al. 2012). When DBT is compared to active treatments, its efficacy as a psychotherapeutic intervention for suicidal behavior is even more compelling. Compared to treatment by experts and supportive psychotherapy, DBT is more effective in reducing reattempt risk and current suicidality (Clarkin et al. 2007; Linehan et al. 2006; Turner 2000). DBT is similarly effective in reducing suicidality and recurrent suicidal behavior as general psychiatric management plus psychodynamic psychotherapy (Clarkin et al. 2007; McMain et al. 2009). Panos et al. (2013) conducted a meta-analysis of five of the above RCTs and concluded that DBT is moderately more effective in reducing suicidal behavior and non-suicidal self-injury than other treatments, including TAU, supportive psychotherapy or manualized psychodynamic, or client centered therapy.

Furthermore, the reduction in suicidal behavior as a result of DBT appears to persist posttreatment. Linehan et al. (2006) in the aforementioned trial found that participants who received DBT were also less likely to make a suicide attempt during the year following treatment than those receiving treatment by experts. Similarly, McMain et al. (2012) found that the reduction of suicidal and non-suicidal self-injurious behaviors in participants who received either DBT or psychopharmacological treatment persisted for 2-years following treatment.

13.2.2 Cognitive Therapy to Prevent Suicide Attempts

Cognitive Therapy (CT) for the prevention of suicide attempts (Brown et al. 2002) is another treatment with empirical support for the prevention of suicide attempt. CT is based on cognitive theory, which posits that the manner in which an individual thinks about and interprets situations determines the emotional and behavioral response to said situation (Beck 1976). Thus, CT focuses on changing maladaptive thought patterns, including those of hopelessness and helplessness, that lead to suicidal behavior. The 10-session intervention is divided into three phases. During the first three sessions, the focus is on treatment engagement, orientation to the cognitive model, and identification of target problems and treatment goals. During the next four sessions, suicidal behavior is targeted through cognitive restructuring and behavioral change and includes such interventions as coping cards and hope kits. The final three sessions focus is on relapse prevention, during which guided imagery is used to help the patient understand the index suicide attempt as well as likely triggers and components of a future suicidal crisis, with an emphasis on using skills acquired during the treatment to avoid acting on a suicidal urge (Berk et al. 2004).

Brown et al. (2005) conducted a RCT of CT versus enhanced usual care (enhanced TAU). One hundred twenty recent suicide attempters were assigned to either CT or enhanced TAU and were followed for 18 months following the 10-

session CT intervention. Individuals in the CT group had significantly fewer suicide attempts than those in the usual care group. In fact, they were half as likely to attempt suicide in the follow-up period than their counterparts. Though Brown et al. (2005) provided the largest and most rigorous test of CT to prevent suicide attempt, prior tests of 5 to 10-session CT-based approaches to prevent the recurrence of suicide attempt have been similarly promising, showing reductions in suicidal ideation and trends toward lower incidence of suicide attempt among participants receiving CT but not TAU.

13.2.3 Mindfulness-Based Cognitive Therapy to Prevent Suicide

We (Latorre et al. n.d.) recently combined and adapted Mindfulness-Based Cognitive Therapy (MBCT; Segal et al. 2002, 2013) with the Safety Planning Intervention (SPI; Stanley and Brown 2008, 2012) to treat outpatients who present with current suicidal thoughts and recent suicide-related behavior despite ongoing pharmacotherapy and Veterans transitioning to outpatient treatment post-hospitalization for suicide-related concerns. MBCT is an 8-week group treatment that includes mindfulness training and some CT techniques, namely psychoeducation about depressive symptoms and relapse prevention planning. SPI, described below, is a one-session CT-based intervention focused on identifying individual warning signs and internal and external resources for managing suicidal crisis. Patients leave with a written individualized crisis survival plan for reference when suicidal thoughts and urges reemerge.

MBCT was originally designed to address the cognitive reactivity, or the onset of biased thinking subsequent to mild mood deterioration (Teasdale and Dent 1987), that makes individuals with a history of recurrent depression vulnerable to depressive relapse (Teasdale et al. 2000). In MBCT, individuals practice, through repeated in-class experiential exercises and home meditations, relating to experience with awareness, nonjudgment and non-reactivity, i.e., mindfully. In this manner, ruminative responding is impeded, or at least, identified. Mindfulness training proceeds by first, i.e., during weeks one to four, increasing attention and awareness of internal experience, including feelings, thoughts, and body sensations. Then, in the second half of MBCT, improved focus, awareness and non-reactivity to difficult feelings and thoughts, and open-monitoring of experience is attempted (Segal et al. 2013). CT techniques include psychoeducation about depression, symptoms of depression and depressogenic cognitions as well as discussion of the cognitive model of depression, and relapse prevention planning (Segal et al. 2013). CT techniques complement the mindfulness training. They serve to increase awareness of experience as opposed to change it, as in traditional CT.

Given known deficits in cognitive control among suicide attempters (Keilp et al. 2013), we thought to adapt and test MBCT-S as an add-on treatment to prevent recurrent suicide attempt among individuals at acute suicide risk. Our rationale for developing and testing MBCT-S was also bolstered by: 1. additional overlap between other mechanisms of treatment gains in MBCT and deficits specific to suicide attempters, namely blunted physiological arousal in response to social stress (Chesin et al. 2014, for a review); 2. studies showing MBCT is effective in the treatment of acute depression (Hofmann et al. 2010), and 3. studies showing slightly adapted MBCT was well-tolerated and effective for preventing depressive relapse among remitted individuals with a past suicide attempt (Barnhofer et al. 2009; Williams et al. 2013).

Adaptations to the MBCT curriculum in MBCT-S include identifying warning signs for suicide and crisis coping skills early in treatment using SPI and systematically working with suicide-related concerns and suicidal thoughts and behavior with mindfulness and CT exercises throughout treatment. To date, data from a few pilot trials (Chesin et al. 2014) suggest MBCT-S is feasible, acceptable, and helpful to outpatients and Veterans with recent suicidal behavior and current suicidal ideation.

13.2.4 A CT Intervention for Suicidal Children and Adolescents: Cognitive Behavior Therapy for Suicide Prevention

Adolescents have been found to be at significant risk for suicidal behavior (Ting et al. 2012). To address the need for a targeted intervention for suicidal behavior in adolescence, Cognitive Behavior Therapy for Suicide Prevention (CBT-SP) was developed and manualized for adolescent suicide attempters, though its authors suggest that is can also be used for adolescents who experience acute suicidal ideation (Stanley et al. 2009). CBT-SP is based on a stress-diathesis model of suicidal behavior (Mann et al. 1999) where stressors, such as interpersonal conflicts or academic difficulties, may trigger a suicidal crisis in an individual who possesses a diathesis (e.g., sex, gender, genetic predisposition) for suicidal behavior. The therapist and patient work collaboratively in this treatment to identify treatment strategies specifically tailored to the patient's proximal risk factors and stressors.

CBT-SP is divided into an acute phase and a continuation phase. During the acute phase, the patient is seen for 12–16 weekly sessions, and treatment consists of mostly individual sessions and up to six family sessions. The initial phase of acute treatment involves the following: (1) a chain analysis of the index suicide attempt; (2) safety planning; (3) psychoeducation; (4) identifying reasons for living; and (5) case conceptualization. During the middle phase of treatment, behavioral and cognitive skills are taught during individual and family therapy sessions. The final phase of acute treatment focuses on relapse prevention. During the continuation phase, the patient is seen for up to six more sessions over the course of 12 weeks. In these sessions, the focus is on generalizing the use of skills. Stanley et al. (2009)

found that CBT-SP participants found the intervention to be acceptable and helpful. Further, 86 % of adolescent participants reported that they would recommend the intervention to a friend.

13.3 Brief Interventions

Despite the promise of longer-term psychotherapeutic treatment approaches to suicidal behavior, the majority of suicidal individuals do not seek or maintain in outpatient or voluntary mental health treatment (see Lizardi and Stanley (2010) for a review; Hamdi et al. (2008)). Thus, some very brief crisis interventions have been designed to address and prevent the recurrence of suicidal behavior among patients presenting with suicidal ideation or behavior. Such interventions require at most one face-to-face individual session and can be delivered by professionals or trained paraprofessionals. These brief interventions help clinicians meet some needs of suicidal patients and attend to their legal and professional duties (American Psychiatric 2003) while respecting limits to patient willingness and ability to engage in and sometimes pay for longer-term treatment.

Brief interventions to prevent suicidal behavior can be broadly categorized into contact- and CT-based interventions. Most have been implemented and tested among patients presenting with suicidal behavior to acute care settings.

13.4 Contact Interventions

Motto and Bostrom (Motto 2001) developed a stand-alone, low-level contact intervention for individuals at high risk for suicide. Specifically, patients who refused treatment following an inpatient hospitalization for suicidal behavior or depression were sent up to 24 personalized and unique letters from inpatient staff for a period of 5 years. The letters were brief and simply offered well wishes and the opportunity for the patient to respond, if he or she felt so inclined. In a RCT, Motto and Bostrom (2001) found that the patient group who received this brief, cost-effective contact intervention had significantly lower rates of suicide for 2 years post-discharge compared to a control group who received no further follow-up contact.

Subsequent studies have not found as robust results for a contact intervention. Carter et al. (2005) tested a contact intervention where patients who presented to an emergency department for self-poisoning, regardless of suicidal intent, were sent monthly and then bi-monthly postcards for 1 year. They found that this intervention significantly reduced the incidence of self-harm behaviors. However, the proportion of individuals reengaging in self-harm behavior did not differ between those in the intervention and control groups. Beautrais et al. (2010), meanwhile, found that differences in rates of acute care visits for self-harm behaviors did not differ between those who received a contact intervention and those who did not once the number of visits for self-harm behaviors in the year prior to the index event was considered. They concluded that the contact intervention may only be efficacious for a subset of individuals who engage in suicidal behavior.

Despite these mixed findings, contact interventions continue to be implemented and tested internationally. Chen et al. (2010) developed an intervention where individuals who were seen in an emergency department or inpatient unit for self-harm behaviors received weekly supportive text messages. This intervention was found to be acceptable and was perceived to be helpful by participants. Fleischmann et al. (2008) conducted a multinational RCT of a combined intervention that consisted of a 1-hour psychoeducational session prior to discharge from the ED and brief follow-up contacts. The psychoeducational session focused on identifying risk factors and coping skills to manage suicidal urges. The authors found that suicide attempters who received the combined intervention were significantly less likely to commit suicide during an 18-month follow-up period.

13.5 CT-Based Brief Interventions

Safety Planning Intervention (SPI; Stanley and Brown 2008, 2012) is a very brief (20–45 min) manualized, single session intervention developed from evidence-based CT strategies. This intervention was developed as a stand-alone intervention for patients who present for suicidal behavior at acute care settings and remain at some suicide risk at discharge. In SPI, the patient and clinician collaboratively develop a written, customized safety plan that is given to the patient at the end of the session for patient reference in future crises. This written, personalized plan focuses on increasing the patient's crisis survival skills and restricting access to means for suicide.

The written safety plan includes six strategies for reducing suicide risk and lists (1) crisis warning sign; (2) internal coping strategies/distraction techniques; (3) social distractions; (4) friends and family members who can be called for help; (5) a personalized list of mental health professionals/agencies; and (6) a plan for restricting access to means for suicide. The first step of the SPI, identifying warning signs, is done alongside a thorough understanding of the index suicide event. Warning signs can be thoughts, feelings, behaviors, images, events, or situations and identifying specific, personal warning signs are emphasized. The next four steps include individual internal and external resources to manage suicidal crises. These steps are presented in a hierarchical fashion such that internal resources are presented before external resources (e.g., friends who may distract and friends, family, and professionals who may help in crisis). Thus, self-efficacy in the management of suicidal urges is encouraged. Patients are, however, specifically instructed to bypass the initial steps and reach out for help if they feel they are at imminent risk for suicide (Stanley and Brown 2012). SPI has been implemented in a variety of acute care settings, including many emergency departments nationwide.

The intervention has been found to be acceptable and helpful in managing suicidal urges by both staff and patients at moderate risk for suicidal behavior (AAS meeting 2013). SPI has been identified as a best practice by the American Foundation for Suicide Prevention and the Suicide Prevention Resource Center Registry for Suicide Prevention (www.sprc.org).

Several other brief crisis interventions exist, primarily focusing on psychoeducation (King et al. 2009; Kruesi et al. 1999; McManus et al. 1997) and treatment engagement (Rotheram-Borus et al. 2000) For example, "Means Restriction Education" (Kruesi et al. 1995) is a brief, stand-alone intervention for children and adolescents who are seen in EDs for psychiatric concerns. The intervention involves informing parents of their child's suicide risk, providing psychoeducation on how means restriction can reduce this risk, and developing a plan to limit access to lethal means in their home. The authors found that the intervention was useful in improving parental restriction of various lethal means, including firearms, prescription drugs, and over- the-counter medications, at 2 months follow-up (Kruesi et al. 1999). Rotheram-Borus et al. (1996) developed an intervention for adolescent female suicide attempters who presented to an emergency department. The "specialized emergency department care" intervention included three key components: (1) staff education; (2) a 20-min orientation video introducing the ED and its practices and emphasizing the importance of follow-up treatment; and (3) a structured family session to address management of future suicidal crises and to gain commitment to aftercare. Researchers found that those who received the specialized ED care intervention were significantly more likely to engage in outpatient psychotherapy, and trended toward attending more sessions and completing the full course of psychotherapy, compared to those who received TAU in the ED (Rotheram-Borus et al. 1996). Ward-Ciesielski (2013) developed a novel intervention targeting suicidal community members who possibly were not engaged in any psychiatric treatment. Suicidal community members were provided a single stand-alone session of DBT-based group treatment. The pilot study found reductions in suicidal ideation and increased use of coping skills in the month following the intervention.

In a somewhat different approach to preventing suicide among high suicide-risk adolescents, King et al. (2009), through the Youth-Nominated Support Team-Version II (YST-II), trained youth-nominated adults in means restriction, suicide warning signs, and crisis resources. Then, the adult checked-in weekly with the nominating, at-risk adolescent to provide hope and support and encourage the adolescent to maintain in treatment. King et al. (2009) conducted a RCT comparing YST-II + TAU to TAU and found that adolescents who made multiple suicide attempts and received YST-II + TAU demonstrated quicker decreases in suicidal ideation post-hospitalization. However, at follow-up, treatment gains did not persist: The control and treatment groups did not differ significantly in suicidal ideation at 6 weeks post-discharge (King et al. 2009).

13.6 Summary

The findings of these various interventions are mixed and suggest that contact interventions and targeted, brief interventions provided in acute care settings may potentially reduce suicidal behavior in the short-term when compared to TAU. However, further study is required to confirm these results.

13.7 Future Directions

Rigorous outcome studies of MBCT-S are needed. Given difficulties engaging and maintaining suicidal individuals in treatment (Lizardi and Stanley 2010, for a review), providing a brief psychosocial intervention at the time and place suicidal individuals present allows for psychoeducation and coping skills training that may otherwise be unavailable or not provided to individuals who need it. A few promising brief interventions exist, but development and testing of additional such interventions and more rigorous testing of the most promising available brief interventions, e.g., SPI, are needed. Meanwhile, an evidence base supporting CT and DBT for suicidal behavior is available. Thus, empirically grounded CT and DBT treatment refinement and empirically supported personalization of treatment, i.e., matching suicidal individuals to specific treatments based on empirical evidence of what works for whom, become the logical next steps in providing efficient and cost-effective psychosocial treatment to suicidal individuals.

Treatment refinement can be informed by dismantling and mediational studies which provide information on treatment components or changes driving treatment gains. Both CT for depression and MBCT to prevent the recurrence of depression among previously depressed patients have been subjected to dismantling studies, with no additive benefit discerned for the defining aspect of either treatment (i.e., training and practice in challenging thoughts and meditation, respectively) (Jacobson et al. 1996; Williams et al. 2013). Active ingredients of DBT, adapted CT, MBCT, or effective brief interventions to prevent suicide among high suicide-risk individuals are unknown. An effort to identify whether skills training, individual therapy, or both are the necessary and active ingredient(s) in DBT, however, is underway (Lynch et al. 2007). Similarly, few meditational studies positing and testing mechanisms of treatment gains among suicidal patients have been conducted. Lynch et al. (2006) posited DBT reduces suicidal behavior and non-suicidal self-injury by increasing mindfulness, including attentional control, and decreasing maladaptive or ineffective emotion regulation. Perroud et al. (2012) recently found increased acceptance without judgment, an aspect of mindfulness, explained decreased BPD symptomatology among DBT participants.

Where meditational or dismantling studies can determine effective components or refine targets of existing treatment, moderational studies may help determine what works for whom. Suicide attempters are a heterogeneous group, with findings from multiple studies showing, for example, differences in trajectories to suicide attempt between individuals with impulsive-aggressive traits and those who are chronically and persistently depressed (Carballo et al. 2008). Though most CT-based interventions, including DBT, CT to prevent suicide attempt and SPI, are somewhat personalized, matching individuals with either impulsive-aggressive traits or pessimistic tendencies, for example, to the most appropriate and likely effective treatment from the outset requires formal study of the effect of these traits on treatment outcome. To date, predictors of treatment response have been investigated in a only a few empirical studies of suicidal populations (Koerner 2013). Verheul et al. (2003) found individuals with more lifetime episodes of NSSI randomized to DBT as opposed to TAU had fewer suicide attempts during treatment. Williams et al. (2013) found individuals who were previously depressed and in most cases had made a lifetime suicide attempt benefited equally, in terms of time to relapse, from slightly adapted MBCT + TAU, 8 weeks of group Cognitive Psychological Education (Williams et al. 2010) + TAU, and TAU. However, participants with more significant histories of childhood abuse and neglect responded better to the addition of MBCT (Williams et al. 2013). Thus, third-wave behavioral treatments, i.e., those that incorporate mindfulness such as DBT and MBCT-S, offered in addition to medication management may be indicated for suicidal individuals with significant histories of deliberate self-harm or childhood adversity, though more studies are needed to determine whether MBCT-S works for acutely suicidal populations before predictor studies of MBCT-S are undertaken. Further, additional predictor studies of DBT and predictor studies of CT for suicide prevention and brief interventions are needed.

13.8 Conclusions

In this chapter, we have outlined longer-term and very brief psychosocial interventions to prevent suicide. We have also reviewed the evidence base for these treatments and suggested directions for future research aimed at providing appropriate, efficient, and thus hopefully effective psychosocial treatment to suicidal individuals.

References

American Psychiatric A (2003) American psychiatric association practice guidelines for the treatment of patients with suicidal behavior: Compendium 2003. American Psychiatric Association, Washington

Association AP (2000) Diagnostic and statistical manual of mental disorder, 4th edn. APA, Washington

Barnhofer T, Crane C, Hargus E, Amarasinghe M, Winder R, Williams JMG (2009) Mindfulness-based cognitive therapy as a treatment for chronic depression: a preliminary study. Behav Res Ther 47(5):366–373. doi:10.1016/j.brat.2009.01.019

Beautrais AL, Gibb SJ, Faulkner A, Fergusson DM, Mulder RT (2010) Postcard intervention for repeat self-harm: randomised controlled trial. Br J Psychiatry 197(1):55–60
Beck AT (1976) Cognitive therapy and the emotional disorders. Meridian, New York
Berk MS, Henriques GR, Warman DM, Brown GK, Beck AT (2004) A cognitive therapy intervention for suicide attempters: an overview of the treatment and case examples. Cogn Behav Pract 11(3):265–277. doi: http://dx.doi.org/10.1016/S1077-7229(04)80041-5
Brown GK, Henriques GR, Ratto C et al (2002) Cognitive therapy treatment manual for suicide attempters. University of Pennsylvania, Philadelphia
Brown GK, Ten Have T, Henriques GR, Xie SX, Hollander JE, Beck AT (2005) Cognitive therapy for the prevention of suicide attempts: a randomized controlled trial. J Am Med Assoc 294 (5):563–570. doi:10.1001/jama.294.5.563
Carballo JJ, Akamnonu CP, Oquendo MA (2008) Neurobiology of suicidal behavior. An integration of biological and clinical findings. Arch Suicide Res 12(2):93–110. doi:10.1080/13811110701857004
Carter GL, Clover K, Whyte IM, Dawson AH, D'Este C (2005) Postcards from the EDge project: randomised controlled trial of an intervention using postcards to reduce repetition of hospital treated deliberate self poisoning. Br Med J 331(7520):805–807
Carter GL, Willcox CH, Lewin TJ, Conrad AM, Bendit N (2010) Hunter DBT project: randomized controlled trial of dialectical behaviour therapy in women with borderline personality disorder. Aust NZJ Psychiatry 44(2):162–173. doi:10.3109/00048670903393621
Chen H, Mishara BL, Liu XX (2010) A pilot study of mobile telephone message interventions with suicide attempters in China. Crisis J Crisis Interv Suicide Prev 31(2):109–112. doi:10.1027/0227-5910/a000017
Chesin MS (2014) Scale of suicidal ideation scores pre- and post- MBCT-S. Unpublished raw data
Clarkin JF, Levy KN, Lenzenweger MF, Kernberg OF (2007) Evaluating three treatments for borderline personality disorder: a multiwave study. Am J Psychiatry 164:922–928
Favazza AR (1998) The coming of age of self-mutilation. J Nerv Ment Dis 186(5):259–268
Fleischmann A, Bertolote JM, Wasserman D, De Leo D, Bolhari J, Botega NJ, Thanh HTT (2008) Effectiveness of brief intervention and contact for suicide attempters: a randomized controlled trial in five countries. Bull World Health Organ 86:703–709
Goldsmith S, Pellmar T, Kleinman A, Bunney W (2002) Reducing suicide: a national imperative. National Academy Press, Washington
Hamdi E, Price S, Qassem T, Amin Y, Jones D (2008) Suicides not in contact with mental health services: risk indicators and determinants of referral. J Ment Health 17(4):398–409. doi:10.1080/09638230701506234
Hofmann SG, Sawyer AT, Witt AA, Oh D (2010) The effect of mindfulness-based therapy on anxiety and depression: a meta-analytic review. J Consult Clin Psychol 78(2):169–183. doi:10.1037/a0018555
Jacobson CM, Gould M (2007) The epidemiology and phenomenology of non-suicidal self-injurious behavior among adolescents: a critical review of the literature. Arch Suicide Res 11 (2):129–147. doi:10.1080/13811110701247602
Jacobson NS, Dobson KS, Truax PA, Addis ME, Koerner K, Gollan JK, Prince SE (1996) A component analysis of cognitive-behavioral treatment for depression. J Consult Clin Psychol 64(2):295–304. doi:10.1037/0022-006x.64.2.295
Keilp JG, Gorlyn M, Russell M, Oquendo MA, Burke AK, Harkavy-Friedman J, Mann JJ (2013) Neuropsychological function and suicidal behavior: attention control, memory and executive dysfunction in suicide attempt. Psychol Med 43(03):539–551. doi:10.1017/S0033291712001419
King CA, Klaus N, Kramer A, Venkataraman S, Quinlan P, Gillespie B (2009) The youth-nominated support Teamâ€"Version for suicidal adolescents: a randomized controlled intervention trial. J Consult Clin Psychol 77(5):880–893. doi:10.1037/a0016552
Koerner K (2013) What must you know and do to get good outcomes with DBT? Behav Ther 44 (4):568–579

Koons CR, Robins CJ, Lindsey Tweed J, Lynch TR, Gonzalez AM, Morse JQ, Bastian LA (2001) Efficacy of dialectical behavior therapy in women veterans with borderline personality disorder. Behav Ther 32(2):371–390. doi:10.1016/S0005-7894(01)80009-5

Kruesi M, Grossman G, Hirsch J (1995) Five minutes of your time may mean a lifetime to a suicidal adolescent. Ronald McDonald House Charities, University of Illinois-Chicago, Chicago

Kruesi MJP, Grossman J, Pennington JM, Woodward PJ, Duda D, Hirsch JG (1999) Suicide and violence prevention: parent education in the emergency department. J Am Acad Child Adolesc Psychiatry 38(3):250–255. doi:10.1097/00004583-199903000-00010

Latorre M, Chesin MS, Zanetich K, Kline A (n.d.) Mindfulness-based cognitive therapy for individuals at risk of suicide treatment manual. Department of Psychiatry, Columbia University, New York

Linehan MM (1987) Dialectical behavioral therapy: a cognitive behavioral approach to parasuicide. J Pers Disord 1(4):328–333

Linehan MM (1993) Cognitive-behavioral treatment of borderline personality disorder. Guilford, New York

Linehan MM, Armstrong HE, Suarez A, Allmon D, Heard HL (1991) Cognitive-behavioral treatment of chronically parasuicidal borderline patients. Arch Gen Psychiatry 48(12): 1060–1064. doi:10.1001/archpsyc.1991.01810360024003

Linehan MM, Schmidt H, Dimeff LA, Craft JC, Kanter J, Comtois KA (1999) Dialectical behavior therapy for patients with borderline personality disorder and drug-dependence. Am J Addict 8 (4):279–292. doi:10.1080/105504999305686

Linehan MM, Comtois K, Murray AM et al (2006) Two-year randomized controlled trial and follow-up of dialectical behavior therapy vs therapy by experts for suicidal behaviors and borderline personality disorder. Arch Gen Psychiatry 63(7):757–766. doi: 10.1001/archpsyc.63.7.757

Lizardi D, Stanley B (2010) Treatment engagement: a neglected aspect in the psychiatric care of suicidal patients. Psychiatr Serv 61:1183–1191

Lynch TR, Chapman AL, Rosenthal MZ, Kuo JR, Linehan MM (2006) Mechanisms of change in dialectical behavior therapy: theoretical and empirical observations. J Clin Psychol 62 (4):459–480

Lynch TR, Trost WT, Salsman N, Linehan MM (2007) Dialectical behavior therapy for borderline personality disorder. Ann Rev Clin Psychol 3(1):181–205. doi:10.1146/annurev.clinpsy.2.022305.095229

Mann JJ, Waternaux C, Haas GL, Malone KM (1999) Toward a clinical model of suicidal behavior in psychiatric patients. Am J Psychiatry 156:181–189

McMain SF, Links PS, Gnam WH, Guimond T, Cardish RJ, Korman L, Streiner DL (2009) A randomized trial of dialectical behavior therapy versus general psychiatric management for borderline personality disorder. Am J Psychiatry 166:1365–1374

McMain SF, Guimond T, Streiner DL, Cardish RJ, Links PS (2012) Dialectical behavior therapy compared with general psychiatric management for borderline personality disorder: clinical outcomes and functioning over a 2-year follow-up. Am J Psychiatry 169:650–661

McManus BL, Kruesi MJP, Dontes AE, Defazio CR, Piotrowski JT, Woodward PJ (1997) Child and adolescent suicide attempts: an opportunity for emergency departments to provide injury prevention education. Am J Emerg Med 15(4):357–360. doi:10.1016/s0735-6757(97)90124-8

Motto JABAG (2001) A randomized controlled trial of postcrisis suicide prevention. Psychiatr Serv 52:828–833

National Center for Injury Prevention and Control, C. f. D. C. a. P (2012) Web-based injury statistics query and reporting system (WISQARS). www.cdc.gov/ncipc/wisqars

Panos PT, Jackson JW, Hasan O, Panos A (2013) Meta-analysis and systematic review assessing the efficacy of dialectical behavior therapy (DBT). Res Soc Work Pract. doi:10.1177/1049731513503047

Perroud N, Nicastro R, Jermann F, Huguelet P (2012) Mindfulness skills in borderline personality disorder patients during dialectical behavior therapy: preliminary results. Int J Psychiatry Clin Pract 16(3):189–196. doi:10.3109/13651501.2012.674531

Pistorello J, Fruzzetti AE, MacLane C, Gallop R, Iverson KM (2012) Dialectical behavior therapy (DBT) applied to college students: a randomized clinical trial. J Consul Clin Psychol 80 (6):982–994. doi:10.1037/a0029096

Rotheram-Borus MJ, Piacentini J, Van Rossem R, Graae F, Cantwell C, Castro-Blanco D, Feldman J (1996) Enhancing treatment adherence with a specialized emergency room program for adolescent suicide attempters. J Am Acad Child Adolesc Psychiatry 35(5):654–663. doi:10.1097/00004583-199605000-00021

Rotheram-Borus MJ, Piacentini J, Cantwell C, Belin TR, Song J (2000) The 18-month impact of an emergency room intervention for adolescent female suicide attempters. J Consul Clin Psychol 68(6):1081–1093. doi:10.1037/0022-006x.68.6.1081

Segal ZV, Williams JMG, Teasdale JG (2002) Mindfulness-based cognitive therapy for depression: a new approach to preventing relapse. Guilford, New York

Segal ZV, Williams JMG, Teasdale JD (2013) Mindfulness-based cognitive therapy for depression, 2nd edn. Guilford, New York

Stanley B, Brown GK (2008) Safety plan treatment manual to reduce suicide risk: veteran version. United States Department of Veterans Affairs, Washington

Stanley B, Brown GK (2012) Safety planning intervention: a brief intervention to mitigate suicide risk. Cogn Behav Pract 19(2):256–264

Stanley B, Brown G, Brent DA, Wells K, Poling K, Curry J, Hughes J (2009) Cognitive-behavioral therapy for suicide prevention (CBT-SP): treatment model, feasibility, and acceptability. J Am Acad Child Adolesc Psychiatry 48(10):1005–1013. doi:10.1097/CHI.0b013e3181b5dbfe

Teasdale JD, Dent J (1987) Cognitive vulnerability to depression: An investigation of two hypotheses. Br J Clin Psychol 26(2):113–126. doi:10.1111/j.2044-8260.1987.tb00737.x

Teasdale JD, Segal ZV, Williams JMG, Ridgeway VA, Soulsby JM, Lau MA (2000) Prevention of relapse/recurrence in major depression by mindfulness-based cognitive therapy. J Consul Clin Psychol 68(4):615–623. doi:10.1037/0022-006x.68.4.615

Ting SA, Sullivan AF, Boudreaux ED, Miller I, Camargo CA (2012) Trends in US emergency department visits for attempted suicide and self-inflicted injury, 1993–2008. Gen Hosp Psychiatry 34(5):557–565

Turner RM (2000) Naturalistic evaluation of dialectical behavior therapy-oriented treatment for borderline personality disorder. Cogn Behav Pract 7(4):413–419. doi: http://dx.doi.org/10.1016/S1077-7229(00)80052-8

Verheul R, Van Den Bosch LMC, Koeter MWJ, De Ridder MAJ, Stijen T, Van Den Brink W (2003) Dialectical behaviour therapy for women with borderline personality disorder: 12-month, randomised clinical trial in The Netherlands. Br J Psychiatry 182(2):135–140. doi:10.1192/bjp.02.184

Ward-Ciesielski EF (2013) An open pilot feasibility study of a brief dialectical behavior therapy skills-based intervention for suicidal individuals. Suicide Life Threat Behav 43(3):324–335. doi:10.1111/sltb.12019

Williams JM, Russell I, Crane C, et al (2010) Staying well after depression: trial design and protocol. BMC Psychiatry 10(1):23

Williams JMG, Crane C, Barnhofer T, Brennan K, Duggan D et al (2013) Mindfulness-based cognitive therapy for preventing relapse in recurrent depression: a randomized dismantling trial. http://oxfordmindfulness.org/science/publications/

World Health Organization (2012) Public health action for the prevention of suicide: A framework. World Health Organization, Geneva

Chapter 14
Cognitive Therapy with Suicidal Patients

Michael E. Thase

Abstract Cognitive Therapy is both the best-studied time-limited psychotherapy for treatment of depressive disorders and one of the few forms of psychotherapy that has been specifically adapted for treatment of acutely suicidal individuals. In Cognitive Therapy for Suicide Prevention the primary targets for intervention are hopelessness, suicidal ideations, and the behaviors that have been associated with suicide attempts in the past. Acute suicidal risk is mitigated by collaboratively developing a safety plan and hopelessness explicitly counteracted by identifying and strengthening reasons for living and social support. In the one controlled study conducted to date, patients randomly allocated to Cognitive Therapy for Suicide Prevention were significantly less likely to make another suicide attempt than were those receiving usual care.

14.1 Introduction

Cognitive Therapy, which was developed more than 30 years ago by Aaron T. Beck and colleagues (Beck 1976; Beck et al. 1979), is the best-studied time-limited treatment for depression (Cuijpers et al. 2008). In Cognitive Therapy, the therapist helps the depressed patient learn to identify and modify the automatic negative thoughts that can trigger and sustain dysphoric mood states. Grouped within a broader class of interventions known as Cognitive Behavior Therapy (CBT), treatment also usually incorporates behavioral activation and other related interventions to address maladaptive behaviors and improve coping skills. For the purposes of this chapter, these terms will be used interchangeably. As most depressed patients have some thoughts about hopelessness, death, and/or suicidal

M.E. Thase (✉)
Department of Psychiatry, Perelman School of Medicine, University of Pennsylvania and Philadelphia Veterans Affairs Medical Center, 3535 Market Street, Suite 670, Philadelphia, PA 19104, USA
e-mail: thase@mail.med.upenn.edu

K.E. Cannon and T.J. Hudzik (eds.), *Suicide: Phenomenology and Neurobiology*,
DOI 10.1007/978-3-319-09964-4_14

ideations, it is common to therapists to address these symptoms, typically beginning within the first few minutes of the very first session. Nevertheless, in conventional Cognitive Therapy hopelessness and suicidal ideations are but one of the constellation of signs and symptoms of the depressive syndrome. A more focused intervention—Cognitive Therapy for Suicide Prevention (Wenzel et al. 2009)—was therefore developed specifically to treat individuals in suicidal crises. Cognitive Therapy for Suicide Prevention focuses on suicidal ideations and suicidal behaviors as the principal targets of therapy. Thus, in Cognitive Therapy of Suicide Prevention, the therapist helps the patient to recognize the various triggers and risk factors that are proximally related to suicidal ideation or behavior and then to practice specific coping and problem-solving strategies that are intended to prevent or attenuate subsequent suicidal crises. This chapter will provide an overview of Cognitive Therapy for Suicide Prevention, as well as a brief summary of the results of research using this approach to treatment.

14.1.1 Methods of Cognitive Therapy for Suicide Prevention

As briefly described below, Cognitive Therapy for Suicide Prevention consists of four phases: (a) the early phase of treatment, (b) the cognitive case formulation, (c) the middle phase of treatment, and (d) the later phase of treatment.

14.1.1.1 Early Phase of Treatment

The first phase of Cognitive Therapy for Suicide Prevention is the most important because it is focused on ensuring patient safety and because it sets the tone for all that follows. Like other forms of Cognitive Therapy, the therapist fosters a "collaborative empirical" atmosphere and is entrusted to engage the patient into a psychoeducational treatment process. Without overpromising (i.e., Cognitive Therapy doesn't help everyone), the therapist engenders a cautiously optimistic attitude, drawing upon the knowledge that this approach to treatment has helped many people in similar or even worse circumstances. Beyond starting to teach about therapy and how it helps to prevent suicide, the therapist must conduct an assessment of suicide risk and develop a Safety Plan in the initial session. Consistent with the psychoeducational nature of therapy, the therapist teaches the patient about the limits of privacy and confidentiality, the potential risks, and benefits of treatment, provides an overview of the methods used in therapy. If the patient has a past treatment history, it is helpful discuss what aspects of therapy were—and were not—helpful in the past. It is the therapist's responsibility to obtain the patient's commitment to give treatment a chance to work, including agreement to consistently attend sessions, actively participate, and complete homework assignments.

The assessment suicide risk includes both narrative and psychometric sources, as well as information from tools such as the Beck Hopelessness Scale. Mindful of the time available and multiple competing priorities, it is almost always helpful for the patient to have the opportunity to tell his or her own story. Most patients will describe a suicidal crisis that has been provoked or at least temporally preceded by an adverse life event. Enculturation to Cognitive Therapy methods typically begins seamlessly as the therapists asks about the patient's reactions—thoughts, feelings, and actions—that accompanied the life event and subsequent crisis.

For a patient who has attempted to end his or her life, it is important to try to clarify the point or moment at which suicide was chosen as the course of action. By focusing on this moment, the therapist may be able to elicit characteristic automatic negative thoughts that help to justify or underpin this decision. A question such as "what was going through your mind" "when you decided to kill yourself" is likely to lead to uncovering self-statements such as "I can't stand this pain any longer" or "This situation is intolerable", along with the accompanying emotions of despair or intense sadness. As relatively few suicidal people can easily differentiate thoughts and feelings, therapy becomes an iterative process to learn to accept feelings as an understandable consequence of thoughts and, once detached (at least to some extent) from overwhelmingly strong feelings, to test the accuracy of the thoughts.

In addition to identifying the thoughts, feelings and actions that preceded the crisis, the therapist should try to elicit the patient's reactions to surviving the attempt.

As regret about surviving a suicide attempt may be associated with an increased likelihood of subsequent attempts, it is important to have this information early on.

Novice Cognitive Therapists sometimes compromise the therapeutic alliance by overzealously challenging the accuracy or reasonableness of the patient's story early in the narrative process. Instead, it is more useful to first listen, carefully and empathically, so that the patient feels understood. Likewise, even good advice about ways to cope better can have an oft-putting effect if timed too early in the interaction. To ensure that a collaborative alliance is developing, the therapist periodically solicits feedback about the patient's perception of how the session is going and whether or not the patient is feeling understood.

14.1.1.2 Safety Planning

Following the suicide risk assessment, developing a Safety Plan is the next priority during the first session of treatment. The Safety Plan is an explicit, written list of strategies that the suicidal patient agrees to do, as well as a list of resources that the patients agrees to use if he or she develops a suicidal crisis (Stanley and Brown 2013). Whenever possible, the plan should be written in patients' own words and kept close at hand so that it can be accessed on a moment's notice. For example, an individual may keep a hard copy of the plan in his or her purse or wallet and an electronic copy on his or smart phone and/or laptop. A well-crafted Safety Plan should include the following elements:

(1) a way to recognize warning signs that might precede a suicidal crisis;
(2) a summary of coping strategies that can be used without the help of another person;
(3) a list of people—friends and family members—who may be able to help in a crisis;
(4) therapists, psychiatrists, and other mental health professionals, as well as after-hours services and agencies; and
(5) an agreement to remove access to lethal means of completing suicide.

The therapist collaborates with the patient to identify actions that have worked in previous crises and to develop a personalized hierarchy of coping strategies. The proximal goal is to "ride out" a crisis by following each step of the Safety Plan until the crisis is resolved. There likewise should be an explicit discussion about making the environment safe, recognizing that some patients are very reluctant to part with their firearms. The right to keep a firearm sometimes conflates a strongly held political belief with an often unspoken lethal escape fantasy, namely that the individual finds is oddly comforting to know that the gun can always be used to end one's misery if things get too bad. Nevertheless, given the fact that guns are commonly used in suicide attempts and have high lethality, it is the therapist's obligation to ensure that all guns and ammunition are removed whenever practicable. It is sometimes more agreeable if the firearm/ammunition is kept by a trusted person, such as a family member or trusted friend, who shares the patient's values about firearm rights. The potentially touchy topic about when (and if) the property can be returned should be deferred for another day.

The Safety Plan should be continuously revised throughout the course of Cognitive Therapy for Suicide Prevention as new information is learned and as new skills are learned. Although best thought of as part of a fully developed intervention, the Safety Plan can be used as a stand-alone intervention in acute care settings such as emergency rooms or crisis intervention services (Stanley and Brown 2008, 2012).

14.1.2 Research

Surprisingly few intervention studies have been conducted in suicidal individuals and, to date, only one randomized controlled trial has evaluated the utility of Cognitive Therapy for Suicidal Patients. In this study, which was conducted by investigators at the University of Pennsylvania (Brown et al. 2005), consenting patients who presented to a medical or psychiatric emergency department following a suicide attempt were randomized to receive Usual Care with or without Cognitive Therapy for Suicidal Patients. This study included 120 individuals age 16 and older; about two-thirds of the study group was female. Although the study was not limited to patients with Major Depressive Disorder (MDD), most (92 %) met criteria for MDD, and 68 % had a comorbid substance use disorder. The majority of participants (58 %) had recently attempted suicide by overdose of pills. Cognitive Therapy for Suicide Prevention was provided by experienced therapists; on average participants received about 10 sessions of individual therapy across 6 months of protocol treatment. After treatment ended, participants entered a naturalistic follow-up was extended for an additional 12 months.

Across the full 18 month study period, 42 % of the participants assigned to the Usual Care control condition made another suicide attempt, as compared to only 24 % of the group that received Cognitive Therapy for Suicide Prevention (Brown et al. 2005). This nearly 50 % reduction in the risk of suicidal behavior was both clinically meaningful and statistically significant. Participants who received Cognitive Therapy for Suicide Prevention also had significantly lower scores on the Beck Depression Inventory and the Beck Hopelessness Scale as compared to those who received only Usual Care (Brown et al. 2005). Although Cognitive Therapy for Suicide Prevention did not fully eradicate suicidality in this high-risk sample, it did significantly reduce the risk of repeat suicidal behavior and resulted in significant improvements in symptomatic status.

A second study is underway evaluating Cognitive Therapy for Suicide Prevention in an extremely high-risk population, namely older men presenting for treatment with depression and suicidal ideation. Although it will be several years before the results of this study are available, the findings will provide and important replication and extension of this model of treatment in a patient group that is truly in need of effective treatment.

Another related line of research pertains to the model of therapy developed by Marsha Linehan, Dialectical Behavior Therapy (Linehan 1993). Although originally developed primarily for treatment of parasuicidal behaviors among individuals with borderline personality disorder (Linehan et al. 1991, 2006), this model of treatment has recently been adapted to work with individuals with more chronic, treatment resistant depressive disorders (see, e.g., Kahl et al. 2012). It therefore would be worthwhile to compare the merits of these differently targeted psychosocial interventions, including patients with and without significant personality pathology.

14.1.3 Conclusions

Suicide is potentially preventable cause of death and effective treatment depression is one of the most important ways to reduce the risk of suicide. Among the several strategies that have been specifically developed to work with suicidal patients, Cognitive Therapy for Suicidal Patients builds upon 30+ years of research to provide an efficient and targeted form of individual therapy that directly addresses both the proximal and more remote factors that are associated with the risk suicide.

References

Beck AT (1976) Cognitive therapy and the emotional disorders. Meridian, New York

Beck AT, Rush AJ, Shaw BF, Emery G (1979) Cognitive therapy of depression. Guilford, New York

Brown GK, Tenhave T, Henriques GR, Xie SX, Hollander JE, Beck AT (2005) Cognitive therapy for the prevention of suicide attempts: a randomized controlled trial. J Am Med Assoc 294:563–570

Cuijpers P, van Straten A, van Oppen P, Andersson G (2008) Are psychological and pharmacologic interventions equally effective in the treatment of adult depressive disorders? A meta-analysis of comparative studies. J Clin Psychiatry 2008(69):1675–1685

Kahl KG, Winter L, Schweiger U (2012) The third wave of cognitive behavioural therapies: what is new and what is effective? Curr Opin Psychiatry 25:522–528

Linehan MM (1993) Cognitive-behavioral treatment of borderline personality disorder. Guilford Publications, New York

Linehan MM, Armstrong HE, Suarez A et al (1991) Cognitive-behavioral treatment of chronically parasuicidal borderline patients. Arch Gen Psychiatry 48:1060–1064

Linehan MM, Comtois KA, Murray AM et al (2006) Two-year randomized controlled trial and follow-up of dialectical behavior therapy vs. therapy by experts for suicidal behavior and borderline personality disorder. Arch Gen Psychiatry 63:757–766

Stanley B, Brown GK (2012) Safety planning intervention: a brief intervention to mitigate suicide risk. Cogn Behav Pract 19(2):256–264

Stanley B, Brown GK (with Karlin B, Kemp J, von Bergen H) (2008) Safety plan treatment manual to reduce suicide risk: Veteran version. United States Department of Veterans Affairs, Washington, DC

Wenzel A, Brown GK, Beck AT (2009) Cognitive therapy for suicidal patients: scientific and clinical applications. American Psychological Association, Washington, DC

Part IV
Clinical and Preclinical Neurobiology

Chapter 15
Human Imaging Studies of Suicidal Behavior and its Risk Factors

Kees van Heeringen, Stefanie Desmyter and Stijn Bijttebier

Abstract This chapter reviews neuroimaging studies of suicidal behavior and its major risk factors, and discusses the relevance of the findings for the understanding, prediction, and prevention of suicide. Functional and structural imaging studies show a reduced prefrontal perfusion or metabolism and a blunted increase in activation when challenged in association with a history of suicide attempts. Moreover, impairment of the prefrontal serotonergic system in association with suicidal behavior is demonstrated in a number of studies. Recent structural and functional imaging studies show changes in cortical and subcortical areas and their connections in association with suicidal behavior and risk factors, such as hopelessness, impulsivity, and aggression. The global picture that emerges from these studies reflects the involvement of a fronto-cingulo-striatal network in the development of suicidal behavior. The relevance of these findings for our understanding of suicidal behavior is supported by findings from neuropsychological studies in suicide attempters, showing dysfunctions in neuropsychological domains, which involve similar neuroanatomical regions. Further study is needed to translate the increasing knowledge from neuroimaging studies in clinical tools for the prediction and prevention of suicidal behavior.

In spite of increasing evidence, the prevention of suicide still poses major challenges at societal and individual levels. Clinicians are unable to predict the occurrence of suicidal behavior at the level of the individual. Depressed patients are very often frightened by their suicidal thoughts, because patient prediction of future suicidal behavior based on current thoughts appears impossible. In addition, when suicide risk is considered high, its management is challenging because of the poor evidence base. For instance, we cannot predict the individual response to treatment in terms of decrease in suicide risk, and interventions, be it pharmacological or psychotherapeutic, may even be associated with an increased risk of suicidal behavior. Even if there is a positive response to treatment in terms of a reduction in

---

K. van Heeringen (✉) · S. Desmyter · S. Bijttebier
Unit for Suicide Research, Department of Psychiatry and Medical Psychology, University Hospital, 1K12F de Pintelaan 185, 9000 Gent, Belgium
e-mail: cornelis.vanheeringen@ugent.be

K.E. Cannon and T.J. Hudzik (eds.), *Suicide: Phenomenology and Neurobiology*,
DOI 10.1007/978-3-319-09964-4_15

suicide risk, we do not know how and why this happens. Limitations at the level of assessment of risk and prediction of treatment response thus constitute two major barriers to effective suicide prevention. This chapter will discuss the potential contribution of brain imaging to suicide prevention through the identification of markers of risk and targets of treatment.

15.1 Imaging Studies of Suicidal Behavior

15.1.1 Structural Imaging

Structural imaging studies of suicidal behavior, using MRI, have focused on changes in white and gray matter.

Six studies demonstrated an association between suicidal behavior and white matter hyperintensities, i.e., deep white matter hyperintensities, periventricular hyperintensities, or subcortical matter hyperintensities (Ahearn et al. 2001; Ehrlich et al. 2004, 2005; Pompili et al. 2007, 2008; Serafini et al. 2011). Noteworthy is the study by Serafini et al. (2011), in which the relationship was studied between affective temperamental profiles, white matter hyperintensities, and suicidal behavior in patients with mood disorders. They found that patients with higher dysthymia and lower hyperthymia were more likely to have white matter hyperintensities and recent suicide attempts.

Monkul et al. (2007) (compared fronto-limbic brain structures between females diagnosed with a unipolar mood disorder and a history of one or more suicide attempt(s), unipolar females without such a history and female healthy controls. The presence of a history of suicide attempt(s) was associated with smaller bilateral orbitofrontal gray matter volumes and larger right amygdala volumes. There were no differences in gray matter volumes between unipolar patients without a history of suicide attempt(s) and healthy controls.

Three studies investigated gray and white matter in the brains of patients suffering from schizophrenia in association with suicidal behavior. Male patients with a history of suicide attempt(s), compared to those without such a history, showed a significant reduction in gray matter density in the left superior temporal gyrus and the left orbitofrontal cortex (Aguilar et al. 2008). Rusch et al. (2008) found significantly larger bilateral inferior frontal (and posterior orbital) white matter volumes in patients with a history of suicide attempts as compared to patients without such a history and to healthy controls. No other significant white or gray matter volume differences were observed. Spoletini et al. (2011) studied selected subcortical regions and found a significant increase in right amygdala volumes in association with a history of suicide attempts in individuals suffering from schizophrenia when compared to such individuals without a history of suicide attempts and healthy controls.

Numbers of suicidal behaviors and pituitary gland volume were correlated in young patients diagnosed with borderline personality disorder and with minimal exposure to treatment Jovev et al. (2008). Studying the association between a history of attempted suicide and anterior corpus callosum volumes, Matsuo et al. (2010) found no differences between bipolar patients with a history of suicide and those without such a history. Cyprien et al. (2011) however, studied the association between corpus callosum size and suicidal behavior in a large general population sample of elderly persons. While controlling for age, gender, childhood trauma, head trauma, and total brain volume, the area of the posterior third of the corpus callosum was significantly smaller in suicide attempters than in affective controls and healthy controls. Diminished interhemispheric connectivity may thus play a role in the pathophysiology of suicidal behavior.

Caplan et al. (2010) studied frontotemporal volumes in pediatric epilepsy patients according to the presence or absence of suicidal ideation. Suicidal ideation was associated with smaller right orbitofrontal gyrus white matter volumes and larger left temporal lobe gray matter volumes.

A history of suicide attempts in elderly male patients with late-onset depression was associated with decreased volumes of gray matter and white matter in the frontal, temporal, and parietal regions and the insula, lentiform nucleus, midbrain, and the cerebellum when compared to healthy controls. A particularly marked regional volume reduction was noticed in the dorsal medial prefrontal cortex (Hwang et al. 2010). Goodman et al. (2011) studied the volume of the anterior cingulate gyrus in adolescent patients with borderline personality disorder and comorbid depression and in healthy controls. They found smaller gray but not white matter volumes in the patients than in the controls, while, in the patient group, a greater number of suicide attempts was associated with smaller volumes of the anterior cingulate region.

Baldacara et al. (2011) found no effect of a history of suicide attempts on cerebellar volumes in euthymic bipolar type 1 patients.

Benedetti et al. (2011) studied gray matter volumes in currently depressed bipolar patients, some of whom had a history of suicide attempts, while others were treated with lithium. Suicide attempters showed reduced gray matter volumes in several brain areas, including the dorsolateral prefrontal cortex, orbitofrontal cortex, anterior cingulate, superior temporal cortex, parieto-occipital cortex, and basal ganglia. Noteworthy is the finding that long-term lithium treatment was associated with increased gray matter volumes in the same areas in which suicide attempters showed decreased gray matter volumes.

Wagner et al. (2011, 2012) (used a different approach to study the vulnerability to suicidal behavior by comparing voxel-based morphometric properties in the brains of depressed patients at high risk of suicide (as indicated by a personal or familial history of suicidal behavior), depressed patients without such a risk and matched healthy controls. Patients with a high risk of suicide showed significantly decreased gray matter density in a fronto-striato-limbic network when compared to the healthy controls and in caudate and rostral anterior cingulate cortex when compared to nonhigh risk patients. The same research group investigated prefrontal cortical thickness in similar study groups (Wagner et al. 2011, 2012). Patients with high risk of suicide showed a significantly thinner cortex in the left dorsolateral, ventrolateral prefrontal cortex, and the anterior cingulate in contrast to nonhigh risk patients. Taken together, the findings provide evidence for structural brain alterations in depressed patients at high risk of suicide in the fronto-cingulo-striatal network that is strongly involved in reward processing and emotional control.

Within a group of persons with borderline personality disorders, those with a history of suicide attempts showed significantly decreased gray matter in the left insula when compared to nonattempters. High-lethality attempters had significant decreases in the right temporal gyrus, right orbitofrontal gyrus, right insular cortex, and right parahippocampal gyrus when compared to low-lethality attempters (Soloff et al. 2012).

Gray matter changes in brain regions in association with suicidal behavior in psychotic patients were studied by Giakoumatos et al. (2013)

Compared to nonattempters, attempters had significantly less gray matter volume in bilateral inferior temporal and superior temporal cortices, left superior parietal, thalamus and supramarginal regions, right insula, and superior frontal and rostral middle frontal regions. Among attempters, a history of high lethality attempts was associated with significantly smaller volumes in the left lingual gyrus and right cuneus. Compared to nonattempters, low-lethality attempters had significant decreases in the left supramarginal gyrus, thalamus, and the right insula.

15.1.2 Functional Imaging

Oquendo et al. (2003) published a pivotal functional imaging study of the involvement of the serotonergic neurotransmission system in suicidal behavior using ^{18}F-FDG PET. Depressed high-lethality and low-lethality suicide attempters were scanned after a single-blind placebo and after the serotonin agonist fenfluramine hydrochloride administration on a second day. Secondary and proportional to the postsynaptic serotonin receptor stimulation, the anterior pituitary gland releases prolactin in the circulation following fenfluramine administration. Depressed high-lethality suicide attempters showed relative hypometabolism compared to low-lethality attempters in the ventral, medial, and lateral prefrontal cortex. This difference was more pronounced after fenfluramine administration. Lethality of the attempt appeared to be inversely correlated with metabolism in the ventromedial prefrontal cortex after challenge with fenfluramine. A lower rCMRglu correlated with higher lethality of suicidal behavior. They found a lower rCMRglu in high versus low-lethality suicide attempters. This hypometabolism in frontal cortex structures was related to the degree of suicide intent and impulsivity and not to depression.

Leyton et al. (2006) studied regional serotonin synthesis in the brain with PET and α-(^{11}C)-Methyl-L-Tryptophan trapping in high-lethality suicide attempters and in healthy controls. Suicide attempters showed reduced serotonin synthesis in the orbital and ventromedial prefrontal cortices, and α-(^{11}C)-Methyl-L-tryptophan trapping in these regions correlated negatively with suicide intent. Low serotonin synthesis in the prefrontal cortex may thus lower the threshold for suicidal behavior.

Four studies of suicidal behavior using SPECT have been published. Using ^{123}I-5-I-R91150, Audenaert et al. (2001) (studied 5-HT_{2a} receptor binding in the brains of recent suicide attempters and healthy controls. They found a significantly reduced binding index in the frontal cortex in the patient group. The binding index was significantly lower in the deliberate self-injury patients compared to the deliberate self-poisoning subjects. In a split-dose ^{99m}Tc-ECD SPECT activation paradigm using a verbal fluency task, Audenaert et al. (2002) further studied recent suicide attempters. Attempters showed a blunted increase during verbal fluency tasks in perfusion in the left gyrus frontalis inferior, right gyrus parietalis inferior and bilateral gyrus cinguli anterior, the left and right gyrus temporalis medius, and the hypothalamic region.

Brain ^{99m}Tc HMPAO SPECT scans of individuals who committed suicide between 10 days and 36 months after the SPECT scan were compared to the SPECT scans of depressed and healthy controls in two studies in a partly overlapping study population (Amen et al. 2009; Willeumier et al. 2011). Resting-state activity was lower in the suicide victims than in the controls in the premotor and primary motor cortex, corpus callosum, subgenual cingulate, and anterodorsal cortex. A significant area of low activity was the nucleus accumbens, extending into the ventromedial prefrontal cortex and the left and right putamen. During the Continuous Performance Test, the baseline perfusion deficits were attenuated in the depressed group and exacerbated in the suicide group during concentration.

Marchand et al. (2012) studied functional connectivity characteristics in association with attempted suicide. A network involving the bilateral striatum and anterior cortical midline structures was found to be associated with depressive symptom severity. Current suicidal ideation was associated with a similar but less extensive circuit in the left hemisphere. A distinct striatal motor/sensory network was associated with self-harm behaviors. Thus, a striatal-anterior cortical midline circuit likely plays a significant role in the expression of depressive symptoms and suicidal ideation. In contrast, a striatum-motor/sensory cortex network may be a trait marker of suicide-related behaviors.

15.2 Imaging Studies of Suicide Risk Factors

Suicidal behavior is the consequence of the interaction between proximal and distal risk factors (Hawton and van Heeringen 2009). Proximal risk factors, or state-dependent characteristics associated with an increased risk of suicidal behavior, include psychiatric disorders including depression, schizophrenia, and substance use disorders. As the vast majority of individuals suffering from these disorders will not show suicidal behavior, the specificity of these disorders with regard to suicide risk is limited. The imaging literature concerning these disorders will therefore not be reviewed in this chapter. However, particular state-dependent characteristics are more specifically associated with an increased risk of suicidal behavior, including mental pain (or 'psychache') and hopelessness. Imaging studies of these state-dependent clinical correlates of suicidal behavior will therefore be reviewed below, as they may inform suicide risk assessment and treatment.

Distal risk factors include trait-dependent characteristics such as impulsivity, sensitivity to social stressors and disturbances in decision-making. A number of imaging studies have addressed these potential markers of suicide risk in studies of suicide attempters and will therefore be reviewed in this chapter.

15.2.1 Mental Pain

Two studies have assessed brain correlates of mental pain in relation to suicidal behavior. Using ^{99m}Tc-ECD SPECT, van Heeringen et al. (2010) (examined the effect of psychological pain severity on resting-state activity in patients with major depressive disorder (MDD) by comparing patients who scored high in psychological pain to those who scored low. Mental pain (measured with the Orbach and Mikulincer Mental Pain Scale), suicidal ideation (measured using the Hamilton Rating Scale for Depression), hopelessness (measured using Beck's Hopelessness Scale), and regional cerebral blood flow as measured with single photon emission computed tomography were assessed in depressed individuals. Levels of mental pain were significantly and positively associated with suicidal ideation and levels of hopelessness. When compared with patients with low levels of mental pain, those with high levels of mental pain showed relatively increased perfusion in the right dorsolateral prefrontal cortex, occipital cortex and inferior frontal gyrus and in the left inferior temporal gyrus, and relatively decreased perfusion at the medulla. Reisch et al. (2010) tested the hypothesis that negative emotions experienced as psychological pain would exhibit decreased neural activity in the frontal cortex. Studying women who had attempted suicide in the two months prior to the study, the authors reported decreased prefrontal activity. Thus, Reisch et al. (2010) reported decreased PFC activity (left BA46, right BA10), whereas van Heeringen et al. (2010) (reported increased activity in the right PFC (BA9, BA44). Both studies used the Orbach and Mikulincer Mental Pain questionnaire to assess psychological pain, which has been shown to be reliable and have a high degree of validity, but it should be noted that different reference conditions were used.

15.2.2 Hopelessness

Two other imaging studies investigated hopelessness, and its association with serotonergic disturbances. Using SPECT, van Heeringen et al. (2003) (studied the binding index of 5-HT$_{2a}$ receptors in the frontal cortex of attempted suicide patients and normal controls using [I-123]5-I-R91150, a highly selective 5-HT$_{2a}$ receptor ligand. Moreover, they measured personality characteristics (using Cloninger's Temperament and Character Inventory) and levels of hopelessness (using Beck's

Hopelessness Scale), and studied the association between 5-HT_{2a} receptor binding index, hopelessness and these personality dimensions. When compared to normal controls, attempted suicide patients had a significantly lower binding potential of frontal 5-HT_{2a} receptors, a higher level of hopelessness, a higher score on the temperament dimension harm avoidance and lower scores on the character dimensions self-directedness and cooperativeness. A significant correlation was found between harm avoidance, hopelessness and binding index in the population of suicide attempters. Lower central serotonergic function, hopelessness and harm avoidance are interrelated phenomena, which may increase the probability of the occurrence of attempted suicide.

Meyer et al. (2004) used PET in order to measure the relationship between brain serotonin transporter binding potential with carbon 11-labeled DASB and negativistic dysfunctional attitudes during depression. Dysfunctional attitudes are negatively biased assumptions and beliefs regarding oneself, the world, and the future. Depressed subjects with highly negativistic dysfunctional attitudes had significantly higher 5-HTT binding potential compared with healthy subjects in brain regions mainly sampling serotonergic nerve terminals (prefrontal cortex, anterior cingulate, thalamus, bilateral caudate, and bilateral putamen). Increased 5-HTT binding potential was strongly associated with more negativistic dysfunctional attitudes in brain regions primarily sampling serotonergic nerve terminals (prefrontal cortex, anterior cingulate, thalamus, caudate, and putamen). The magnitude of regional 5-HTT binding potential thus may provide a vulnerability to low levels of extracellular serotonin and symptoms of extremely negativistic dysfunctional attitudes.

15.2.3 Impulsivity

Yurgelun-Todd et al. (2011) studied the association between frontal white matter integrity and measures of impulsivity and suicidal ideation in male veterans with mild traumatic brain injury (n = 15) using DTI. Total and right cingulum fractional anisotropy values (reflecting fiber density, axonal diameter, and myelination in white matter) were found to correlate with current suicidal ideation. Mahon et al. (2012) used DTI to study white matter in the brains of bipolar patients with a history of suicide attempts, bipolar patients without such a history and healthy controls. Lower fractional anisotropy values were found in the left orbital frontal white matter in association with a history of suicide attempts, correlating with levels of motor impulsivity.

Using SPECT and the mixed monoamine transporter tracer ^{123}I-β-CIT, Lindstrom et al. (2004) examined whole brain binding potentials of the SERT and DAT in suicide attempters and matched healthy controls. No significant differences in binding potential between study groups were found. In attempters, but not in controls, there was a significant correlation between whole brain 5-HTT and DAT binding potential and between high impulsiveness and low SERT-binding potential. Ryding et al. (2006) further analyzed these data, examining regional serotonin reuptake (5-HTT) and dopamine reuptake (DAT) capacity. They observed no significant difference concerning the regional levels of SERT or DAT binding potential. However, they did find regional significant negative correlations between SERT-binding potential and impulsiveness among suicide attempters but not in controls. Significant correlations between the level of impulsivity and local 5-HTT binding potential in suicide attempters were found in the right inferior frontal (orbital) and bilateral temporal cortical regions, subcortically in the midbrain, thalamic, and bilateral basal ganglia regions and in the left cerebellar hemisphere. Furthermore, the patients showed a significant negative correlation between whole brain DAT binding potential and mental energy. Regional significant correlations were found solely in bilateral basal ganglia regions. These correlations were not found in controls.

Pan et al. (2011) examined impaired response inhibition in adolescent suicidal behavior by comparing adolescent suicide attempters with a history of depression to adolescent nonattempters with a history of depression and to adolescent healthy controls. Using a go-no-go task, they found a significantly higher activation in the right anterior cingulate gyrus in nonattempters, compared to the suicide attempters. No other significant differences in whole brain activity were observed when comparing suicide attempters to nonattempters and healthy controls. The findings showed that adolescent suicidal behavior cannot be associated with abnormal neuronal activation in the response inhibition circuit.

15.2.4 Sensitivity to Social Stressors

Jollant et al. (2008) were the first to use fMRI to elucidate the functional neural basis of the neurobiological abnormalities underlying the vulnerability to suicidal behavior. They measured neural activity in response to angry and happy versus neutral faces in currently euthymic men with a history of MDD and suicidal behavior and currently euthymic men with a history of MDD but not of suicidal acts (affective comparison subjects) and healthy male comparison subjects. Relative to affective comparison subjects, suicide attempters showed greater activity in the right lateral orbitofrontal cortex (Brodmann's area 47) and decreased activity in the right superior frontal gyrus (area 6) in response to prototypical angry versus neutral faces, greater activity in the right anterior cingulate gyrus (area 32 extending to area 10) to mild happy versus neutral faces, and greater activity in the right cerebellum to mild angry versus neutral faces. However, activation in these frontal regions did not differ between healthy individuals and either patient group. Relative to healthy comparison subjects, both patient groups showed reduced activity in the right cerebellum to neutral faces and to mild happy versus neutral faces. Suicide attempters were distinguished from nonsuicidal patients by responses to angry and happy faces that may suggest increased sensitivity to others' disapproval, higher propensity to act on negative emotions, and reduced attention to mildly positive stimuli. These patterns of neural activity and cognitive processes may represent vulnerability markers of suicidal behavior in men with a history of depression.

A subsequent fMRI study (Pan et al. 2011, 2013a, b) investigated neural reactivity to neutral, mild, or intense emotion face morphs in adolescent suicide attempters, affective controls, and healthy volunteers. To 50 % intensity angry faces, attempters showed significantly greater activity than affective controls in anterior cingulate gyral-dorsolateral prefrontal cortical attentional control circuitry, primary sensory and temporal cortices; and significantly greater activity than healthy volunteers in the primary sensory cortex, while affective controls had significantly lower activity than healthy volunteers in the anterior cingulate gyrus and ventromedial prefrontal cortex. To neutral faces during the angry emotion-processing run, attempters had significantly lower activity than affective controls in the fusiform gyrus. Attempters also showed significantly lower activity than healthy volunteers to 100 % intensity happy faces in the primary sensory cortex, and to neutral faces in the happy run in the anterior cingulate and left medial frontal gyri (all $p < 0.006$, corrected). Psychophysiological interaction analyses revealed significantly reduced anterior cingulate gyral-insula functional connectivity to 50 % intensity angry faces in attempters versus affective controls or healthy volunteers. Thus, elevated activity in attention control circuitry, and reduced anterior cingulate gyral-insula functional connectivity, to 50 % intensity angry faces in attempters than other groups suggest that attempters may show inefficient recruitment of attentional control neural circuitry when regulating attention to mild intensity angry faces, which may represent a potential biological marker for suicide risk.

15.2.5 Decision-Making

Suicide can be viewed as an escape from unendurable punishment at the cost of any future rewards (Dombrovski et al. 2012, 2013). Could faulty estimation of these outcomes predispose to suicidal behavior? In behavioral studies, many of those who have attempted suicide misestimate expected rewards on gambling and probabilistic learning tasks. Neuropsychological studies have indeed demonstrated a link between impairments in decision-making and suicidal behavior. Subsequent studies have applied neuroimaging techniques to further understand the neurocognitive mechanisms of these impairments, which could facilitate the development of effective treatments.

Dombrovski et al. (2012) demonstrated that elderly depressed suicide attempters had lower putamen but not caudate or pallidum gray matter voxel counts than elderly depressed nonattempters and nondepressed controls. Suicide attempters with lower putamen gray matter voxel counts displayed higher delay discounting but not delay aversion. A second study by Dombrovski et al. (2013) showed that depressed elderly participants displayed two distinct disruptions of control over reward-guided behavior. First, impulsivity and a history of suicide attempts (particularly poorly planned ones) were associated with a weakened expected reward signal in the paralimbic cortex, which in turn predicted the behavioral insensitivity to contingency change. Second, depression was associated with disrupted cortico-striato-thalamic encoding of unpredicted rewards, which in turn predicted the behavioral oversensitivity to punishment. These results were robust to the effects of possible brain damage from suicide attempts, depressive severity, co-occurring substance use and anxiety disorders, antidepressant and anticholinergic exposure, lifetime exposure to electroconvulsive therapy, vascular illness, and incipient dementia. Thus, altered paralimbic reward signals and impulsivity and/or carelessness may facilitate unplanned suicidal acts. This pattern, also seen in gambling and cocaine use, may reflect a primary deficit in the paralimbic cortex or in its mesolimbic input. The over-reactivity to punishment in depression may be caused in part by a disruption of appetitive learning in cortico-striato-thalamic circuits.

In a controlled study of the involvement of decision-making in adolescent attempted suicide, (Pan et al. 2011, 2013a, b) assessed decision-making and learning-related neural activity during Iowa Gambling Task (IGT) performance. Attempters performed best on the IGT. During low-risk decisions nonattempter controls, but not attempters, showed greater left hippocampal and middle temporal activation than healthy controls. During high-risk decisions, attempters showed less activation in the right thalamus, and during low-risk decisions, attempters showed greater activation in the left caudate. Thus, nonattempters but not attempters were differentiated from healthy controls during performance of the IGT. Functional abnormalities in neural circuitry implicated in learning in the context of risk may underlie risk for MDD, but not risk for suicide attempt, in adolescence.

Jollant et al. (2010) explored the neural and cognitive basis of poor decision-making ability associated with the vulnerability to suicidal behavior. A group of currently not depressed males, some of whom had a history of suicidal acts (suicide attempters), while others had none (affective controls), performed an adapted version of the IGT during fMRI. Task-related functional Regions-of-Interest were independently defined in 15 male healthy controls performing the same task. In comparison to affective controls, suicide attempters showed (1) poorer performance on the gambling task (2) decreased activation during risky relative to safe choices in left lateral orbitofrontal and occipital cortices (3) no difference for the contrast between wins and losses. Altered processing of risk under conditions of uncertainty, associated with left lateral orbitofrontal cortex dysfunction, could explain the decision-making deficits observed in suicide attempters. These impaired cognitive and neural processes may represent future predictive markers and therapeutic targets in a field where identification of those at risk is poor and specific treatments are lacking. These results also add to our growing understanding of the role of the orbitofrontal cortex in decision-making and psychopathology.

15.3 Discussion

Suicidal behavior constitutes an important public health problem and poses a major challenge to health care because of difficulties in its prediction and treatment, and, consequently, its prevention. This chapter reviews studies of the association between structural or functional brain characteristics and suicidal behavior. Such a review is relevant as knowledge of neural characteristics may contribute to our understanding, and thus to the prediction and prevention of suicidal behavior.

The findings from this review can be summarized as follows. Gray and white matter hyperintensities are comparatively more frequent in suicide attempters. With regard to *inferior frontal and orbitofrontal areas*, white matter volumes are increased, while gray matter volumes of the orbitofrontal cortex of suicide attempters appear to be reduced. Serotonin synthesis is negatively correlated with suicidal intent. A history of attempted suicide is associated with greater activity in the right orbitofrontal cortex in response to angry (versus neutral) faces and with a reduction in activation in the left lateral orbitofrontal cortex during disadvantageous choices is found.

Serotonin synthesis and glucose uptake are decreased in the *ventromedial prefrontal cortex*, both correlating negatively with suicidal intent. Ventromedial glucose uptake also correlates negatively with lethality of suicide attempts but positively with impulsivity. With regard to *dorsolateral prefrontal areas*, a history of suicidal behavior is associated with a reduction in 5-HT_{2A} receptor binding particularly among violent attempters, a blunted increase in perfusion during activation using a verbal fluency task, reduced glucose uptake particularly among high-lethality attempters, and less activation following exposure to angry faces.

A history of suicidal behavior is associated with larger right amygdala volumes, increased activity in the right insular cortex, anterior cingulate cortex and putamen, and increased serotonin synthesis in the hippocampal gyrus and left thalamus. Lethality of the most serious lifetime suicide attempt correlates negatively with glucose uptake after fenfluramine administration in the anterior cingulate gyrus.

Preceding a discussion of these findings, a number of methodological issues need to be addressed. The comparability of findings from different studies is limited because of variations in imaging and analytic techniques. Radioligands differ in their binding specificity, and, in spite of the use of Statistical Parametric Mapping in many studies, anatomical localization of findings is often imprecise. Small sample sizes, whether or not due to high dropout rates, limit the power of studies to detect small group differences or can tend to amplify individual differences due to biological heterogeneity. Other potential biases may be due to the lack of (e.g., healthy or psychiatric) comparison groups. In many studies, patients and controls are not matched for potentially biasing characteristics, such as demographic variables, psychiatric (co-) morbidity, nature and severity or chronicity of associated disorders, treatment, and exposure to risk and protective factors. Generalizability of findings may be limited due to inclusion of only male or female individuals or patients with particular disorders such as schizophrenia. Finally, in the majority of studies, assessment of imaging is not blind to behavioral history.

This chapter confirms and updates the conclusions from our recent reviews of neuroimaging studies of suicidal behavior published between 1990 and 2010 (Desmyter et al. 2013; van Heeringen et al. 2011), i.e., that involved brain areas constitute a fronto-cingulo-striatal network. Recent neurobiological research outside the suicidological domain has clearly demonstrated the major role of this network in the process of decision-making. Decision-making is a complex process involving different components such as the recognition of the present state, the evaluation of action candidates (or options) in terms of how much reward a choice would bring, and the selection of an action in reference to one's needs. A neural basis for each of these components has been demonstrated in terms of the brain regions constituting the FCS network (Doya 2008). Not coincidentally, recent neuropsychological studies in suicide attempters have also identified changes in decision-making processes as crucial characteristics of the predisposition to suicidal behavior.

Taken together with the results from recent functional MRI studies, these findings suggest, first, that suicidal behavior is associated with disturbances in the attribution of importance to stimuli, i.e., undue importance to signals of others' disapproval and insufficient importance to risky choices. Secondly, changes in the prefrontal–striatal network are associated with changes in the representation of value to different outcome options, which may lead to the choice of immediate reward over abstract and delayed reward in the process of decision-making. The development of unbearable emotional pain following perception of signals of others' disapproval may be associated with a choice for immediate alleviation of pain, not taking into account the possibility of a better future. Disturbed intertemporal reward discounting may thus play an important role in the vulnerability to suicidal behavior. As the serotonergic neurotransmission system is involved in the modulation of this process of delay discounting, this may explain the demonstrated association between prefrontal serotonergic dysfunctioning and levels of hopelessness in suicide attempters.

This review and discussion of neuroimaging studies indicates that knowledge of neural network substrates of suicidal behavior is rapidly increasing. Potential contributions of neuroimaging to suicide prevention may therefore include improved risk assessment and treatment planning, which are two major limitations in suicide prevention as discussed in the introductory section of this chapter.

With regard to risk assessment, neuroimaging correlates of suicidal behavior are currently defined in terms of differences between groups depending on the presence or absence of a history of suicidal behavior. To date, no (neurobiological or any other) measures can identify risk of future suicidal behavior at an individual level. The next step therefore will be the application of computer-based techniques that allow automatic discovery of patterns in imaging data, which then can be used to classify individuals into risk groups. These 'machine learning' techniques have been successfully used in the study of psychiatric disorders, and fMRI studies of suicidal behavior using such algorithms are currently being conducted.

With regard to the contribution of neuroimaging to the treatment of suicide risk, the more detailed delineation of brain regions and networks involved in suicide risk parallels the development of interventions, which target specific regions and networks. Findings from recent imaging studies showing orbitofrontal dysfunction in relation to suicidal behavior may inform cognitive-behavioral treatments of suicide risk by showing that inappropriate use of positive feedback and insensitivity to risk may be more relevant to the development of suicidal behavior than aggression and impulsivity.

With respect to the treatment of suicidal behavior, transcranial magnetic stimulation could be a method of choice. Continuous theta burst stimulation of the right dorsolateral prefrontal cortex influence functional activity in, among others, the orbitofrontal cortex and reduces myopia for the future, so that delayed rewards are favored instead of immediate reward (Cho et al. 2012).

While it clearly is too early to use neuroimaging in the management of suicide risk, this chapter shows that imaging studies may shed new light on our understanding of the reasons why people may become suicidal when confronted with particular adversities. New insights in the role of dysfunctional brain networks may thereby increase our possibilities to identify risk, inform current therapies, and lead to the implementation of new treatment approaches.

References

Aguilar EJ et al (2008) Left orbitofrontal and superior temporal gyrus structural changes associated to suicidal behavior in patients with schizophrenia. Prog Neuropsychopharmacol Biol Psychiatry 32(7):1673–1676 Print

Ahearn EP et al (2001) MRI correlates of suicide attempt history in unipolar depression. Biol Psychiatry 50(4):266–270 Print

Amen DG et al (2009) A comparative analysis of completed suicide using high resolution brain spect imaging. J Neuropsychiatry Clin Neurosci 21(4):430–439 Print

Audenaert K et al (2002) Spect neuropsychological activation procedure with the verbal fluency test in attempted suicide patients. Nucl Med Commun 23(9):907–916 Print

Audenaert K et al (2001) Decreased frontal serotonin 5-Ht2a receptor binding index in deliberate self-harm patients. Eur J Nucl Med 28(2):175–182 Print

Baldacara L et al (2011) Is cerebellar volume related to bipolar disorder? J Affect Disord 135(1-3):305–309 Print

Benedetti F et al (2011) Opposite effects of suicidality and lithium on gray matter volumes in bipolar depression. J Affect Disord 135(1-3):139–147 Print

Caplan R et al (2010) Suicidality and brain volumes in pediatric epilepsy. Epilepsy Behav 18 (3):286–290 Print

Cho SS et al (2012) Effect of continuous theta burst stimulation of the right dorsolateral prefrontal cortex on cerebral blood flow changes during decision making. Brain Stimulation 5 (2):116–123 Print

Cyprien F et al (2011) Suicidal behavior is associated with reduced corpus callosum area. Biol Psychiatry 70(4):320–326 Print

Desmyter S, Bijttebier S, Heeringen KV (2013) The role of neuroimaging in our understanding of the suicidal brain. CNS Neurol Disord Drug Targets 12(7):921–929 Print

Dombrovski AY et al (2012) The temptation of suicide: striatal gray matter, discounting of delayed rewards, and suicide attempts in late-life depression. Psychol Med 42(6):1203–1215 Print

Dombrovski AY et al (2013) Reward signals, attempted suicide, and impulsivity in late-life depression. Jama Psychiatry 70(10):1020–1030 Print

Doya K (2008) Modulators of decision making. Nat Neurosci 11(4):410–416 Print

Ehrlich S et al (2005) White matter hyperintensities and their association with suicidality in depressed young adults. J Affect Disord 86(2-3):281–287 Print

Ehrlich S et al (2004) White matter hyperintensities and their associations with suicidality in psychiatrically hospitalized children and adolescents. J Am Acad Child Adolesc Psychiatry 43 (6):770–776 Print

Giakoumatos CI et al (2013) Are structural brain abnormalities associated with suicidal behavior in patients with psychotic disorders? J Psychiatr Res 47(10):1389–1395 Print

Goodman M et al (2011) Anterior cingulate volume reduction in adolescents with borderline personality disorder and co-morbid major depression. J Psychiatr Res 45(6):803–807 Print

Hawton K, van Heeringen K (2009) Suicide. Lancet 373(9672):1372–1381 Print

Hwang JP et al (2010) Cortical and subcortical abnormalities in late-onset depression with history of suicide attempts investigated with MRI and voxel-based morphometry. J Geriatr Psychiatry Neurol 23(3):171–184 Print

Jollant F et al (2008) Orbitofrontal cortex response to angry faces in men with histories of suicide attempts. Am J Psychiatry 165(6):740–748 Print

Jollant F et al (2010) Decreased activation of lateral orbitofrontal cortex during risky choices under uncertainty is associated with disadvantageous decision-making and suicidal behavior. Neuroimage 51(3):1275–1281 Print

Jovev M et al (2008) An MRI study of pituitary volume and parasuicidal behavior in teenagers with first-presentation borderline personality disorder. Psychiatry Res Neuroimag 162 (3):273–277 Print

Leyton M et al (2006) Alpha-[C-11]methyl-L-tryptophan trapping in the orbital and ventral medial prefrontal cortex of suicide attempters. Eur Neuropsychopharmacol 16(3):220–223 Print

Lindstrom MB et al (2004) Impulsivity related to brain serotonin transporter binding capacity in suicide attempters. Eur Neuropsychopharmacol 14(4):295–300 Print

Mahon K et al (2012) Relationship between suicidality and impulsivity in bipolar i disorder: a diffusion tensor imaging study. Bipolar Disord 14(1):80–89 Print

Marchand WR et al (2012) Striatal and cortical midline circuits in major depression: implications for suicide and symptom expression. Prog Neuropsychopharmacol Biol Psychiatry 36 (2):290–299 Print

Matsuo K et al (2010) Anterior genu corpus callosum and impulsivity in suicidal patients with bipolar disorder. Neurosci Lett 469(1):75–80 Print

Meyer JH et al (2004) Brain serotonin transporter binding potential measured with carbon 11-labeled dasb positron emission tomography—effects of major depression episodes and severity of dysfunctional attitudes. Arch Gen Psychiatry 61(12):1271–1279 Print

Monkul ES et al (2007) Fronto-limbic brain structures in suicidal and non-suicidal female patients with major depressive disorder. Mol Psychiatry 12(4):360–366 Print

Oquendo MA et al (2013) Positron emission tomography of regional brain metabolic responses to a serotonergic challenge and lethality of suicide attempts in major depression. Arch Gen Psychiatry 60(1):14–22 Print

Pan LA et al (2011) Dissociable patterns of neural activity during response inhibition in depressed adolescents with and without suicidal behavior. J Am Acad Child Adolesc Psychiatry 50 (6):602–611 Print

Pan LA et al (2013a) Differential patterns of activity and functional connectivity in emotion processing neural circuitry to angry and happy faces in adolescents with and without suicide attempt. Psychol Med 43(10):2129–2142 Print

Pan L et al (2013b) Preserved hippocampal function during learning in the context of risk in adolescent suicide attempt. Psychiatry Res Neuroimag 211(2):112–118 Print

Pompili M et al (2007) White matter hyperintensities and their associations with suicidality in patients with major affective disorders. Eur Arch Psychiatry Clin Neurosci 257(8):494–499 Print

Pompili M et al (2008) Periventricular white matter hyperintensities as predictors of suicide attempts in bipolar disorders and unipolar depression. Prog Neuropsychopharmacol Biol Psychiatry 32(6):1501–1507 Print

Reisch T et al (2010) An fMRI study on mental pain and suicidal behavior. J Affect Disord 126(1-2): 321–325 Print

Rusch N et al (2008) Inferior frontal white matter volume and suicidality in schizophrenia. Psychiatry Res Neuroimag 164(3):206–214 Print

Ryding E et al (2006) Regional brain serotonin and dopamine transporter binding capacity in suicide attempters relate to impulsiveness and mental energy. Psychiatry Res Neuroimag 148 (2-3):195–203 Print

Serafini G et al (2011) Affective temperamental profiles are associated with white matter hyperintensity and suicidal risk in patients with mood disorders. J Affect Disord 129(1-3): 47–55 Print

Soloff PH et al (2012) Structural brain abnormalities and suicidal behavior in borderline personality disorder. J Psychiatr Res 46(4):516–525 Print

Spoletini I et al (2011) Suicidal attempts and increased right amygdala volume in schizophrenia. Schizophr Res 125(1):30–40 Print

van Heeringen C, Bijttebier S, Godfrin K (2011) Suicidal brains: a review of functional and structural brain studies in association with suicidal behaviour. Neurosci Biobehav Rev 35 (3):688–698 Print

van Heeringen K et al (2003) Prefrontal 5-Ht2a receptor binding index, hopelessness and personality characteristics in attempted suicide. J Affect Disord 74(2):149–158 Print

van Heeringen K et al (2010) The functional neuroanatomy of mental pain in depression. Psychiatry Res Neuroimag 181(2):141–144 Print

Wagner G et al (2011) Structural brain alterations in patients with major depressive disorder and high risk for suicide: evidence for a distinct neurobiological entity? Neuroimage 54 (2):1607–1614 Print

Wagner G et al (2012) Prefrontal cortical thickness in depressed patients with high-risk for suicidal behavior. J Psychiatr Res 46(11):1449–1455 Print

Willeumier K, Taylor DV, Amen DG (2011) Decreased cerebral blood flow in the limbic and prefrontal cortex using spect imaging in a cohort of completed suicides. Transl Psychiatry 1:e28

Yurgelun-Todd DA et al (2011) Neuroimaging correlates of traumatic brain injury and suicidal behavior. J Head Trauma Rehabil 26(4):276–289 Print

Chapter 16
Using Awake Animal Imaging to Fingerprint Drugs for CNS Liability: Risk of Suicide?

Craig F. Ferris

Abstract Awake animal imaging has become an important tool in preclinical drug discovery. Noninvasive ultra-high field, functional magnetic resonance imaging (fMRI) provides a window to the mind making it possible to image changes in brain activity across distributed, integrated neural circuits with high temporal and spatial resolution. Awake animal imaging offers the ability to record signal changes across the entire brain in seconds. When combined with the use of 3D segmented, annotated, brain atlases, and computational analysis, it is possible to reconstruct distributed, integrated neural circuits, or "fingerprints" of brain activity. These fingerprints can be used to characterize the activity and function of new psychotherapeutics in preclinical development and to study the neurobiology of integrated neural circuits controlling cognition and emotion. In this chapter, we briefly describe the methods used to image awake animals and its application toward the study of drugs with black box warnings for suicidal ideation and self-harm.

16.1 Introduction

Awake animal imaging has become an important tool in preclinical drug discovery (Borsook 2006). Noninvasive ultra-high field, functional magnetic resonance imaging (fMRI) provides a window to the functioning central nervous system, making it possible to image changes in brain activity across distributed, integrated neural circuits with high temporal and spatial resolution. Awake animal imaging offers the ability to record signal changes across the entire brain in seconds. When combined with the use of 3D segmented, annotated, brain atlases, and computational analysis, it is possible to reconstruct distributed, integrated neural circuits, or "fingerprints" of brain activity. These fingerprints can be used to characterize the activity

C.F. Ferris (✉)
Departments of Psychology and Pharmaceutical Sciences, Northeastern University, Boston, MA, USA
e-mail: C.Ferris@neu.edu

K.E. Cannon and T.J. Hudzik (eds.), *Suicide: Phenomenology and Neurobiology*,
DOI 10.1007/978-3-319-09964-4_16

and function of new psychotherapeutics in preclinical development and to study the neurobiology of integrated neural circuits controlling cognition and emotion.

A major area of effort in preclinical drug development is safety pharmacology, particularly in the area of CNS. In toxicology and safety pharmacology studies, careful observation of potentially drug-related behavioral changes, as well as histopathology have the potential to identify brain areas sensitive and potentially vulnerable to novel psychotherapeutics. Yet, there is no way to predict unwanted emotional or cognitive effects with high fidelity. Studies on animal behavior are limited in their ability to predict such states as anger, aggression, suicidal ideation, and self-harm. Given the limitations of observational behaviors in preclinical species, it is possible that fMRI in awake animals can provide complimentary information to assist in predicting such undesired effects. This notion is addressed in the present paper by assessment of the effects of drugs with "Black Box" warnings for suicidal behavior in pharmacological fMRI (phMRI) studies. The drugs under study are: (1) venlafaxine, serotonin-norepinephrine reuptake inhibitor used to treat depression, (2) rimonabant, an inverse agonist for the CB1 cannabinoid receptor used to treat obesity, and (3) gabapentin, a GABA analog acting on voltage-dependent calcium channels used to treat epilepsy and neuropathic pain. While these drugs have different indications, mechanisms of action, and structures, they all carry a warning for suicidal ideation and self-harm. As such, one starts with the presupposition that these drugs share some similarity in brain activity. If so, phMRI can be used to identify brain activity common to these drugs. This common brain activity can then be compared to drugs used to treat suicidal and aggressive behaviors helping to identify mutually exclusive brain areas as the fingerprint of a putative neural circuit involved in suicidal ideation and self-harm. In this chapter, we briefly describe the methods used to image awake animals and its application toward the study of drugs with black box warnings.

16.2 Awake Animal Imaging

The field of awake animal imaging was pioneered by the first publication in 1998, assessing the effects of foot shock upon brain activity. (Lahti et al. 1998). Since then, numerous studies have been conducted including a variety of behavioral and neurological models ranging from sexual arousal in monkeys (Ferris et al. 2004), pup suckling in rat dams (Ferris et al. 2005b; Febo et al. 2005) generalized absence seizures in rats and monkeys (Tenney et al. 2004a, b), aggressive and sexual motivation in rats (Ferris et al. 2008), and nongenomic effects of stress hormone (Ferris and Stolberg 2010).

16.2.1 Setup

There are multiple technical and methodological issues to overcome in order to perform awake animal imaging. The first and foremost is the issue of head restraint and motion artifact. Any minor head movement distorts the image and may also create a change in signal intensity that can be mistaken for stimulus-associated changes in brain activity (Hajnal et al. 1994). To minimize motion artifacts, studies are performed using a custom-designed head holder and restraining system for adult rats (Animal Imaging Research, LLC, MA). In brief, just prior to the imaging session, animals are lightly anesthetized with 2–3 % isoflurane. Their head is fitted into a restrainer with molded, padded side panels, which when compressed minimize movement. This head restrainer is placed into a quadrature transmit/receive volume coil optimized for brain imaging. The body of the animal is placed into a body restrainer with attachments for stabilizing the shoulders and neck. The coil/head holder and body restrainer are attached to a carriage that can be inserted into the bore of the magnet.

16.2.2 Acclimation Prior to Imaging

The stress associated with head restraint, restricted movement in the body tube, noise from the gradient coil and the duration of the imaging session are all concerns when imaging awake animals. To address these problems, protocols have been developed for acclimating animals to the environment of the MR scanner and imaging procedure leading to a reduction in stress hormones levels and measures of autonomic activity regulated by the sympathetic nervous system (Zhang et al. 2000; King et al. 2005). Acclimation protocols have been used to prepare awake animals for a range of behavioral, neurological, and pharmacological imaging studies, many of which are noted above. In all cases, acclimation to the scanning session is achieved by putting subjects through several simulated imaging studies. For example, on each day of acclimation, animals are lightly anesthetized with 2–3 % isoflurane, while being secured into the restraint system. When fully conscious, the restraint system is placed into a black opaque box "mock scanner" for 30–60 min with a tape-recording of an MRI pulse sequence to simulate the bore of the magnet and an imaging protocol. A significant decline in respiration, heart rate, motor movements, and plasma corticosterone has been measured when the first and last acclimation periods are compared (King et al. 2005). The reduction in autonomic and somatic measures of arousal and stress improve the signal resolution and quality of the MR images. Critical in acclimation is the finding that unacclimated and acclimated animals show no difference in baseline cerebral blood flow, a key determinant in BOLD fMRI (King et al. 2005).

16.2.3 Data Processing and Analysis

Imaging data are corrected for motion and drift. Each image is spatially smoothed to improve signal-to-noise. Spin echo EPI is used to reduce distortion in field homogeneity and susceptibility artifacts. The functional images are registered to a segmented, annotated 3D MRI atlas for rats. The fully segmented 3D rat brain atlas has the potential to delineate and analyze 154 distinct anatomical volumes within the brain. The alignment process is facilitated by an interactive graphic user interface. The affine registration involves translation, rotation, and scaling in all three dimensions, independently. The matrices that transformed the subject's anatomy to the atlas space were used to embed each slice within the atlas. Details of the alignment of scans to the rat brain atlas have been published elsewhere (Ferris et al. 2005a).

An initial voxel-based analysis is followed by Region of Interest (ROI)-based analyses using Medical Image Visualization and Analysis (MIVA) software. The scanning sessions described here lasted 35 min. The control window was the first 5 min with 50 scan repetitions (6 s/acquisition), drug administration, followed by 30 min with 300 scan repetitions. Statistical t tests are performed on each voxel (ca, 16,000 in number) of each subject within their original coordinate system. The baseline threshold is set at 2 % based on data showing that BOLD signal changes above this threshold are reliably above noise levels for awake rat imaging (Brevard et al. 2003). The t test statistics use a 95 % confidence level, two-tailed distributions, and heteroscedastic variance assumptions. As a result of the multiple t test analyses performed, a false-positive detection controlling mechanism is introduced (Genovese et al. 2002). This subsequent filter guarantees that, on average, the false-positive detection rate is below our cutoff of 0.05. Statistical differences between experimental conditions are determined using Newman-Keuls multiple comparisons test (alpha value was set at 5 %). Tests are done separately for each ROI.

16.3 Pharmacological MRI

The study presented is preliminary and tested the feasibility of characterizing drugs at risk for suicidal ideation and self-harm. A schematic of the experimental design and predicted outcome is shown in Fig. 16.1. Five hypothetical drugs (A–E) with black box warnings were screened for brain activity using phMRI. While each drug has its own unique activity represented in red lines and patches, they all presumably have something in common related to their potential to influence thoughts of suicide and self-injury. This putative neural circuit is indicated in the black spots. Statistical analysis between these five hypothetical drugs identifies areas of common brain activity. The remaining areas shown in red (second brain down on the far right) are general patterns of nonspecific brain activity common to each drug but not common to suicidal ideation or self-harm. To help screen for this neural circuit, a parallel phMRI study was run characterizing drugs used to treat suicidal ideation and self-harm. The hypothesis was that these drugs are effective treatments because they block the neural circuit at risk (blue dots in Drugs F & D). The commonality is found between the treatment drugs. This list of brain areas is compared to the common list of brain areas for drugs at risk. The difference between them reflects the activity in brain areas with potential liability.

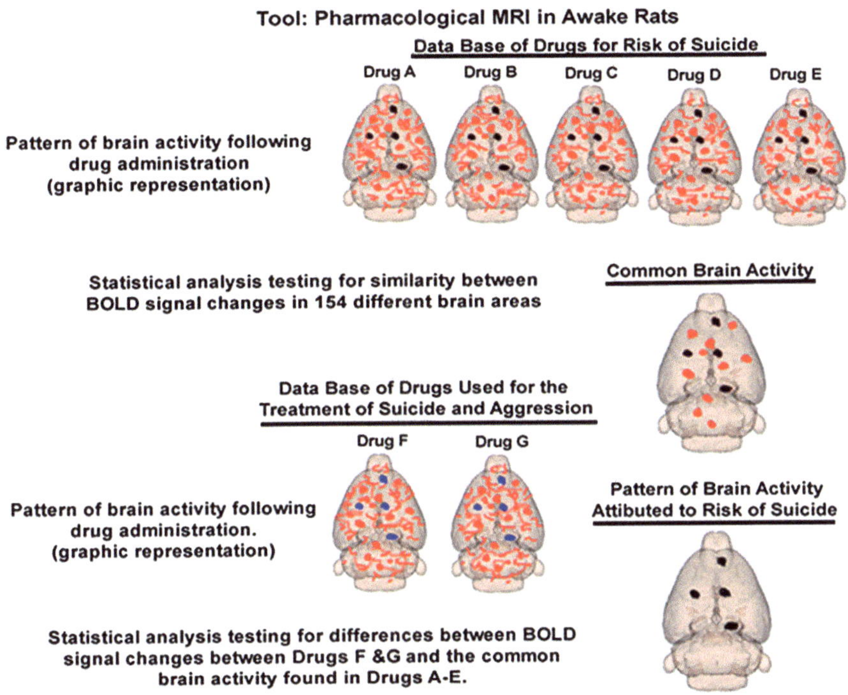

Fig. 16.1 Schematic of experimental design. Shown are the steps using phMRI to identify common brain activity in drugs at risk, and those for treating suicidal ideation and self-harm. Finding the difference between the two drug conditions identifies the vulnerable neural circuit

The three candidate drugs with black box warnings are shown in Table 16.1 and highlighted for their indication, mechanism of action, and chemical structure. Each drug was given i.v. in a single dose (rimonabant 1 mg/kg; venlafaxine 10 mg/kg; gabapentin 10 mg/kg). These drugs were compared to two test drugs used to treat suicidal ideation (clozapine 3 mg/kg) and aggressive behavior (buspirone 10 mg/kg) shown in Table 16.2. Clozapine was chosen because it is approved for the treatment of suicidal ideation in schizophrenics. Busprione was chosen because it is used to treat inappropriate aggressive behavior (Kavoussi et al. 1997), considered to be a risk factor for suicidal behavior. In fact, approximately 21 % of highly aggressive men diagnosed with Intermittent Explosive Disorder commit suicide (McCloskey et al. 2008).

All animals were imaged continuously for 35 min starting with a 5 min baseline followed by 30 min post i.v. injection of test drugs.

Figure 16.2 shows 3D activation maps for each of the test drugs. The red is the average significant positive BOLD signal change in over 16,000 voxels from the sample size shown beneath each figure. Starting with 154 brain areas that comprise the rat atlas, 67 were found to be common, or not significantly different from one another. Those areas that were common to clozapine and buspirone (data not

Table 16.1 Drugs with black box warnings for suicidal ideation and self-harm

Drugs with black box warnings for suicidal ideation and self-harm	
Venlafaxine—used to treat depression. Functions as a serotonin–norepinephrine reuptake inhibitor	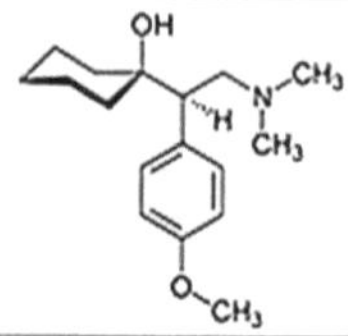
Rimonabant—used to treat obesity. Functions as an inverse agonist for the cannabinoid receptor CB1	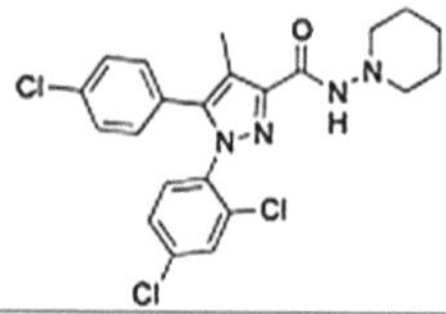
Gabapention—used to treat epilepsy and neuropathic pain. Functions as a GABA analog acting on voltage-dependent calcium channels	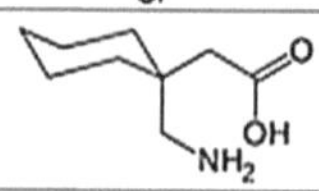

Table 16.2 Drugs used to treat suicidal ideation and aggression

Drugs used to treat suicidal ideation and self-harm	
Colzapine—used to treat schizophrenia. Functions as an atypical antipsychotic acting on multiple signaling systems. FDA approved for the treatment of suicide risk inschizophrenics	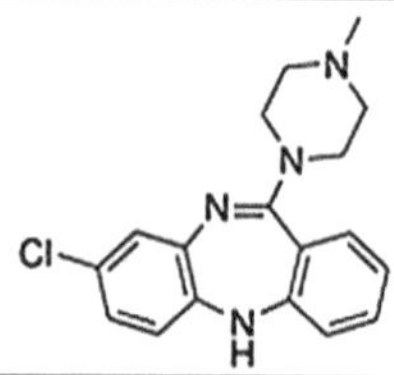
Buspirone—used primarily to treat anxiety. Also, indicated for treatment of aggression associated with head injury. Functions as serotonin 5-HT_{1A} partial agonist	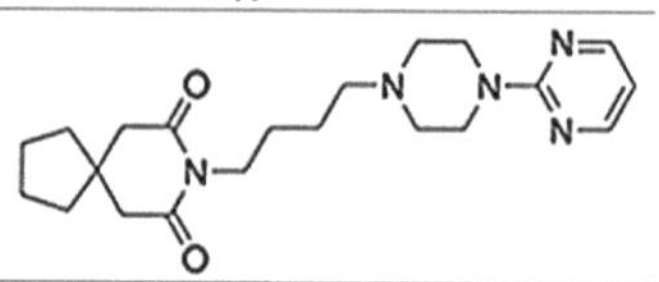

shown) were compared to the 67 brain areas of the black box drugs. Seventeen brain areas were identified in the risk drugs that were not found in the treatment drugs. These areas constitute the putative neural circuit that has the potential when activated to arouse thoughts of suicide and self-harm.

This pattern of brain activity was generated, reconstructed as an integrated neural circuit, and visualized as a 3D volume of activation and 2D activation maps as shown in Fig. 16.3. The 3D localization of these brain areas are shown in color with labels. These areas were coalesced into a single volume shown in yellow in the glass brain below. The average significant change in BOLD signal in these areas is shown in red using the rimonabant data as the example. These same data are presented in 2D activation maps to the right showing the localization of activated voxels within axial sections of the rat brain atlas.

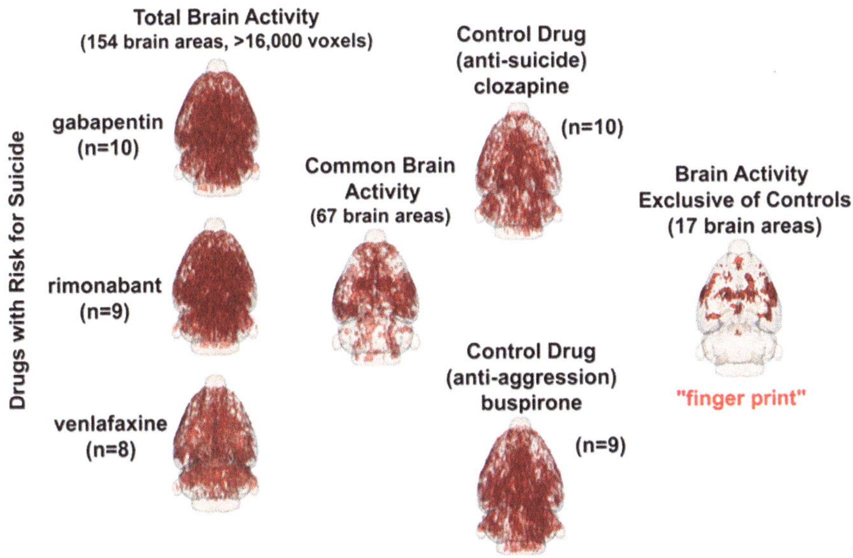

Fig. 16.2 Brain activity in the whole brain for each test drug shown are glass brains for each test drug and the location of the average significant change in BOLD signal from 154 brain areas and over 16,000 voxels. The *parenthesis* beneath each shows the sample size. Finding brain areas that were not significantly different between drugs at risk reduced the possible areas to 67. Identifying areas not common to the treatment drugs clozapine and buspirone reduced the brain areas to 17

The areas of the brain most represented in this integrated neural circuit is the thalamus followed by cortex, particularly limbic cortex, with contributions from hippocampus. Ostensibly absent from the list is amygdala, hypothalamus, periaqueductal gray, primary olfactory system, and basal ganglia, e.g., substantia nigra, ventral tegmental area, accumbens, globus pallidus, ventral pallidum, caudate/putamen. Indeed, the dorsomedial striatum is the only representative from this key neural network.

Prior to the start of these studies, there was no previous notion as to which, if any, brain areas would be associated with these drugs having a black box warning. Interestingly, the areas identified do have a general relationship to neural circuits involved in executive function and working memory as depicted in Fig. 16.4. Highlighted in black are major nodes recognized from human imaging studies as associated with cognitive dysfunction in schizophrenia (Eisenberg and Berman 2010). These areas starting with the prefrontal cortex have outputs to hippocampus, limbic cortex, and basal ganglia, all of which ultimately communicate with the thalamus and from there, back to prefrontal cortex (Little et al. 2010). Highlighted in red are the analogous areas in the rat identified with phMRI. Perhaps the activation of this distributed integrated neural circuit can affect cognitive function, which in some individuals may lead to thoughts and potentially actions of self-harm. As noted above, the scheme of integrated brain areas in Fig. 16.4 is associated with cognitive dysfunction in schizophrenia. Indeed, one in ten schizophrenics will commit suicide and one in four will attempt suicide.

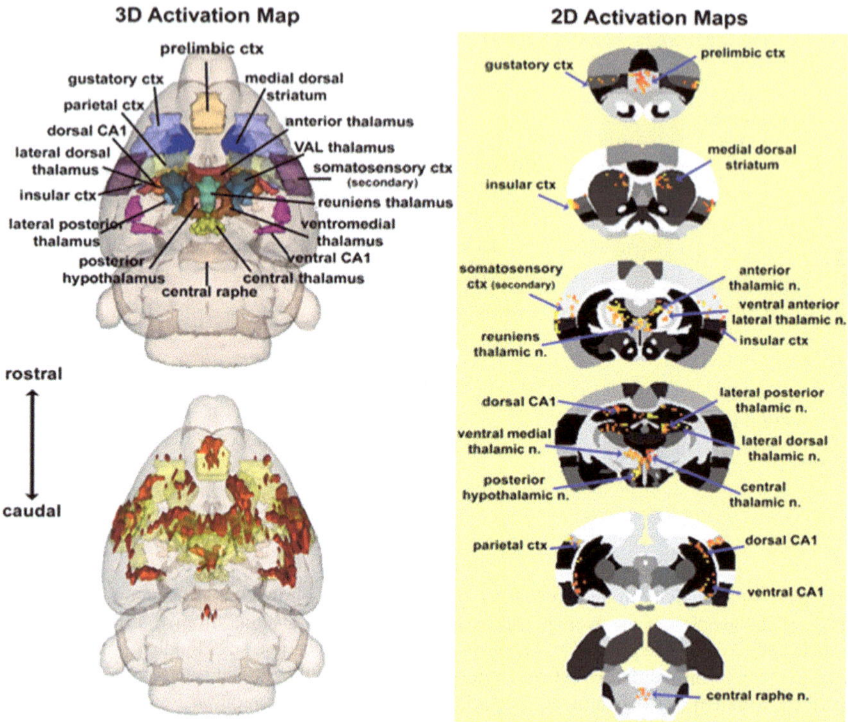

Fig. 16.3 Putative neural circuit associated with suicidal ideation and self-harm. Shown on the left is a 3D color representation of the different brain areas comprising the putative neural circuit associated with suicidal ideation and self-harm. The segmented, annotated illustration is a coronal view. The *yellow/gold* illustration below is confluence of the segmented brain areas showing the location of the average, significant increase (*red*) in BOLD signal for nine rats, 20–30 min post rimonabant injection. The panel of 2D axial images on the far *left* depict the location of significant increase in BOLD signal (*red*) in brain slices from the rat atlas

16.4 Discussion

Do drugs that carry a black box warning for suicidal ideation activate a common neural circuit in the brain? The data is suggestive, not conclusive, and invites more questions than answers. As noted in the introduction, this was a preliminary study to examine the feasibility of using phMRI in awake animals to fingerprint drugs with common black box warnings. In this case, the example was suicidal ideation and self-harm. The limitations in study design are many. Brain activity was assessed in response to a single dose of test drug, at a single time point (30 min), to drug naive rats. A comprehensive study would include a dose-response for each test drug, pharmacokinetics to correlate brain activity with drug levels, and a 28-day treatment regimen. Indeed, the profile of brain activity may be very different in response to acute and chronic drug exposure. For phMRI to have a future role in the

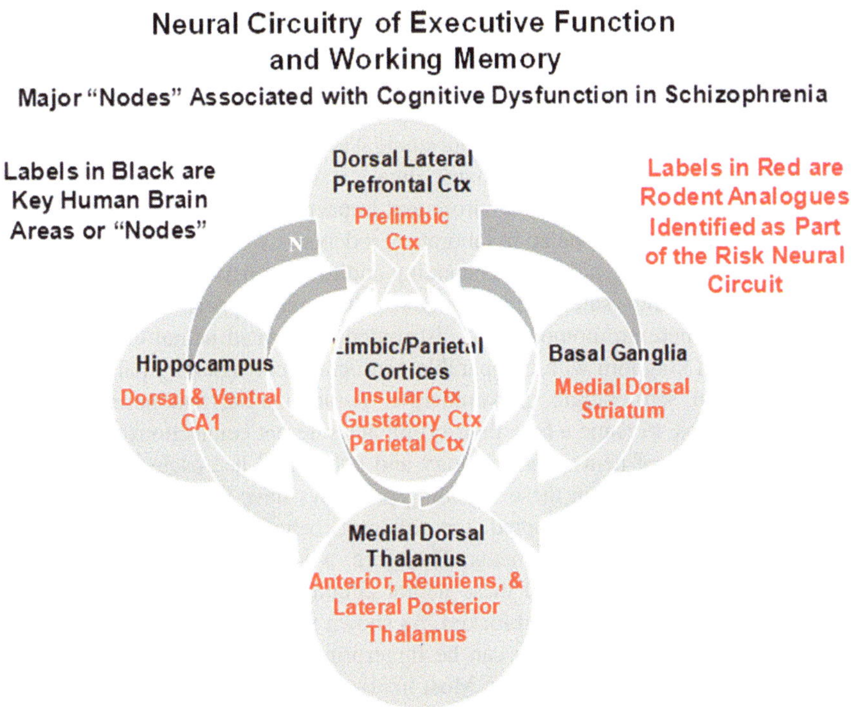

Fig. 16.4 Schematic of brain areas involved in executive function and working memory. Shown are different brain areas clustered into brain regions that have been identified as participating in executive function and working memory. Areas highlighted in *black* come from the imaging studies on patients diagnosed with schizophrenia (Eisenberg and Berman 2010). Those in *red* come from the phMRI studies identifying the putative neural circuit associated with suicidal ideation and self-harm

field of CNS safety, it will be necessary to develop a large database drawn from multiple classes of drugs with unwanted emotional and cognitive side effects. From this database of brain activation, pattern recognition software can be used to screen novel psychotherapeutics for potential liability.

Three drugs were chosen from the literature, picked because of their differences in mechanism of action. One could have simply characterized the class of serotonin reuptake inhibitors but this would have created the dilemma of parsing out neural circuits helping depression from those involved in thoughts and action of self-harm. This point is raised because it addresses the larger picture of integrated neural circuits as templates for animal and human behavior. If you adopt this notion, then one could ask if there are analogous neural circuits subserving similar functions in animals and humans as suggested in Fig. 16.4. Do we learn anything from the distributed neural circuitry identified in this preliminary study as it relates to human mental health, i.e., does this preclinical work translate to the human condition? One could argue that rodent behavior does not translate but brain activity may. It should be emphasized that the patterns of brain activity elicited by venlafaxine, gabapentin, and rimonabant are not to be associated with, or reflective of, any adverse "self-destructive" behavioral phenotype in the rat. Rats do not commit suicide. In these studies, the rat brain is simply an "inkblot" for comparing the patterns of brain activity across different drugs. It is unlikely we can learn anything about suicidal ideation, depression, and self-harm from the behavior of rodents. Psychiatric illness is a complex interaction over time between multiple genes and the environment impacting perception, cognition, and emotion that cannot be modeled in laboratory rodents.

Animal imaging may aid in understanding and treating psychiatric illness, and in potentially predicting safety-related signals that may appear later in clinical development. There are homologous, distributed, integrated neural circuits across the mammalian kingdom with comparable neurochemical signaling pathways. The conservation of serotonergic, dopaminergic, noradrenergic, and neuropetidergic signaling systems, to name a few, their origin and efferent connections in the brain, are the foundation of neuropharmacology and behavioral neuroscience. Over millions of years of evolution, these signaling pathways have been conserved across mammalian species but co-opted for different behaviors that have selective advantages in different environments. Therefore, what translates across species is the activation or suppression of these neural circuits with drugs—not necessarily the behaviors that are elicited or blocked. As shown here, drugs designed to interact with specific signaling pathways can be fingerprinted in the rat and compared to identify common areas of activation. Most likely these same signaling pathways are being activated in humans and they share common areas of activation. How this common brain activity translates into behavior encouraging self-harm is unknown. Given the complexity of the human psyche forged by genes, environment, and experience, it may not generalize to the population but only to the individual.

References

Borsook D, Becerra L, Hargreaves R (2006) A Role for fMRI in optimizing CNS drug development. Nat Rev Drug Discov 5.5:411–424

Brevard ME et al (2003) Changes in MRI signal intensity during hypercapnic challenge under conscious and anesthetized conditions. Magn Reson Imaging 21.9:995–1001

Eisenberg DP, Berman KF (2010) Executive function, Neural circuitry, and genetic mechanisms in schizophrenia. *Neuropsychopharmacology* 35.1:258–277

Febo M, Numan M, Ferris CF (2005) Functional magnetic resonance imaging shows oxytocin activates brain regions associated with mother-pup bonding during sucking. J Neursoci 25:11637–11644

Ferris CF et al (2005a) Pup suckling is more rewarding than cocaine: evidence from functional magnetic resonance imaging and three-dimensional computational analysis. J Neurosci 25.1:149–156

Ferris CF et al (2004) Activation of neural pathways associated with sexual arousal in non-human primates. J Magn Reson Imaging 19.2:168–175

Ferris CF, Stolberg T (2010) Imaging the immediate Non-genomic effects of stress hormone on brain activity. Psychoneuroendocrinology 35:5–14

Ferris CF et al (2005b) Pup suckling is more rewarding than cocaine: evidence from fMRI and 3D computational analyses. J Neurosci 25:149–156
Ferris CF et al (2008) Imaging the neural circuitry and chemical control of aggressive motivation. BMC Neuroscience 9:111
Genovese CR, Lazar NA, Nichols T (2002) Thresholding of statistical maps in functional neuroimaging using the false discovery rate. NeuroImage 15:870–878
Hajnal JV et al (1994) Artifacts due to stimulus correlated motion in functional imaging of the brain. Magn Reson Med 31:283–291
Kavoussi R, Armstead P, Coccaro E (1997) The neurobiology of impulsive aggression. Psychiatr Clin North Am 20.2:395–403
King JA et al (2005) Procedure for minimizing stress for fMRI studies in conscious rats. J Neurosci Methods 148.2:154–160
Lahti KM et al (1988) Imaging brain activity in conscious animals using functional MRI. J Neurosci Methods 82.1:75–83
Little DM et al (2010) Thalamic integrity underlies executive dysfunction in traumatic brain injury. Neurology 74.7:558–564
McCloskey MS et al (2008) Prevalence of suicidal and self-injurious behavior among subjects with intermittent explosive disorder. Psychiatry Res 158.2:248–250
Tenney JR et al (2004a) fMRI of brain activation in a genetic rat model of absence seizures. Epilepsia 45.6:576–582
Tenney JR et al (2004b) fMRI of generalized absence status epilepticus in conscious marmoset monkeys reveals corticothalamic activation. Epilepsia 45.10:1240–1247
Zhang Z et al (2000) Functional MRI of apomorphine activation of the basal ganglia in awake rhesus monkeys. Brain Res 852.2:290–296

Chapter 17
microRNA Function and Dysregulation in Depression and Suicide

Yogesh Dwivedi

Abstract Major depressive disorder and suicide are major public health concerns. Thus, there is a desperate need for identifying risk factors and noninvasive, reliable biomarkers that can be used for early detection of depression, suicidality, and treatment response. Recently, microRNAs (miRNAs) have emerged as an important class of small noncoding RNAs that by binding to 3′UTR of mRNAs, suppress the translation and/or stability of specific target genes. Since miRNAs show a highly regulated expression, they contribute in the development and maintenance of a specific transcriptome and thus have the unique ability to influence a wide range of physiological and disease phenotypes. Recent studies demonstrating involvement of miRNAs in several aspects of neural plasticity, stress response, and more direct studies in human postmortem brain and peripheral blood cells provide strong evidence that miRNAs not only can play a critical role in major depression and suicide pathogenesis but can also open new avenues for the development of therapeutic targets. In this chapter, these aspects have been discussed in a comprehensive manner.

Major depression is one of the most prevalent psychiatric disorders. It affects about 17 % of Americans during their lifetime (Kessler et al. 1994) and is associated with psychosocial impairment, poor quality of life, and significant disability (Murray and Lopez 1997). Major depression is being diagnosed at early ages, and about 25 % of people diagnosed with major depression are under 19 years old (Burke et al. 1991). Although, much work has been done to characterize depressive disorder, about 40 % of depressed patients do not respond sufficiently to the currently available medications (Fava and Davidson 1996). In addition, major depression is frequently associated with suicidal behavior, which is a major cause of death and morbidity worldwide (Mulrow et al. 1999). Nevertheless, the molecular and cellular mechanisms underlying major depression and suicidal behavior are still not well understood.

Y. Dwivedi (✉)
Department of Psychiatry and Behavioral Neurobiology, University of Alabama at Birmingham, SC711 Sparks Center, 1720 2nd Avenue South, Birmingham, AL, USA
e-mail: ydwivedi@uab.edu

K.E. Cannon and T.J. Hudzik (eds.), *Suicide: Phenomenology and Neurobiology*,
DOI 10.1007/978-3-319-09964-4_17

Alterations have been consistently shown in expression of genes that are critical in synaptic and structural plasticity in depression and suicide (Dwivedi et al. 2001, 2006, 2009a; Leistedt and Linkowski 2013; Ota and Duman 2013). In addition, altered structural and functional plasticity (Ongur et al. 1998; Cotter et al. 2001), changes in the synaptic circuitry (Aganova and Uranova 1992), impaired synaptic connectivity (Honer 1999), changes in number and shape of dendritic spines (Toni et al. 1999), altered dendritic morphology of neurons in hippocampus, and decreased length and number of apical dendrites (McEwen 2000) have been reported during stress, depression, and in suicidal subjects. The molecular mechanisms that underlie such compromised neural plasticity and structural impairments in these disorders are not clearly understood and no single mechanism appears to be responsible for its etiopathogenesis; however, it is becoming increasingly evident that these disorders may result from disruptions across whole cellular signaling networks, leading to aberrant information processing in the circuits that regulate mood, cognition, and neurovegetative functions (Leistedt and Linkowski 2013).

In recent years, the emergence of small noncoding RNAs as a meta controller of gene expression has gained much attention in various disease pathophysiologies. Among a number of noncoding RNAs, miRNAs are the most studied and well characterized and have emerged as a major regulator of neural plasticity and higher brain functioning (Dwivedi et al. 2011a; Im and Kenny 2012). miRNAs regulate about 60 % of total mammalian RNAs and are involved in virtually all biological functions (Malphettes and Fussenegger 2006). These miRNAs are expressed highly in neurons, and because they can regulate the expression of a large number of target mRNAs, neuronal miRNA pathways can create an extremely powerful mechanism to dynamically alter the protein content of neuronal compartments (Schratt 2009; Hussain 2012).

A large body of evidence demonstrates the role of miRNAs in neuropsychiatric diseases, such as schizophrenia, autism, Parkinson's disease, Huntington's disease, Tourette's syndrome, Fragile X syndrome, DiGeorge syndrome, and Alzheimer's disease. The role of miRNAs in depression and suicidal behavior is still in its infancy; however, several lines of evidence, including clinical and preclinical, demonstrate that miRNAs may play a major role in the development of stress-related disorders including depression and suicidal behavior. An understanding of how miRNAs can contribute to CNS disorders begins with knowledge of their biogenesis.

17.1 miRNA Biogenesis

miRNA biogenesis occurs in the nucleus (Fig. 17.1). miRNAs are encoded within primary miRNA (pri-miRNA) gene transcripts that could be inter- or intragenic. miRNA genes are transcribed to long primary miRNA by RNA polymerase II or III. The pri-miRNAs are then processed by RNase III enzyme Drosha to form small hairpin miRNA precursors (pre-miRNAs) that are generally 60–100 nt long and

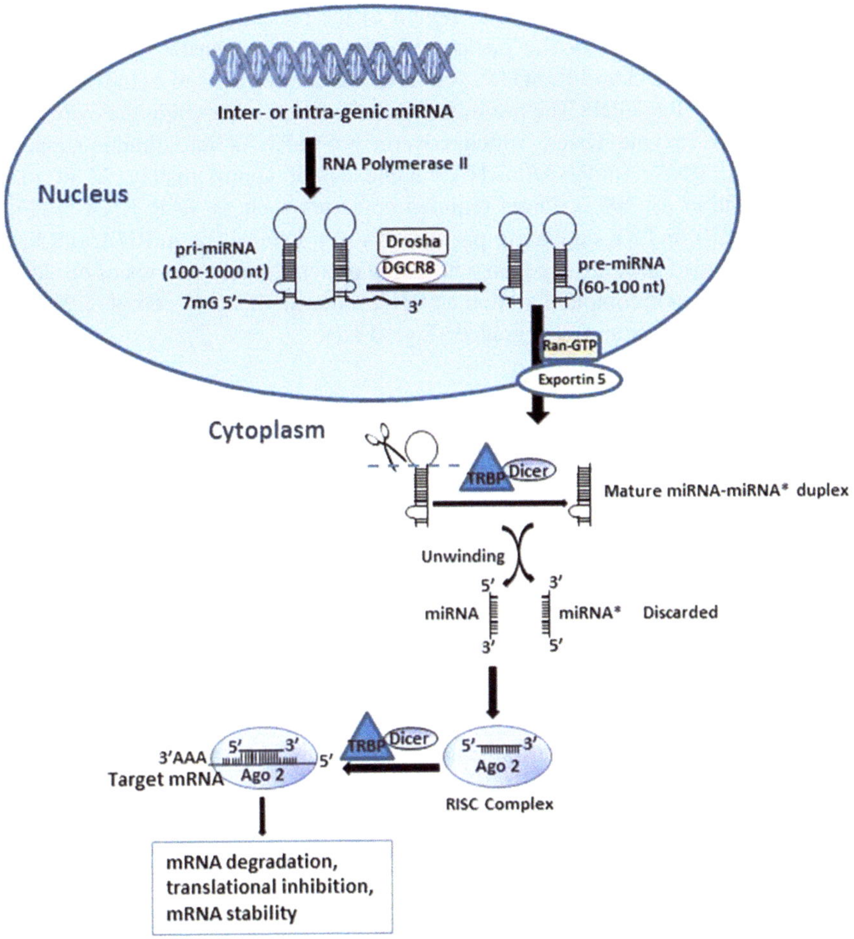

Fig. 17.1 miRNA biogenesis. miRNAs are encoded in the genome (inter or intragenis) and transcribed by RNA polymerase II to generate primary microRNA (pri-miRNA). These pri-miRNAs are taken up by Drosha/DGCR8, which catalyzes the formation of precursor miRNA (pre-miRNA). pre-miRNA is then exported to cytoplasm by Exportin5 in conjunction with Ras-related nuclear protein, RanGTP. In the cytoplasm, pre-miRNA is cleaved into miRNA:miRNA* duplex by Dicer/Tar RNA-binding protein (*TRBP*) or PKR activating protein (*PACT*). One of these miRNA/miRNA* duplexes is discarded and the other one is loaded onto an Argonaute homolog protein (Ago, isoforms of eIF2c) to generate the effector complex, known as RNA-induced silencing complex (*RISC*). The RISC complex directs miRNA to specific "short-seed" sequences located predominantly within the 3-UTR region of the target mRNA. This leads to degradation or translational inhibition

fold into a stem-loop structure. This process requires DiGeorge syndrome critical region 8 (DGCR8) protein as a cofactor. Together with DiGeorge, Drosha forms a large complex known as the "microprocessor complex." Drosha removes the flanking segments and $\sim$11 bp stem region of the pri-miRNA. The pre-miRNAs are then transported out of the nucleus via the exportin transfer system, which consists of Exportin 5 and RanGTP. Pre-miRNAs are released to cytoplasm upon hydrolysis of GTP to GDP. The pre-miRNAs are further processed in the cytoplasm by RNase III enzyme Dicer, which coverts pre-miRNAs into double-stranded mature small RNAs (miRNA/miRNA* duplexes) of approximately 22 nt long (Chendrimada et al. 2005). Dicer requires cofactors such as TAR RNA-binding protein (TRBP) or PKR-activating protein (PACT). One of the miRNA/miRNA* duplexes is loaded onto an Argonaute homolog protein (Ago, isoforms of eIF2c) to generate the effector complex, known as RNA-induced silencing complex (RISC). The other miRNA* strand is degraded (Fig. 17.1).

17.2 Possible Mechanisms of miRNA Regulation of Target Genes

RISC is critical in recognizing specific "short-seed" sequences located predominantly within the 3′ untranslated region (3′UTR) of target mRNAs. The binding of RISC to these short-seed sequences leads to interference in the translation of mRNA. miRNA-mediated translational inhibition also depends upon the 5′cap region of the target mRNA. Ago proteins can stimulate miRNA-dependent inhibition of translation by competing with elongation factor eIF4E for the 5′cap binding site, thus preventing circularization of mRNA and lowering initiation efficiency (Mathonnet et al. 2007). Because the RISC/miRNA complex recognizes target mRNA on a seed region containing 2–8 nucleotides at the 5′end of mRNA, it provides a mechanism by which one miRNA can target several mRNAs (Brodersen and Voinnet 2009). RISC can also associate with 60S ribosome and eIF6 (Chendrimada et al. 2007). eIF6 regulates the formation of the transnationally active 80S subunit. By regulating eIF6, miRNAs can modify polysome formation and expose target mRNAs for degradation (Chendrimada et al. 2007). In certain cases, miRNAs may actually enhance, rather than inhibit, translation (Vasudevan et al. 2007). miRNA-mediated regulation of mRNA stability is another mechanism by which miRNAs suppress expression of specific mRNA (Wu et al. 2006).

Besides regulating translational process, it has been shown that miRNA can also regulate gene transcription by targeting transcription factors. In this case, levels of transcription factors are downregulated by miRNAs, which in turn cause less expression of mRNA, leading to reduced protein synthesis (Kosik 2006; Michalak 2006). miRNA biogenesis can also be regulated at the epigenetic level (Tardito et al. 2013). For example, inhibitors of DNA methylation and histone deacetylases can affect expression of several miRNAs (Chuang and Jones 2007). On the other hand, a subset of miRNAs can control the expression of epigenetic regulators, such as DNA methyltransferases, histone deacetylases, and polycomb group genes, leading to transcriptional activation of protein coding gene sequences (Sato et al. 2011).

Table 17.1 miRNAs implicated in depression and suicide

miRNAs	Effects	References
Restraint stress	Frontal cortex: miR-9, miR-9*, miR-26b, miR-29b, miR-30b, miR-30c, miR-30e, miR-125a, miR-126-3p, miR-129-3p, miR-207, miR-212, miR-351, miR-423, miR-487b, miR-494, miR-690, miR-691, miR-709, miR-711, and Let-7 a-e let-7a, miR-9, miR-26a/b, miR-30b/c, and miR-125a	Rinaldi et al. (2010)
Immobilization stress	Hippocampus CA1, amygdala: miR-134, miR-183, miR-132, Let-7a-1, miR-9-1, and miR-124a-1	Meerson et al. (2010)
Unpredictable chronic mild stress	Hippocampus: miR298, miR-130b, miR-135a, miR-323, miR-503, miR-15b, miR-532, and miR-125a and up-regulating miRNAs miR7a, miR-212, miR-124, miR-139, and miR-182	Cao et al. (2013)
Animal model of behavioral depression	Learned helpless versus control: mmu-miR-184, mmu-miR-197, mmu-miR-107, mmu-miR-329, mmu-miR-125a-5p, mmu-miR-872, mmu-miR-181c, mmu-miR-18a*, mmu-miR-29b*, mmu-let-7a*, rno-let-7e*, rno-miR-20a*	Smalheiser et al. (2011)
Postmortem brain study in depressed suicide subjects	Prefrontal cortex: downregulation of hsa-miR-142-5p, hsa-miR-33a, hsa-miR-137, hsa-miR-489, hsa-miR-148b, hsa-miR-101, hsa-miR-324-5p, hsa-miR-301a, hsa-miR-146a, hsa-miR-335, hsa-miR-494, hsa-miR-20b, hsa-miR-376a*, hsa-miR-190, hsa-miR-155, hsa-miR-660, hsa-miR-552, hsa-miR-453, hsa-miR-130a, hsa-miR-27a, hsa-miR-497, hsa-miR-10a, hsa-miR-20a, hsa-miR-142-3p	Smalheiser et al. (2012)
Postmortem brain study in suicide completers	Hsa-miR-185 inversely correlated with TrkB.T1	Maussion et al. (2012)
Postmortem brain study in suicide completers	miR-139-5p, miR-320c, inversely correlated with polyamine gene SAT1 and miR34c-5p and miR-320c inversely correlated with polyamine gene SMOX	Lopez et al. (2014)
Blood mononuclear cell study in depressed patients	Differential regulation of has-miR-107, miR-133a, miR-148a, miR-200c, miR-381, miR-425-3p, miR-494, miR-517b, miR-579, miR-589, miR-636, miR-652, miR-941, and miR-1243	Belzeaux et al. (2012)
Whole blood cells (12 weeks of treatment with escitalopram)	Differential regulation of Hsa-miR-130b, hsa-miR-505, hsa-miR-29b-2, hsa-miR-26b, hsa-miR-22, hsa-miR-26a, hsa-miR-664, hsa-miR-494, hsa-let-7d, hsa-let-7 g, hsa-let-7e, hsa-miR-34c-5p, hsa-let-7f, hsa-miR-	Bocchio-Chiavetto et al. (2013)

(continued)

Table 17.1 (continued)

miRNAs	Effects	References
	629, hsa-miR-106b, hsa-miR-103, hsa-miR-191, hsa-miR-128, hsa-miR-502-3p, hsa-miR-374b, hsa-miR-132, hsa-miR-30d, hsa-miR-500, hsa-miR-770-5p, has-miR-589, hsa-miR-183, hsa-miR-574-3p, hsa-miR-140-3p, hsa-miR-335, hsa-miR-361-5p	
Serum of depressed patients	miR-132 and miR-182 were inversely correlated with BDNF gene expression	Li et al. (2013)
Genetic studies in depression and suicide subjects	DGCR8 rs3757 was associated with increased risk of suicidal tendency and improvement response to antidepressant treatment, whereas the variant of AGO1 rs636832 showed decreased risk of suicidal tendency, suicidal behavior, and recurrence. DGCR8 rs3757 and AGO1 rs636832 were found to have significant association with depression	He et al. (2012)

17.3 miRNAs and Synaptic Plasticity

17.3.1 Synaptic Plasticity and Regulation of BDNF and CREB by miRNAs

miRNAs play a critical role in regulating synaptic plasticity, a putative core feature of depression pathophysiology. Knocking down the RNase III enzyme Dicer leads to reduction in neuronal size, and branching, as well as aberrant axonal pathfinding (Davis et al. 2008; De Pietri Tonelli et al. 2008; Schaefer et al. 2007). DGCR8 knockout mice show a loss of synaptic connectivity, reduced number, and size of the dendritic spines (Olde Loohuis et al. 2012; Stark et al. 2008), and interestingly, impaired spatial working memory-dependent tasks (Stark et al. 2008). Such memory deficits are often associated with depressive symptoms. FMRP, which regulates protein synthesis in dendritic spines after binding with specific sites within the 3′UTR of certain mRNAs in concert with RISC components Ago1and Dicer (Jin et al. 2004; Qurashi et al. 2007), is also associated with learning, memory, and associated long-term potentiation (LTP). For example, the RISC protein armitage is essential for LTP and synaptic protein synthesis and is cleaved during the learning process (Ashraf et al. 2006).

FMRP is associated with miR-132 and miR-125b in the brain. miR-132 over-expresion increases dendritic protrusion as well as branching (Wayman et al. 2008), whereas miR-125b targets NR2A mRNA and regulates synaptic plasticity in a negative fashion (Edbauer et al. 2010). Similar negative regulation of the size of dendritic spines in rat hippocampal neurons has been shown to be associated with miR-138 as well as miR-134. miR-138 controls the expression of acyl protein thioesterase 1 (APT1), an enzyme regulating the palmitoylation status of proteins that are known to function at the synapse (Siegel et al. 2009). miR-134 additionally inhibits translation of Lim-domain-containing protein kinase 1 (Limk1) (Schratt et al. 2006), a protein that regulates dendritic spine growth (Meng et al. 2004). Exposure to BDNF relieves the suppression of Limk1 translation caused by miR-134. miR-134 can also promote denditogenesis by inhibiting translational repressor Pumilio2 (Fiore et al. 2009). This is consistent with the finding that BDNF has been shown to be lower in brains of depressed suicide subjects (Dwivedi et al. 2003a, 2009a).

Several studies have demonstrated that CREB, a key transcription factor regulating synaptic plasticity and whose expression is lower in depressed and suicidal brain (Dwivedi et al. 2003b) is one of the major targets of several miRNAs (Vo et al. 2005). Conversely, many miRNAs have binding sites in their promoter regions for CREB (Wu and Xie 2006). Expression of miR-132, which enhances neurite outgrowth, dendritic morphogenesis, and spine formation (Vo et al. 2005; Impey et al. 2010), is induced by BDNF via CREB. Another miRNA, miR-124, which plays a significant role in maintaining neuronal cell identity, is a major target of CREB. Interestingly, miR-124 is rapidly and robustly regulated by 5-HT, which selectively affects mature miR-124 levels, without affecting its precursor, suggesting that the miR-124 level may be regulated during Dicer processing or RISC incorporation and stabilization by Ago (Rajasethupathy et al. 2009). miR-124 responds to serotonin by de-repressing CREB and thereby enhances serotonin-dependent long-term facilitation (Rajasethupathy et al. 2009). More recently, it has been shown that expression of *SIRT1* gene, which modulates synaptic plasticity and memory formation, is altered via posttranscriptional regulation of CREB by miR-134 (Gao et al. 2010). Conversely, *SIRT1* inhibits the expression of miR-134 via a repressor complex containing the transcription factor YY1. Unchecked miR-134 expression after *SIRT1* deficiency may result into the reduced expression of CREB and BDNF, whereas knocking down miR-134 rescues LTP and memory impairment caused by *SIRT1* deficiency (Gao et al. 2010).

CREB- and activity-regulated miR132 is necessary for hippocampal spine formation (Impey et al. 2010). Expression of the miR-132 target, p250GAP, is inversely correlated with miR-132 and spinogenesis. Knockdown of p250GAP increases spine formation while introduction of a p250GAP mutant unresponsive to miR132 attenuates this activity. Inhibition of miR132 decreases both mEPSC frequency and the number of GluR1-positive spines, while knockdown of p250GAP has the opposite effect. Additionally, miR132/p250GAP circuit regulates Rac1 activity and spine formation by modulating synapse-specific Kalirin7-Rac1 signaling. These studies suggest that neuronal activity regulates spine formation, in part, by increasing miR132 transcription, which in turn activates a Rac1-Pak actin remodeling pathway (Impey et al. 2010). Behaviorally, it has been shown that overexpression of miR-132 in the rat perirhinal cortex impairs short-term recognition memory, which is associated with a reduction in both long-term depression and long-term potentiation (Scott et al. 2012).

17.3.2 Synaptic miRNAs: Direct Regulator of Plasticity

Synaptic efficacy is critically dependent upon regulation of specific protein synthesis near or within synapse (Weiler et al. 1997; Todd et al. 2003; Sutton and Schuman 2005). miRNAs provide fascinating mechanisms of regulating synaptic efficacy and plasticity by modifying translational control of protein synthesis locally at the synapse. Synaptic enrichment of miRNAs in mouse forebrain synaptosomes has extensively been characterized (Lugli et al. 2005; Smalheiser 2008). These studies show that a significant subset of miRNAs is highly enriched in synaptic fractions relative to total homogenate. These synaptic-enriched miRNAs were biologically distinct from synaptic-depleted miRNAs, both in their expression patterns (synaptic-enriched miRNAs are expressed primarily in pyramidal neurons, whereas synaptic-depleted miRNAs tend to have widespread and abundant tissue expression) and in their evolutionary histories (synaptic-enriched miRNAs tend to be evolutionarily new, often mammalian-specific, whereas the synaptic-depleted miRNAs tend to be highly conserved across vertebrates). Interestingly, the synaptic enrichment was not simply related to specificity of miRNA expression within neurons, rather, they arise from precursors that are expressed in the synaptic fractions and associated tightly with post-synaptic density (PSD) (Smalheiser 2008). Furthermore, synaptic enrichment of miRNAs has been shown to be related to structural features of their precursors, suggesting a basis by which pre- or pri-miRNA may be selectively and stably transported to dendrites (Budhu and Wang 2010). Because both dicer and pre-RNAs are expressed in synaptic fractions and are strongly associated with PSDs, it suggests that at least a portion of the mature miRNAs is locally processed near synapses. Because of the critical feature of miRNAs to regulate gene circuitry locally at the synapse in an activity-dependent fashion, one can modulate synaptic efficacy by modulating miRNA functions at the synapse and consequently synaptic plasticity. This provides unique opportunity at therapeutic level, where regulation of miRNA can be used to control plasticity at the synapse.

17.4 miRNAs and Stress

Glucocorticoids regulate the hypothalamic-pituitary adrenal axis through a negative feedback mechanism while binding to soluble glucocorticoid receptors (GRs) in the pituitary and the hypothalamus and inhibit the release of corticotropin-releasing factor and adrenocorticotropic hormone. Expression of GRs are downregulated in depressed individuals (Pariante and Miller 2001). GR protein is under constant regulation by miRNAs (Vreugdenhil et al. 2009); specifically, miR-124a and miR-18a bind to 3′UTR of GR gene and downregulate its expression (Vreugdenhil et al. 2009). Overexpression of miR-18a attenuates glucocorticoid-induced leucine zipper, a gene induced by stress-like levels of glucocorticoid. Interestingly, Uchida et al. (2008) found that miR-18a-mediated downregulation of GR translation is important in susceptibility to stress. Turner et al. (2010) recently predicted several possible miRNA binding sites within the GR first exon, suggesting regulation of GR genes by miRNAs.

Several types of stressors have been utilized to examine how miRNAs respond to these stressors. Using unpredictable chronic mild stress combined with separation, Cao et al. (2007) found changes in 13 specific miRNAs in rat hippocampus. These include: downregulating miRNAs miR298, miR-130b, miR-135a, miR-323, miR-503, miR-15b, miR-532, and miR-125a and upregulating miRNAs miR7a, miR-212, miR-124, miR-139, and miR-182. Among these, miR-125a and miR-182 recovered to normal after intervention with antidepressant medication.

Acute and chronic restrained stress cause differential changes in expression of miRNAs in a brain region-specific manner (Rinaldi et al. 2010). For example, acute stress induces a transient increase in the expression of miR-9, miR-9*, miR-26b, miR-29b, miR-30b, miR-30c, miR-30e, miR-125a, miR-126-3p, miR-129-3p, miR-207, miR-212, miR-351, miR-423, miR-487b, miR-494, miR-690, miR-691, miR-709, miR-711, and Let-7 a-e in the frontal cortex but not in hippocampus. Some of these miRNAs (let-7a, miR-9, miR-26a/b, miR-30b/c, and miR-125a) show increase in their expression 5 days after acute stress. Interestingly, their expression levels are not altered after repeated restraint. These results suggest that acute stress modulates miRNA expression rapidly to external stimuli, which could be due to altered synaptic efficacy through regulation of localized mRNA translation.

Using chronic immobilization stress paradigms, Meerson et al. (2010) also found that the expression of several miRNAs was differentially altered in the central amygdala and the CA1 region of the hippocampus of rats during acute and chronic stress; chronic stress causing much larger changes than acute stress. Some of the miRNAs that were altered during acute and chronic stress include: miR-134, miR-183, miR-132, Let-7a-1, miR-9-1, and miR-124a-1. Interestingly, except for miR-Let-7a-1, the expression of stress-responsive miRNAs were different in the two analyzed brain regions. In the CA1 region, miR-376b and miR-208 increased whereas miR-9-1 decreased under both acute and chronic stress conditions. Stress-responsive miR-134 and miR-183 target many splicing factors, such as SC35, SRP46, and SFRS11. SC35 promotes the alternative splicing of acetylcholinesterase from the synapse-associated isoform AChE-S to soluble AChE-R protein and the expression of SC35 is increased during stress. Thus, by regulating splicing factors and their targets, miR-183 and miR-134 may modify both alternative splicing and cholinergic neurotransmission in the stressed brain. In addition, one of the targets of miR-183 is profilin 2 mRNA, which regulates dendritic spine morphology in neurons. Interestingly, neurotransmitter homeostasis and behavior are severely affected in profilin 2 knockdown mice (Witke 2004) and PFN2 expression is increased in lymphoblastoid cell lines of monozygotic twin pairs discordant for bipolar disorder (Matigian et al. 2007).

17.5 miRNAs in Animal Models Depression-Like Behaviors

An individual's ability to cope with stress is critical in the development of depression. miRNA expression was recently examined in frontal cortex of rats which developed behavior (learned helpless [LH]) that resembles stress-induced depression and in at those which did not develop depression-like symptoms (non-learned helpless [NLH]) despite similar exposure to inescapable shock (Smalheiser et al. 2011). NLH rats showed a robust adaptive miRNA response to inescapable shocks whereas LH rats showed a markedly blunted miRNA response. One set of miRNAs showed large, significant, and consistent alterations in NLH rats, consisting of miR-96, miR-141, miR-182, miR-183, miR-183*, miR-198, miR-200a, miR-200a*, miR-200b, miR-200b*, miR-200c, and miR-429. All were downregulated in NLH rats relative to tested controls (no-shock group), and all showed a blunted response in LH rats. These miRNAs were encoded at a few shared polycistronic loci, suggesting that their downregulation was coordinately controlled at the level of transcription. Most of these miRNAs have previously been shown to be enriched in synaptic fractions (Lugli et al. 2008). Moreover, almost all of these miRNAs share 5′-seed motifs with other members of the same set, suggesting that they will hit similar or overlapping sets of target mRNAs. Interestingly, half of this set are predicted to hit CREB1 as a target, and binding sites for CREB lie upstream of miR-96, miR-182, miR-183, miR-200a, miR-200b, miR-200c, miR-220a*, and miR-200b*. This suggests that a similar feedback loop arrangement may also exist for CREB as well, similar to what has been described for other CREB-stimulated miRNAs and target genes (Wu and Xie 2006). Because these miRNAs are downregulated in NLH rats, but not LH rats, this can be interpreted as a homeostatic response intended to minimize repressive effects on CREB1. In addition, a large core coexpression module was identified (Smalheiser et al. 2011), consisting of miRNAs that are strongly correlated with each other across individuals of the LH group, but not either the NLH or tested control group. The presence of such a module implies that the normal homeostatic miRNA response to repeated inescapable shock is not merely absent or blunted in LH rats; rather, gene expression networks are actively reorganized in LH rats, which may support their distinctive persistent phenotype.

In further support of the suggestion that miRNAs can affect depressive-like behavior, Enoxacin, a fluoroquinolone used clinically as an antibacterial compound that also enhances the production of miRNAs in vitro and in peripheral tissues in vivo, can affect depressive behavior. Treatment of rats with 10 or 25 mg/kg enoxacin for 1 week increased the expression of miRNAs in frontal cortex and decreased the proportion of rats exhibiting learned helpless behavior following inescapable shock, suggesting that enoxacin may ameliorate depressive behavior, possibly due to upregulation of miRNAs (Smalheiser et al. 2014).

17.6 miRNAs in Depression and Suicide: Human Postmortem Brain Studies

The role of miRNAs in depression and suicide is still in infancy and so far, there have been only a handful of studies investigating the role of miRNAs in depression and suicide. miRNA expression in prefrontal cortex of depressed subjects who died by suicide was recently characterized (Smalheiser et al. 2012), finding that 21 miRNAs were significantly downregulated in the MDD group. 24 additional miRNAs were downregulated by 30 %. Although not statistically significant, the findings suggest a global downregulation of miRNAs levels in the MDD group. When analyzed individually, almost half of the downregulated miRNAs were encoded at chromosomal loci near another miRNA and are possibly transcribed by the same pri-miRNA gene transcripts (miR-142-5p and 142-3p; miR-494, 376a*, 496, and 369-3p; miR-23b, 27b, and 24-1*; miR-34b* and 34c; miR-17* and 20a). In addition, three pairs of miRNAs were encoded at distances greater than 100 kb but still found to lie within the same chromosomal region (miR-424 and 20b at Xq26.2-3, 377 kb apart; miR-142 and 301a at 17q22, 820 kb apart; miR-324-5p and 497 at 17p13.1, 205 kb apart). This suggests that at least some of the downregulated miRNA expression is due to decreased transcription. Many of the downregulated miRNAs also shared 5′-seed sequences that are involved in target recognition. For example, identical seed sequences are shared by (a) miR-20a and 20b; (b) miR-301a and 130a; and (c) miR-424 and 497. As well, a 6-mer nucleotide motif is shared by miR-34a, 34b*, and 34c, and strikingly, a 5-mer motif (AGUGC) within the 5′-seed is shared by five of the affected miRNAs (miR-148b, 301a, 130a, 20a, and 20b) that is predicted to bind Alu sequences within the 3′-UTR region of target mRNAs. This suggests that the downregulated miRNAs should exhibit extensive overlap among their mRNA targets.

When pair-wise correlations were made (a complementary method of analyzing the miRNA expression data is to identify pairs of miRNAs that are co-regulated in their expression, up or down, across individuals within a single group), a set of 29 miRNAs were identified, none of which were pair-wise correlated in the normal control group, but which formed a very extensive interconnected network in the depressed group. Several of the miRNAs (let-7b, miR-132, 181b, 338-3p, 486-5p, and 650) were "hubs" correlated with four to nine other miRNAs in the network. Target analysis revealed that many of the targets are transcription factors, and nuclear, transmembrane, and signaling proteins. Intriguingly, four different downregulated miRNAs target VEGFA (miR-20b, 20a, 34a, and 34b*), a molecule implicated in depression in both humans and in animal models. Other validated targets include BCL2 (miR-34a), DNMT3B (miR-148b), and MYCN (miR-101, 34a). Among predicted targets, estrogen receptor alpha, ESR1, was predicted to be targeted by three different downregulated miRNAs (miR-148b, 301a, and 496). Others targeted by three or more affected miRNAs include ubiquitin ligases (UBE2D1 and UBE2 W), signal transduction mediators (CAMK2G, AKAP1), the splicing factor NOVA1 that regulates brain-specific alternative splicing; the

GABA-A receptor subunit GABRA4; calcium channel CACNA1C; and brain-active transcription factors including SMAD5, MITF, BACH2, MYCN, and ARID4A. Several of these predicted targets interact with validated targets; for example, ARIA4A binds E2F1; SMAD5 binds RUNX1; and estradiol treatment decreases E2F1 levels in prefrontal cortex (Wang et al. 2004). BACH2 transcription factor binding sites have been identified upstream of many brain-expressed miRNAs (Wu and Xie 2006). Retinoblastoma binding protein 1 (ARIA4A) is of interest because it recruits histone deacetylases and regulates gene expression via chromatin-based silencing.

Selected target proteins such as DMNT3b, VEGFA, and BCL2 were studied by examining their expression in depressed suicide brain. DMNT3b was strongly upregulated in the depressed suicide group, whereas BCL2 was downregulated. Several miRNAs that were coregulated with their targets showed a strong positive correlation with DMNT3b and BCL2. A variety of factors such as transcription factor activity and turnover rate, as well as possible regulatory effects of other miRNAs may also be responsible for changes in mean expression levels of these target proteins. In addition, DNMT3b levels showed an extremely strong positive correlation with miR-148b across subjects ($r = 0.91$ in controls, $r = 0.94$ in the depressed suicide group). Similarly, BCL2 was strongly and positively correlated with miR-34a ($r = 0.92$ in healthy controls, $r = 0.82$ in the depressed suicide group). The correlation of miR-34a was positive in healthy controls, but inverse in the depressed suicide group, presumably reflecting a reorganization of miRNA-target networks (Smalheiser et al. 2012).

Previous studies indicate that TrkB-T1, a BDNF receptor lacking a tyrosine kinase domain that is highly expressed in astrocytes and regulates BDNF-evoked calcium transients, is downregulated in frontal cortex of suicide subjects (Ernst et al. 2009, 2011). In a recent study, Maussion et al. (2012) examined whether this TrkB-T1 gene is regulated by miRNAs. The investigators found that Hsa-miR-185* and Hsa-miR-491-3p were upregulated in suicide completers with low expression of TrkB.T1 (P(nominal): 9.10(−5) and 1.8.10(−4), respectively; FDR-corrected $p = 0.031$). Bioinformatic analyses revealed five putative binding sites for the DiGeorge syndrome-linked miRNA Hsa-miR-185*in the 3′UTR of TrkB-T1, but none for Hsa-miR-491-3P. The increase of Hsa-miR-185* in frontal cortex of suicide completers was validated then confirmed in a larger, randomly selected group of suicide completers, where an inverse correlation between Hsa-miR-185* and TrkB-T1 expression was observed ($R = -0.439$; $p = 0.001$). Silencing and overexpression studies performed in human cell lines confirmed the inverse relationship between hsa-mir-185* and trkB-T1 expression. Luciferase assays demonstrated that Hsa-miR-185* binds to sequences in the 3′UTR of TrkB-T1. These results suggest that an increase of Hsa-miR-185* expression levels regulates, at least in part, the TrkB-T1 decrease observed in the frontal cortex of suicide completers and further implicate the 22q11 region in psychopathology.

Alterations in metabolic enzymes of the polyamine system have been reported to play a role in predisposition to suicidal behavior (Fiori et al. 2011). Recently, Lopez et al. (2014) examined whether dysregulation of polyamine genes in depressed suicide completers could be influenced by miRNA post-transcriptional regulation. These investigators identified several miRNAs that target the 3′UTR of polyamine genes SAT1 and SMOX. When the expression of 10 miRNAs in the prefrontal cortex of suicide completers and controls using qRT-PCR were profiled, they found that several miRNAs showed significant up-regulation in the prefrontal cortex of suicide completers compared to psychiatrically-healthy controls (miR-124, miR-139-5p, miR-195, miR-198, miR-320c, miR-33b, miR-34a, miR-34c-5p, miR-497, miR-873). However, they found that only miR-139-5p, miR-320c were inversely correlated with polyamine gene SAT1 whereas miR34c-5p and miR-320c were inversely correlated with polyamine gene SMOX. These results suggest a relationship between miRNAs and polyamine gene expression in the suicide brain, and postulate a mechanism for SAT1 and SMOX down-regulation by post-transcriptional activity of miRNAs.

17.7 miRNAs in Clinical Diagnosis of Depression and Suicidal Behavior: Role of Circulating miRNAs

miRNA can be detected in circulating biological fluids such as serum, plasma, urine, saliva, and CSF (Cogswell et al. 2008; Hanke et al. 2010; Weber et al. 2010). Under healthy conditions, these miRNAs are stably expressed in blood cells; however, under pathological conditions, the profile of miRNAs changes significantly, suggesting that peripheral miRNAs can possibly be used as a reliable biomarker under disease conditions. Recently, blood cell miRNAs have been shown to be extremely useful for detecting and following the course of human cancer, myocardial infarction, and neurodegenerative conditions, including Alzheimer's disease, Parkinson disease, Huntington disease, and prion disease (Chen et al. 2008; Fichtlscherer et al. 2010; Ma et al. 2013; Dorval et al. 2013; Jin et al. 2013).

Circulating miRNAs arise from heterogeneous sources and are expressed within different compartments of blood. For neuropsychiatric perspective, it is imperative to characterize miRNAs in blood cells that are brain derived. In this respect, it has been shown that miRNAs can be released actively or passively from neurons into the circulating blood (Fichtlscherer et al. 2010). These miRNAs are enclosed in exosomes or microvesicles and are protected by RNA-binding proteins.

The use of miRNAs as peripheral biomarker in depression is gaining momentum. Belzeaux et al. (2012) examined the miRNA expression profile in peripheral blood mononuclear cells (PBMCs) collected from 16 severely depressed patients and 13 matched controls at baseline, 2 and 8 weeks after treatment. miRNAs that showed changes between depressed and controls at baseline included: has-miR-107, miR-133a, miR-148a, miR-200c, miR-381, miR-425-3p, miR-494, miR-517b, miR-579, miR-589, miR-636, miR-652, miR-941, and miR-1243. Only 2 miRNAs showed stable overexpression in depressed patients during the 8-week follow-up compared with controls (miR-941 and miR-589). They also identified miRNAs exhibiting significant variations of expression among patients with clinical improvement (7 upregulated and 1 downregulated). Fourteen dysregulated miRNAs had putative mRNA targets that were differentially expressed in depressed subjects, suggesting a common RNA regulatory network functions in depression. These results also suggest the potential utility of miRNA signatures as markers of depressive episode evolution.

Bocchio-Chiavetto et al. (2013) conducted a whole-miRNome quantitative analysis in the blood of 10 MDD subjects after 12 weeks of treatment with escitalopram. They found that 30 miRNAs were differentially expressed after the escitalopram treatment: 28 miRNAs were upregulated, and 2 miRNAs were downregulated. Thirteen of them (let-7d, let-7e, miR-26a, miR-26b, miR-34c-5p, miR-103, miR-128, miR-132, miR-183, miR-192, miR-335, miR-494, and miR-22) play a role in the neural plasticity and stress response and in the pathogenetic mechanisms of several neuropsychiatric diseases. miR-132 exerts critical functions in the biological circuits implicated in neurogenesis and synaptic plasticity, stimulating axonal and dendritic outgrowth in different brain areas (Mellios et al. 2011). This miRNA, together with miR-26a, miR-26b, and miR-183, widely contributes to the action of the neurotrophin BDNF in the brain (Wayman et al. 2008; Caputo et al. 2011; Kawashima et al. 2010). miR-132, miR-26a, miR-26b, miR-183, let-7d, let-7e, miR-26b, miR-103, miR-128, miR-494, and miR-22 have been reported to play a role in the pathogenesis of psychiatric disorders and in the mechanism of action of antipsychotic drugs and mood stabilizers. Moreover, postmortem studies in the brains of bipolar disorder patients show increased levels of miR-22* in the prefrontal cortex (Kim et al. 2010). On the other hand, miR-494 and miR-335 are downregulated in the prefrontal cortex of depressed suicide patients (Smalheiser et al. 2012). The target genes of these altered miRNAs include: BDNF, GR, NR3C1, and the nitric oxide synthase NOS1, growth factors (IGF1, FGF1, FGFR1, VEGFa, and GDNF), calcium channels (CACN41C, CACNB4, SLC6A12, and SLC8A3), and neurotransmitter receptors (GABRA4 and 5-HT4), some of which have been implicated depression and in the mechanism of action of antidepressants. These studies suggest that miRNAs can not only be used to diagnose but can also be used for treatment response.

More recently, He et al. (2012) studied an association between miRNA processing gene variants and depression. They genotyped three polymorphisms from three miRNA processing genes (DGCR8, AGO1, and GEMIN4) in a case-control study including 314 patients and 252 matched healthy controls. Frequencies of genotypes and alleles showed significant difference between patients with depression and healthy controls in DGCR8 rs3757 and AGO1 rs636832. An allele frequency was significantly higher in rs3757 and lower in rs636832, respectively. Variant allele of DGCR8 rs3757 was associated with increased risk of suicidal tendency and improvement response to antidepressant treatment, whereas the variant of AGO1 rs636832 showed decreased risk of suicidal tendency, suicidal behavior, and recurrence. Whereas allele frequency showed a significant difference when compared patients with remission to controls, no significant differences were found in GEMIN4 rs7813 between patients and healthy controls. DGCR8 rs3757 and AGO1 rs636832 were found to have significant association with depression, and GEMIN4 rs7813 did not affect susceptibility to depression. These observations suggested that miRNA processing polymorphisms may affect depression risk and treatment.

Depression has been linked with disruption in circadian rhythms, and sleep disturbance is a key symptom in affective disorders (Salgado-Delgado et al. 2011). A SNP in miR-182 has been found to be associated with late insomnia in patients with depression. Patients with this SNP had downregulated expression of genes linked to circadian rhythm like *Clock* that previously had been associated with affective disorders (Serretti et al. 2003).

In a recent study, Li et al. (2013) identified and characterized the roles of BDNF and its putative regulatory miRNAs in depression. They identified that miR-182 may be a putative miRNA that regulates BDNF levels, and characterized the effects of miR-182 on the BDNF levels using cell-based studies, side by side with miR-132 (a known miRNA that regulates BDNF expression). They showed that treatment of miR-132 and miR-182, respectively, decreased the BDNF protein levels in a human neuronal cell model, supporting the regulatory roles of miR-132 and miR-182 on the BDNF expression. Furthermore, they explored the roles of miR-132 and miR-182 on the BDNF levels in depression using human subjects by assessing their serum levels. Compared with the healthy controls, patients with depression showed lower serum BDNF levels and higher serum miR-132 and miR-182 levels. They also found that there was a significant negative correlation between the Self-Rating Depression Scale score and serum BDNF levels, and a positive correlation between the Self-Rating Depression Scale score and miR-132 levels. In addition, a reverse relationship between the serum BDNF levels and the miR-132/miR-182 levels in depression was found. Collectively, this study suggests that miR-182 is a putative BDNF-regulatory miRNA and serum BDNF and its related miRNAs may be utilized as important biomarkers in the diagnosis or as therapeutic targets of depression.

17.8 Conclusion and Future Directions

The measurement and suggested involvement of miRNAs in depression and suicidal behavior is a relatively new field of study. However, the above described studies strongly implicate miRNAs participation in the pathogenesis, expression, severity, and treatment-response in these disorders (Table 17.1). The majority of the studies examined miRNAs linking to individual genes. However, it is now established that a combination of miRNAs is much more powerful regulator than individual miRNAs and differential co-expression of a group of miRNAs not only play a direct role in human disease pathophysiology, but they also help in identifying the nature of disordered pathways implicated in such pathophysiology (Stäehler et al. 2012; Xu et al. 2011; Mo et al. 2009). Thus, by examining sets of miRNAs that are significantly affected in the pathological group, and the corresponding set of mRNAs that are affected in the same samples, will help further clarify this issue.

One can also consider identifying set(s) of miRNAs that are not correlated in expression across individuals in the healthy control group, yet are positively correlated in the pathogenic group and vice versa.

It is important to determine whether the changes in miRNA/mRNA network are similar or different across different brain areas and more so, whether they are cell type-specific, and are reversible. Also important is to examine the potential reasons for altered miRNA expression. Is it because of genetic changes in the promoter region upstream of primary miRNA gene transcripts, the pre-miRNA hairpin, or the mature miRNA or due to RNA editing of transcripts or epigenetic suppression of the chromosomal region encoding the miRNAs? A variety of enzymes are responsible for processing miRNAs. These include drosha, dicer, and cofactors DGCR8, TRBP, and PACT. Several of these proteins have been shown to be modified post-translationally in a dynamic manner. For example, altering the relative expression of eIF2c may change the efficiency of translational arrest produced by a given miRNA (Azuma-Mukai et al. 2008). Recently, it has been shown that dicer is activated by proteolytic cleavage under conditions of elevated calcium levels (Lugli et al. 2005; Smalheiser 2008); and eIF2C undergoes reversible phosphorylation within cells, which is required for its translocation to processing bodies (Zeng et al. 2008). The phosphorylation of eIF2C appears to be due to activation of ERK1/2 (Zeng et al. 2008). Since abnormalities in calcium-sensing proteins and ERK1/2 signaling in the brain of depressed suicide subjects has been shown (Dwivedi et al. 2001, 2006, 2009b, 2011b), it will be worthwhile asking whether dicer cleavage patterns or eIF2C phosphorylation are altered in the these subjects. One can also examine whether there is any genetic link between miRNA and depression and suicide. Such genetic linkage has been reported in specific miRNAs in schizophrenia (Mellios and Sur 2012).

The presence of miRNAs in peripheral tissues, particularly, in blood cells provide promising approach to use miRNAs as potential biomarker for both diagnosis and treatment response. There are several issues that need consideration for the use of circulating miRNAs as biomarker. For example, the source of miRNAs in blood cells is not clear at the present time. In this regard, exosomal miRNAs may be useful in detecting miRNAs of neuronal origin. However, there is a possibility that changes in circulating miRNAs may not be directly related to the changes in the brain. While this complicates the study of circulating miRNAs, miRNAs still appear to have promise to be useful biomarkers, since it is likely that they reflect systemic alterations that accompany the disease process (e.g. chronic stress, inflammatory, and neuroimmune processes) and may therefore be worthy of further study.

Acknowledgment The research was partly supported by grants from National Institute of Mental Health (R01MH082802; R21MH081099; R21MH091509; 1R01MH101890), American Foundation for Suicide Prevention, and University of Illinois at Chicago Center for Clinical and Translational Sciences supported by National Center for Advancing Translational Sciences, National Institutes of Health (Grant # UL1TR000050).

References

Aganova EA, Uranova NA (1992) Morphometric analysis of synaptic contacts in the anterior limbic cortex in the endogenous psychoses. Neurosci Behav Physiol 22:59–65

Ashraf SI, McLoon AL, Sclarsic SM, Kunes S (2006) Synaptic protein synthesis associated with memory is regulated by the RISC pathway in Drosophila. Cell 124:191–205

Azuma-Mukai A, Oguri H, Mituyama T, Qian ZR, Asai K, Siomi H, Siomi MC (2008) Characterization of endogenous human Argonautes and their miRNA partners in RNA silencing. Proc Natl Acad Sci USA 105:7964–7969

Belzeaux R, Bergon A, Jeanjean V, Loriod B, Formisano-Tréziny C, Verrier L, Loundou A, Baumstarck-Barrau K, Boyer L, Gall V, Gabert J, Nguyen C, Azorin JM, Naudin J, Ibrahim EC (2012) Responder and nonresponder patients exhibit different peripheral transcriptional signatures during major depressive episode. Transl Psychiatry 2:e185

Bocchio-Chiavetto L, Maffioletti E, Bettinsoli P, Giovannini C, Bignotti S, Tardito D, Corrada D, Milanesi L, Gennarelli M (2013) Blood microRNA changes in depressed patients during antidepressant treatment. Eur Neuropsychopharmacol 23:602–611

Brodersen P, Voinnet O (2009) Revisiting the principles of microRNA target recognition and mode of action. Nat Rev Mol Cell Biol 10:141–148

Budhu A, Ji J, Wang XW (2010) The clinical potential of microRNAs. J Hematol Oncol 3:37

Burke KC, Burke JD Jr, Rae DS, Regier DA (1991) Comparing age at onset of major depression and other psychiatric disorders by birth cohorts in five US community populations. Arch Gen Psychiatry 48:789–795

Cao MQ, Chen DH, Zhang CH, Wu ZZ (2007) Screening of specific microRNA in hippocampus of depression model rats and intervention effect of Chaihu Shugan San. Zhongguo Zhong Yao Za Zhi 38(10):1585–1589

Cao MQ, Chen DH, Zhang CH, Wu ZZ (2013) Screening of specific microRNA in hippocampus of depression model rats and intervention effect of Chaihu Shugan San. Zhongguo Zhong Yao Za Zhi 38:1585–1589

Caputo V, Sinibaldi L, Fiorentino A (2011) Brain derived neurotrophic factor (BDNF) expression is regulated by microRNAs miR-26a and miR-26b allele-specific binding. PLoSOne 6:e28656

Chen X, Ba Y, Ma L, Cai X, Yin Y, Wang K, Guo J, Zhang Y, Chen J, Guo X, Li Q, Li X, Wang W, Zhang Y, Wang J, Jiang X, Xiang Y, Xu C, Zheng P, Zhang J, Li R, Zhang H, Shang X, Gong T, Ning G, Wang J, Zen K, Zhang J, Zhang CY (2008) Characterization of microRNAs in serum: a novel class of biomarkers for diagnosis of cancer and other diseases. Cell Res 18:997–1006

Chendrimada TP, Gregory RI, Kumaraswamy E, Norman J, Cooch N, Nishikura K, Shiekhattar R (2005) TRBP recruits the Dicer complex to Ago2 for microRNA processing and gene silencing. Nature 436:740–744

Chendrimada TP, Finn KJ, Ji X, Baillat D, Gregory RI, Liebhaber SA, Pasquinelli AE, Shiekhattar R (2007) MicroRNA silencing through RISC recruitment of eIF6. Nature 447:823–828

Chuang JC, Jones PA (2007) Epigenetics and microRNAs. Pediatr Res 61:24R–29R

Cogswell JP, Ward J, Taylor IA, Waters M, Shi Y, Cannon B, Kelnar K, Kemppainen J, Brown D, Chen C, Prinjha RK, Richardson JC, Saunders AM, Roses AD, Richards CA (2008) Identification of miRNA changes in Alzheimer's disease brain and CSF yields putative biomarkers and insights into disease pathways. J Alzheimers Dis 14:27–41

Cotter D, Mackay D, Landau S, Kerwin R, Everall I (2001) Reduced glial cell density and neuronal size in the anterior cingulate cortex in major depressive disorder. Arch Gen Psychiatry 58:545–553

Davis TH, Cuellar TL, Koch SM, Barker AJ, Harfe BD, McManus MT, Ullian EM (2008) Conditional loss of Dicer disrupts cellular and tissue morphogenesis in the cortex and hippocampus. J Neurosci 28:4322–4330

De Pietri Tonelli D, Pulvers JM, Haffner C, Murchison EP, Hannon GJ, Huttner WB (2008) MiRNAs are essential for survival and differentiation of newborn neurons but not for

expansion of neural progenitors during early neurogenesis in the mouse embryonic neocortex. Development 135:3911–3921
Dorval V, Nelson PT, Hébert SS (2013) Circulating microRNAs in Alzheimer's disease: the search for novel biomarkers. Front Mol Neurosci 6:24
Dwivedi Y (2011) Evidence demonstrating role of microRNAs in the etiopathology of major depression. J Chem Neuroanat 42:142–156
Dwivedi Y, Rizavi HS, Roberts RC, Conley RC, Tamminga CA, Pandey GN (2001) Reduced activation and expression of ERK1/2 MAP kinase in the post-mortem brain of depressed suicide subjects. J Neurochem 77:916–928
Dwivedi Y, Rao JS, Rizavi HS, Kotowski J, Conley RR, Roberts RC, Tamminga CA, Pandey GN (2003a) Abnormal expression and functional characteristics of cyclic adenosine monophosphate response element binding protein in postmortem brain of suicide subjects. Arch Gen Psychiatry 60:273–282
Dwivedi Y, Rizavi HS, Conley RR, Roberts RC, Tamminga CA, Pandey GN (2003b) Altered gene expression of brain-derived neurotrophic factor and receptor tyrosine kinase B in postmortem brain of suicide subjects. Arch Gen Psychiatry 60:804–815
Dwivedi Y, Rizavi HS, Conley RR, Pandey GN (2006) ERK MAP kinase signaling in postmortem brain of suicide subjects: differential regulation of upstream Raf kinases Raf-1 and B-Raf. Mol Psychiatry 11:86–98
Dwivedi Y, Rizavi HS, Zhang H, Roberts RC, Conley RR, Pandey GN (2009a) Aberrant extracellular signal-regulated kinase (ERK)1/2 signalling in suicide brain: role of ERK kinase 1 (MEK1). Int J Neuropsychopharmacol 12:1337–1354
Dwivedi Y, Rizavi H, Zhang H, Mondal AC, Roberts RC, Conley RR, Pandey GN (2009b) Neurotrophin receptor activation and expression in human postmortem brain: effect of suicide. Biol Psychiatry 65:319–328
Dwivedi Y, Zhang H, Pandey GN (2011a) Calcium sensing proteins in depressive disorder. Am Coll Neuropsychophramacol Abs 225:S75–S197
Edbauer D, Neilson JR, Foster KA, Wang CF, Seeburg DP, Batterton MN, Tada T, Dolan BM, Sharp PA, Sheng M (2010) Regulation of synaptic structure and function by FMRP-associated microRNAs miR-125b and miR-132. Neuron 65:373–384
Ernst C, Deleva V, Deng X, Sequeira A, Pomarenski A, Klempan T, Ernst N, Quirion R, Gratton A, Szyf M, Turecki G (2009) Alternative splicing, methylation state, and expression profile of tropomyosin-related kinase B in the frontal cortex of suicide completers. Arch Gen Psychiatry 66:22–32
Ernst C, Nagy C, Kim S, Yang JP, Deng X, Hellstrom IC, Choi KH, Gershenfeld H, Meaney MJ, Turecki G (2011) Dysfunction of astrocyte connexins 30 and 43 in dorsal lateral prefrontal cortex of suicide completers. Biol Psychiatry 70:312–319
Fava M, Davidson KG (1996) Definition and epidemiology of treatment-resistant depression. Psychiatr Clin North Am 19:179–200
Fichtlscherer S, De Rosa S, Fox H, Schwietz T, Fischer A, Liebetrau C, Weber M, Hamm CW, Röxe T, Müller-Ardogan M, Bonauer A, Zeiher AM, Dimmeler S (2010) Circulating microRNAs in patients with coronary artery disease. Circ Res 107:677–684
Fiore R, Khudayberdiev S, Christensen M, Siegel G, Flavell SW, Kim TK, Greenberg ME, Schratt G (2009) Mef2-mediated transcription of the miR379-410 cluster regulates activity-dependent dendritogenesis by fine-tuning Pumilio2 protein levels. EMBO J 28:697–710
Fiori LM, Bureau A, Labbe A, Croteau J, Noël S, Mérette C, Turecki G (2011) Global gene expression profiling of the polyamine system in suicide completers. Int J Neuropsychopharmacol 14:595–605
Gao J, Wang WY, Mao YW, Gräff J, Guan JS, Pan L, Mak G, Kim D, Su SC, Tsai LH (2010) A novel pathway regulates memory and plasticity via SIRT1 and miR-134. Nature 466:1105–1109
Hanke M, Hoefig K, Merz H, Feller AC, Kausch I, Jocham D, Warnecke JM, Sczakiel G (2010) A robust methodology to study urine microRNA as tumor marker: microRNA-126 and microRNA-182 are related to urinary bladder cancer. Urol Oncol 28:655–661

He Y, Zhou Y, Xi Q, Cui H, Luo T, Song H, Nie X, Wang L, Ying B (2012) Genetic variations in microRNA processing genes are associated with susceptibility in depression. DNA Cell Biol 31:1499–1506

Honer WG (1999) Assessing the machinery of mind: synapses in neuropsychiatric disorders. J Psychiatry Neurosci 24:116–121

Hussain MU (2012) Micro-RNAs (miRNAs): genomic organisation, biogenesis and mode of action. Cell Tissue Res 349:405–413

Im HI, Kenny PJ (2012) MicroRNAs in neuronal function and dysfunction. Trends Neurosci 35:325–334

Impey S, Davare M, Lasiek A, Fortin D, Ando H, Varlamova O, Obrietan K, Soderling TR, Goodman RH, Wayman GA (2010) An activity-induced microRNA controls dendritic spine formation by regulating Rac1-PAK signaling. Mol Cell Neurosci 43:146–156

Jin P, Zarnescu DC, Ceman S, Nakamoto M, Mowrey J, Jongens TA, Nelson DL, Moses K, Warren ST (2004) Biochemical and genetic interaction between the fragile X mental retardation protein and the microRNA pathway. Nat Neurosci 7:113–117

Jin XF, Wu N, Wang L, Li J (2013) Circulating microRNAs: a novel class of potential biomarkers for diagnosing and prognosing central nervous system diseases. Cell Mol Neurobiol 33:601–613

Kawashima H, Numakawa T, Kumamaru E, Adachi N, Mizuno H, Ninomiya M, Kunugi H, Hashido K (2010) Glucocorticoid attenuates brain-derived neurotrophic factor-dependent upregulation of glutamate receptors via the suppression of microRNA-132 expression. Neuroscience 165:1301–1311

Kessler RC, McGonagle KA, Zhao S, Nelson CB, Hughes M, Eshleman S, Wittchen HU, Kendler KS (1994) Lifetime and 12-month prevalence of DSM-III-R psychiatric disorders in the United States. Results from the National Comorbidity Survey. Arch Gen Psychiatry 51:8–19

Kim AH, Reimers M, Maher B, Williamson V, McMichael O, McClay JL, van den Oord EJ, Riley BP, Kendler KS, Vladimirov VI (2010) MicroRNA expression profiling in the prefrontal cortex of individuals affected with schizophrenia and bipolar disorders. Schizophr Res 124:183–191

Kosik KS (2006) The neuronal microRNA system. Nat Rev Neurosci 7:911–920

Leistedt SJ, Linkowski P (2013) Brain, networks, depression, and more. Eur Neuropsychopharmacol 23:55–62

Li YJ, Xu M, Gao ZH, Wang YQ, Yue Z, Zhang YX, Li XX, Zhang C, Xie SY, Wang PY (2013) Alterations of serum levels of BDNF-related miRNAs in patients with depression. PLoS ONE 8:e63648

Lopez JP, Fiori LM, Gross JA, Labonte B, Yerko V, Mechawar N, Turecki G (2014) Regulatory role of miRNAs in polyamine gene expression in the prefrontal cortex of depressed suicide completers. Int J Neuropsychopharmacol 17(1):23–32

Lugli G, Larson J, Martone ME, Jones Y, Smalheiser NR (2005) Dicer and eIF2c are enriched at postsynaptic densities in adult mouse brain and are modified by neuronal activity in a calpain-dependent manner. J Neurochem 94:896–905

Lugli G, Torvik VI, Larson J, Smalheiser NR (2008) Expression of microRNAs and their precursors in synaptic fractions of adult mouse forebrain. J Neurochem 106:650–661

Ma L, Wei L, Wu F, Hu Z, Liu Z, Yuan W (2013) Advances with microRNAs in Parkinson's disease research. Drug Des Devel Ther 7:1103–1113

Malphettes L, Fussenegger M (2006) Impact of RNA interference on gene networks. Metab Eng 8:672–683

Mathonnet G, Fabian MR, Svitkin YV, Parsyan A, Huck L, Murata T, Biffo S, Merrick WC, Darzynkiewicz E, Pillai RS, Filipowicz W, Duchaine TF, Sonenberg N (2007) MicroRNA inhibition of translation initiation in vitro by targeting the cap-binding complex eIF4F. Science 317:1764–1767

Matigian N, Windus L, Smith H, Filippich C, Pantelis C, McGrath J, Mowry B, Hayward N (2007) Expression profiling in monozygotic twins discordant for bipolar disorder reveals dysregulation of the WNT signalling pathway. Mol Psychiatry 12:815–825

Maussion G, Yang J, Yerko V, Barker P, Mechawar N, Ernst C, Turecki G (2012) Regulation of a truncated form of tropomyosin-related kinase B (TrkB) by Hsa-miR-185* in frontal cortex of suicide completers. PLoS ONE 7:e39301

McEwen BS (2000) Effects of adverse experiences for brain structure and function. Biol Psychiatry 48:713–714

Meerson A, Cacheaux L, Goosens KA, Sapolsky RM, Soreq H, Kaufer D (2010) Changes in brain MicroRNAs contribute to cholinergic stress reactions. J Mol Neurosci 40:47–55

Mellios N, Sur M (2012) The Emerging Role of microRNAs in Schizophrenia and Autism Spectrum Disorders. Front Psychiatry 3:39

Mellios N, Sugihara H, Castro J (2011) miR-132, an experience-dependent microRNA, is essential for visual cortex plasticity. Nat Neurosci 14:1240–1242

Meng Y, Takahashi H, Meng J, Zhang Y, Lu G, Asrar S, Nakamura T, Jia Z (2004) Regulation of ADF/cofilin phosphorylation and synaptic function by LIM-kinase. Neuropharmacology 47:746–754

Michalak P (2006) RNA world - the dark matter of evolutionary genomics. J Evol Biol 19:1768–1774

Mo WJ, Fu XP, Han XT, Yang GY, Zhang JG, Guo FH, Huang Y, Mao YM, Li Y, Xie Y (2009) A stochastic model for identifying differential gene pair co-expression patterns in prostate cancer progression. BMC Genom 10:340

Mulrow CD, Williams JW Jr, Trivedi M, Chiquette E, Aguilar C, Cornell JE, Badgett R, Noel PH, Lawrence V, Lee S, Luther M, Ramirez G, Richardson WS, Stamm K (1999) Treatment of depression-newer pharmacotherapies. Evid Rep Technol Assess (Summ) 7:1–4

Murray CJ, Lopez AD (1997) Alternative projections of mortality and disability by cause 1990–2020: global burden of disease study. Lancet 349:1498–1504

Olde Loohuis NF, Kos A, Martens GJ, Van Bokhoven H, Nadif Kasri N, Aschrafi A (2012) MicroRNA networks direct neuronal development and plasticity. Cell Mol Life Sci 69:89–102

Ongur D, Drevets WC, Price JL (1998) Glial reduction in the subgenual prefrontal cortex in mood disorders. Proc Natl Acad Sci USA 95:13290–13295

Ota KT, Duman RS (2013) Environmental and pharmacological modulations of cellular plasticity: role in the pathophysiology and treatment of depression. Neurobiol Dis 57:28–37

Pariante CM, Miller AH (2001) Glucocorticoid receptors in major depression: relevance to pathophysiology and treatment. Biol Psychiatry 49:391–404

Qurashi A, Chang S, Peng J (2007) Role of microRNA pathway in mental retardation. Sci World J 7:146–154

Rajasethupathy P, Fiumara F, Sheridan R, Betel D, Puthanveettil SV, Russo JJ, Sander C, Tuschl T, Kandel E (2009) Characterization of small RNAs in Aplysia reveals a role for miR-124 in constraining synaptic plasticity through CREB. Neuron 63:803–817

Rinaldi A, Vincenti S, De Vito F, Bozzoni I, Oliverio A, Presutti C, Fragapane P, Mele A (2010) Stress induces region specific alterations in microRNAs expression in mice. Behav Brain Res 208:265–269

Salgado-Delgado R, Tapia Osorio A, Saderi N, Escobar C (2011) Disruption of circadian rhythms: a crucial factor in the etiology of depression. Depress Res Treat 839743

Sato F, Tsuchiya S, Meltzer SJ, Shimizu K (2011) MicroRNAs and epigenetics. FEBS J 278:1598–1609

Schaefer A, O'carroll D, Tan CL, Hillman D, Sugimori M, Llinas R, Greengard P (2007) Cerebellar neurodegeneration in the absence of microRNAs. J Exp Med 204:1553–1558

Schratt G (2009) Fine-tuning neural gene expression with microRNAs. Curr Opin Neurobiol 19:213–219

Schratt GM, Tuebing F, Nigh EA, Kane CG, Sabatini ME, Kiebler M, Greenberg ME (2006) A brain-specific microRNA regulates dendritic spine development. Nature 439:283–289

Scott HL, Tamagnini F, Narduzzo KE, Howarth JL, Lee YB, Wong LF, Brown MW, Warburton EC, Bashir ZI, Uney JB (2012) MicroRNA-132 regulates recognition memory and synaptic plasticity in the perirhinal cortex. Eur J Neurosci 36:2941–2948

Serretti A, Benedetti F, Mandelli L, Lorenzi C, Pirovano A, Colombo C, Smeraldi E (2003) Genetic dissection of psychopathological symptoms: insomnia in mood disorders and CLOCK gene polymorphism. Am J Med Genet B Neuropsychiatr Genet 121B:35–38

Siegel G, Obernosterer G, Fiore R, Oehmen M, Bicker S, Christensen M, Khudayberdiev S, Leuschner PF, Busch CJ, Kane C, Hübel K, Dekker F, Hedberg C, Rengarajan B, Drepper C, Waldmann H, Kauppinen S, Greenberg ME, Draguhn A, Rehmsmeier M, Martinez J, Schratt GM (2009) A functional screen implicates microRNA-138-dependent regulation of the depalmitoylation enzyme APT1 in dendritic spine morphogenesis. Nat Cell Biol 11:705–716

Smalheiser NR (2008) Synaptic enrichment of microRNAs in adult mouse forebrain is related to structural features of their precursors. Biol Direct 3:44

Smalheiser NR, Lugli G, Rizavi HS, Zhang H, Torvik VI, Pandey GN, Davis JM, Dwivedi Y (2011) MicroRNA expression in rat brain exposed to repeated inescapable shock: differential alterations in learned helplessness versus non-learned helplessness. Int J Neuropsychopharmacol 14:1315–1325

Smalheiser NR, Lugli G, Rizavi HS, Torvik VI, Turecki G, Dwivedi Y (2012) MicroRNA expression is down-regulated and reorganized in prefrontal cortex of depressed suicide subjects. PLoS ONE 7:e33201

Smalheiser NR, Zhang H, Dwivedi Y (2014) Enoxacin elevates microRNA levels in rat frontal cortex and prevents learned helplessness. Front Neurogenomics (in press)

Stäehler CF, Keller A, Leidinger P, Backes C, Chandran A, Wischhusen J, Meder B, Meese E (2012) Whole miRNome-wide differential co-expression of microRNAs. Genomics Proteomics Bioinform 10:285–294

Stark KL, Xu B, Bagchi A, Lai WS, Liu H, Hsu R, Wan X, Pavlidis P, Mills AA, Karayiorgou M, Gogos JA (2008) Altered brain microRNA biogenesis contributes to phenotypic deficits in a 22q11-deletion mouse model. Nat Genet 40:751–760

Sutton MA, Schuman EM (2005) Local translational control in dendrites and its role in long-term synaptic plasticity. J Neurobiol 64:116

Tardito D, Mallei A, Popoli M (2013) Lost in translation. New unexplored avenues for neuropsychopharmacology: epigenetics and microRNAs. Expert Opin Investig Drugs 22:217–233

Todd PK, Mack KJ, Malter JS (2003) The fragile X mental retardation protein is required for type-I metabotropic glutamate receptor-dependent translation of PSD-95. Proc Natl Acad Sci USA 100:14374–14378

Toni N, Buchs PA, Nikonenko I, Bron CR, Muller D (1999) LTP promotes formation of multiple spine synapses between a single axon terminal and a dendrite. Nature 402:421–425

Turner JD, Alt SR, Cao L, Vernocchi S, Trifonova S, Battello N, Muller CP (2010) Transcriptional control of the glucocorticoid receptor: CpG islands, epigenetics and more. Biochem Pharmacol 80:1860–1868

Uchida S, Nishida A, Hara K, Kamemoto T, Suetsugi M, Fujimoto M, Watanuki T, Wakabayashi Y, Otsuki K, McEwen BS, Watanabe Y (2008) Characterization of the vulnerability to repeated stress in Fischer 344 rats: possible involvement of microRNA-mediated down-regulation of the glucocorticoid receptor. Eur J Neurosci 27(9):2250–2261

Vasudevan S, Tong Y, Steitz JA (2007) Switching from repression to activation: microRNAs can up-regulate translation. Science 318:1931–1934

Vo N, Klein ME, Varlamova O, Keller DM, Yamamoto T, Goodman RH, Impey S (2005) A cAMP-response element binding protein-induced microRNA regulates neuronal morphogenesis. Proc Natl Acad Sci USA 102:16426–16431

Vreugdenhil E, Verissimo CS, Mariman R, Kamphorst JT, Barbosa JS, Zweers T, Champagne DL, Schouten T, Meijer OC, de Kloet ER, Fitzsimons CP (2009) MicroRNA 18 and 124a down-regulate the glucocorticoid receptor: implications for glucocorticoid responsiveness in the brain. Endocrinology 150:2220–2228

Wang J, Cheng CM, Zhou J, Smith A, Weickert CS, Perlman WR, Becker KG, Powell D, Bondy CA (2004) Estradiol alters transcription factor gene expression in primate prefrontal cortex. J Neurosci Res 76:306–314

Wayman GA, Davare M, Ando H, Fortin D, Varlamova O, Cheng HY, Marks D, Obrietan K, Soderling TR, Goodman RH, Impey S (2008) An activity-regulated microRNA controls dendritic plasticity by down-regulating p250GAP. Proc Natl Acad Sci USA 105:9093–9098

Weber JA, Baxter DH, Zhang S, Huang DY, Huang KH, Lee MJ, Galas DJ, Wang K (2010) The microRNA spectrum in 12 body fluids. Clin Chem 56:1733–1741

Weiler IJ, Irwin SA, Klintsova AY, Spencer CM, Brazelton AD, Miyashiro K, Comery TA, Patel B, Eberwine J, Greenough WT (1997) Fragile X mental retardation protein is translated near synapses in response to neurotransmitter activation. Proc Natl Acad Sci USA 94:5395–5400

Witke W (2004) The role of profilin complexes in cell motility and other cellular processes. Trends Cell Biol 14:461–469

Wu J, Xie X (2006) Comparative sequence analysis reveals an intricate network among REST, CREB and miRNA in mediating neuronal gene expression. Genome Biol 7:R85

Wu L, Fan J, Belasco JG (2006) MicroRNAs direct rapid deadenylation of mRNA. Proc Natl Acad Sci USA 103:4034–4039

Xu J, Li CX, Li YS, Lv JY, Ma Y, Shao TT, Xu LD, Wang YY, Du L, Zhang YP, Jiang W, Li CQ, Xiao Y, Li X (2011) MiRNA-miRNA synergistic network: construction via co-regulating functional modules and disease miRNA topological features. Nucleic Acids Res 39:825–836

Zeng Y, Sankala H, Zhang X, Graves PR (2008) Phosphorylation of Argonaute 2 at serine-387 facilitates its localization to processing bodies. Biochem J 413:429–436

Chapter 18
Animal Models of Risk Factors for Suicidal Ideation and Behaviour

Sarah A. Stuart, Paul Butler and Emma S.J. Robinson

Abstract In order to predict the risk of a drug-induced side effect prior to the start of a clinic trial, studies in valid pre-clinical models are essential. In the area of neuropsychiatric symptoms, animal models are severely limited and novel approaches are essential if such risks are to be identified before expensive clinical studies are initiated. One of the most serious neuropsychiatric side effects is suicidal ideation and behaviour. A major issue with this area as a whole is that the current methods used in pre-clinical drug safety development are not designed to assess neuropsychiatric side effects, and suitable animal models for suicidal ideation and behaviour have not been well validated. Animal models of depression represent a potentially useful starting point as major depressive disorder (MDD) and bipolar disorder carry the highest risk of suicide. Other behavioural traits associated with suicidal behaviour in man, such as impulsivity and aggression, can also be modelled in animals. This chapter considers the different methodological approaches currently available for rodent studies associated with these behaviours. In particular, translational studies investigating whether changes in cognitive processes implicated in depression may also provide a basis for predicting pro-depressant risk will be considered. We also review the available literature relating to animal studies investigating pro-depressant drug treatments to gauge the degree of predictive validity which these animal models can deliver.

S.A. Stuart · E.S.J. Robinson (✉)
School of Physiology and Pharmacology, University of Bristol, University Walk, Bristol BS8 1TD, United Kingdom
e-mail: pmesjr@bris.ac.uk

P. Butler
Global Safety Pharmacology, Pfizer Worldwide Research and Development, La Jolla, San Diego, CA, USA

K.E. Cannon and T.J. Hudzik (eds.), *Suicide: Phenomenology and Neurobiology*,
DOI 10.1007/978-3-319-09964-4_18

18.1 Introduction

Suicidal ideation and behaviour (SIB) has been reported for a number of different therapeutic drugs including antidepressants, antiepileptics, the anti-obesity drug, rimonabant, anti-acne medication, roaccutane and smoking cessation treatment, varenicline (Gartlehner et al. 2011; Stone et al. 2009; Mula et al. 2013; Nathan et al. 2011; Magin et al. 2005; Bremner and McCaffery 2008; Ahmed et al. 2013). In almost all cases, the incidence of neuropsychiatric adverse effects has not become apparent until the drug has completed clinical trials and been licensed for use in the general population (Reith and Edmonds 2007). In these situations, this subsequent evidence of increased risks of depression and/or suicide has a serious impact on the use of the drug, and may lead to withdrawal of the compound or restricted use. The drugs for which SIB has been reported target a diverse range of different pharmacological mechanisms and thus exhibit distinct pharmacological profiles which limit our ability to predict treatment-emergent neuropsychiatric risks based on their site(s) of action (For review see Reith and Edmonds 2007). It is becoming increasingly clear that both pre-clinical and early clinical studies need to be modified if these CNS-related adverse effects are to be predicted more effectively and earlier in the development process. According to the recently revised draft FDA guidance on SIB (Prospective assessment of occurrence in clinical trials, FDA draft guidance, Revision 1, August 2012), prospective monitoring for SIB should be undertaken in all phases of clinical drug development (phase 1 through to phase 4). The scope of these draft guidelines includes drugs for both psychiatric and neurological diseases as well as those for non-psychiatric indications e.g., isotretinoins, other tretinoins, beta blockers, reserpine, smoking cessation drugs and drugs for weight loss. Although these approaches should improve the early detection of SIB in healthy volunteers or patients prior to licensing, it would be a real advantage to the drug development process if a pre-clinical screen were available which could more reliably predict these effects in man. For the majority of pre-clinical safety studies, animal models are employed which have been validated as predictive models for human pharmacology. In the case of SIB, these models have been limited to those associated with suicide-related behavioural traits such as hopelessness, impulsivity and aggression (Malkesman et al. 2009; Preti 2011) as well as animal models of depression (Willner et al. 1984; Cryan and Holmes 2005; McArthur and Borsini 2006; Berton et al. 2012). The following sections discuss these animal models in the context of SIB and consider evidence currently available on the predictive validity of each assay.

18.2 Animal Models: Overview

In psychiatry, an animal model can provide a valuable tool for investigating both the aetiology of a disease and identifying novel drug targets (McKinney 2001; Nestler and Hyman 2010). Animal models are also widely used to try to predict the

Table 18.1 Validity criteria for an animal model in the context of SIB

Validity	Description	Challenges
Face	The animal model should recapitulate one or more of the core symptoms of the disease	Difficult to replicate the features of suicide in a non-human species
Construct	The model should involve similar neurobiological mechanisms as the human condition	No clearly defined neurobiology or genetics No well characterised biomarkers
Predictive	The effects of the drug in humans should be accurately predicted by the animal model	Most models have been validated using conventional antidepressants drugs associated with common sites of action

potential clinical efficacy of a new treatment (McKinney 2001; Nestler and Hyman 2010). The validity of animal models are made against the criteria of *face*, *construct* and *predictive* validity (see Table 18.1) although few, if any models fully recapitulate the characteristics of psychiatric diseases (Geyer and Markou 1995; McKinney 2001; Cryan and Holmes 2005; McArthur and Borsini 2006; Nestler and Hyman 2010). Perhaps the most important aspect of any animal model for psychiatry is how well the findings in animals translate to the clinic (Berton et al. 2012).

Psychiatric conditions are a challenging area to study using animals as their symptoms are difficult to replicate in a non-human species particularly in the most commonly used laboratory animals, rodents (for discussion see Cryan and Holmes 2005; Nestler and Hyman 2010; Hendrie et al. 2013). For most psychiatric disorders, questionnaire-based measures and/or clinical interviews are the most commonly used diagnostic approach for humans (DSM-V 2013) and translational methods in non-human species are therefore not feasible. SIB is characterised by the emergence of suicidal ideation, attempted or completed suicides which can be attributed to the taking of a therapeutic medication. Quantification of these behaviours also depends on questionnaire-based measures and current FDA guidelines recommend using the Columbia-Suicide Severity Rating Scale (C-SSRS) (Pumariega et al. 2011; Posner et al. 2007; 2011) and the Suicidal Behaviours Questionnaire-Revised (SBQ-R) (Osman et al. 2001) for assessment of SIB at screening and/or during clinical trials. Although a specific animal model or test for SIB has not been developed and validated to date, researchers have looked to the closely related psychiatric disorder, MDD as well as behavioural traits associated with SIB including hopelessness, impulsivity and aggression (Cryan and Holmes 2005; Cryan and Slattery 2007; McArthur and Borsini 2006; Malkesman et al. 2009; Preti 2011).

18.3 Animal Models of Depression

Animal models developed to study MDD have been around since the 1960s when behavioural tests which could predict antidepressant efficacy in man were described (Reserpine model, Askew 1963); forced swim test (FST), Porsolt et al. 1977). These assays went on to form the basis for the successful development of all the modern antidepressant drugs including the serotonin-specific re-uptake inhibitors (SSRIs). Animal models for depression form a logical starting point for investigating SIB in non-human species. MDD is associated with an increased risk of suicide with approximately 90 % of suicide attempts associated with a serious mental health condition (Beautrais et al. 1996). Suicidal ideation is also a common feature of MDD and is one of the symptoms included in the DSM-V diagnostic manual (DSM-V 2013). Treatment-induced depressive symptoms are also seen with a number of drug-treatments which have been associated with SIB and therefore may be a major contributing factor (Nathan et al. 2011; Magin et al. 2005; Bremner and McCaffery 2008; Ahmed et al. 2013). An increased risk of SIB linked to treatment-induced depression during interferon-alpha treatment for hepatitis C has also been reported adding to the argument that pro-depressant effects may be an important contributing factor in the development of SIB (Sockalingam et al. 2011). Although not all patients with symptoms of depression go on to attempt suicide, many of those who do commit suicide have a prior history of a mood disorder, either unipolar or bipolar depression (Beautrais et al. 1996).

Although animal models for depression have been used extensively in basic research, their validity has been increasingly questioned and concerns have been raised about how reliable they are in terms of predicting effects in people. These limitations have been discussed in detail in other articles (Willner 1984, 2005; Nestler et al. 2002; Cryan and Holmes 2005; Cryan and Slattery 2007; Nestler and Hyman 2010; Pollak et al. 2010; Berton et al. 2012 reviews) and are therefore only briefly summarised here to put the subsequent discussions about SIB-related studies using these approaches into context.

When considering animal models of depression, the term ‘model’ is often used to describe both methods to induce a depression-like phenotype and those methods used to assay depression-like behaviour. Stress-related paradigms such as chronic mild stress, early life adversity and psychosocial stress have been shown to induce neurobiological and behavioural deficits thought to reflect a depression-like phenotype (Willner et al 1987, 1992; Willner 1997, 2005; Kudryavtseva et al. 1991; Rygula et al. 2005; Mathews et al. 1996; reviwed by Schmidt et al. 2011). Another approach has been to use olfactory bulbectomy to induce depression in rodents (Leonard 1984; Kelly et al. 1997). Although of interest in terms of the roles these models have played in our understanding of the factors which contribute to MDD, these methods largely depend on assays of depression-related behaviour to validate the generated phenotype. Thus, it is these assays of depression-related behaviour which may provide the most suitable predictive assays for evaluation of SIB in drug development. For the majority of non-human studies into depression, the assays used to quantify mood-related symptoms are designed to provide a measure of either behavioural despair e.g. the FST and tail suspension test (TST), or anhedonia e.g. sucrose preference test (SPT) and intracerebral self stimulation (ICSS) (FST: Porsolt et al. 1977; Detke et al. 1995;TST: Steru et al. 1985; reviewed by Cryan et al. 2005a, b; SPT: Willner et al. 1987; Vogel et al. 1986; ICSS: Zacharko and Anisman 1991). A number of more general behavioural symptoms can also be measured in rodents which may relate to depression e.g. poor coat condition, body weight changes and aggression (Cryan and Holmes 2005; Cryan and Slattery 2007; Hendrie et al. 2013).

18.3.1 Behavioural Despair

Assays of behavioural despair were initially developed and validated using prototypical antidepressant drugs (Porsolt et al. 1977) and are now generally considered to provide a valid approach to predicting antidepressant efficacy for drugs acting through monoaminergic systems, but have limited validity for non-monoaminergic targets (Berton and Nestler 2006). In the classical version of the FST, animals are placed into a cylinder of water from which they can't escape. When the procedure is repeated 24hrs later, and the immobility time of the animals is measured to provide an indication of behavioural despair. Pre-treatment with antidepressant-like compounds reduces immobility time in this assay (Porsolt et al. 1977). The assay has subsequently been adapted for mice where the water is replaced with suspension by the tail (Steru et al. 1985). In fact, the first assay used to predict antidepressant-like effects was reserpine-induced behaviours where the monoamine-depleting effects of reserpine treatment were attenuated by imipramine-like compounds (Askew 1963). The FST and TST have shown good predictive validity in terms of antidepressant activity for drugs acting through monoaminergic targets but these assays have also been heavily criticised (Porsolt et al. 1977; Steru et al. 1985; Slattery and Cryan 2012; for reviews see Cryan et al. 2005a, b; Berton and Nestler 2006). The potential issues with these assays may stem from their initial development, which was based on validation using conventional antidepressant drugs such as the tricyclic antidepressants (TCA) and monoamine oxidase inhibitors (MAOI) (Porsolt et al. 1977). The mismatch between the acute time course of effects in the rodent assays and delayed clinical benefits seen in patients following antidepressant drug treatment has also been seen as a limitation of these models. One non-monaminergic antidepressant, ketamine, an NMDA receptor antagonist and rapidly acting antidepressant, acts to reduce immobility time in the FST (e.g. Garcia et al. 2009), however issues relating to the locomotor effects of ketamine are a potential confound (Slattery and Cryan 2012). Locomotor effects in this stress-related paradigm are not only an issue with ketamine, and the original validation data presented for the assay included the caveat that locomotor effects were a potential non-specific confound (Porsolt et al. 1977; Slattery and Cryan 2012). Many researchers now conclude that the FST and TST provide valid models for predicting antidepressant efficacy for monoaminergic drugs and 'me-to' compounds, but are limited in their sensitivity to drugs acting through novel mechanisms such as those associated with SIB. For example rimonabant, a cannabinoid$_1$-receptor antagonist/inverse agonist developed to treat obesity had been shown to be an antidepressant in the FST (Griebel et al. 2005) but was subsequently withdrawn from the European market in 2009 after it was found to induce depression, anxiety and suicidal ideation in obese

Table 18.2 Effects of drugs associated with SIB in animal models of depression (behavioural despair and anhedonia)

Assay	FST/TST	SPT	ICSS	References
Rimonabant	Acute—no effect or ↓ immobility Chronic—↑ immobility	Acute—no effect Chronic—↓ preference	Acute—↑ threshold or no effect Chronic—no info	Adamczyk et al. (2008) Griebel et al. (2005) Gamble-George et al. (2013) Rademacher and Hillard (2007) Beyer et al. (2010) Deroche-Gamonet et al. (2001)
Retinoic acid	Acute—no effect Chronic—immobility or no effect	Chronic; no effect	No info	O'Reilly et al. (2006) Ferguson et al. (2005) Cai et al. (2010) Trent et al. (2009)
IFNα	Acute—↑ immobility Chronic—↑ immobility	Acute—↓ preference Chronic—↓ preference	Acute—no effect Acute (LPS)—↑ threshold	Makino et al. (2000) Sammut et al. (2001) Sammut et al. (2002) Kentner et al. (2007)
Varenicline	Acute—↓ immobility or no effect Chronic—no info	Acute—no info Chronic—no info	Acute—↓ threshold	Caldarone et al. (2011) Turner et al. (2010) Rollema et al. (2009) Igari et al. (2014)
Valproate	Acute—no effect (LiCl—↓ immobility) Chronic—↓ immobility	Acute—no info Chronic—no info	Acute—no effect (LiCl—↑ threshold) Chronic—No info	Tomasiewicz et al. (2006) Semba et al. (1989)
Stress	Acute—no effect Chronic—↑ immobility	Acute—↓ preference Chronic—↑ preference	Chronic—↑ threshold	Platt and Stone (1982) Moreau et al. (1992)

patients (Topol et al. 2010). As summarised in Table 18.2, studies investigating the effects of pro-depressant drugs using behavioural despair methods such as the FST and TST have failed to provide reliable predictive data. Rimonabant was shown to exhibit an antidepressant or neutral profile following acute administration although chronic treatments have been reported to increase immobility time indicative of a pro-depressant effect (Table 18.2). Other pro-depressant drugs have also failed to show effects in these assays although studies are still somewhat limited (see Table 18.2 for details). Overall, the behavioural despair methods appear to lack sensitivity to most pro-depressant drugs following acute administration (Table 18.2). Using a chronic treatment may be a better approach and some evidence for predictive validity has been shown, although this may be restricted to drugs from certain classes. For example, no effects or an antidepressant profile were shown following acute or chronic administration of anti-epileptics drugs such as lithium (Table 18.2). As discussed earlier, one potential issue with the FST and TST may be due to its sensitivity to drugs acting predominantly through monoaminergic pathways (Berton and Nestler 2006). Other sites of action may be associated with pro-depressant effects which are not evident following either acute or chronic treatments in the FST or TST.

18.3.2 Anhedonia

Anhedonia, the reduced sensitivity or experience of reward, is one of the core symptoms of MDD although patients can be diagnosed with MDD in the absence of anhedonia if they exhibit other symptoms such as low mood (DSM-V 2013). Although anhedonia is also commonly seen in other psychiatric disorders, such as schizophrenia and during withdrawal from drugs of abuse. Therefore, drug-induced anhedonia may represent an important pre-clinical screen for assessing risks associated with SIB.

Anhedonia is perhaps one of the more translatable symptoms of emotional dysfunction which can be measured in rodents (for discussion see Anisman and Matheson 2005). To quantify sensitivity to reward using a rodent model, one of the most widely used assays is ICSS (Zacharko and Anisman 1991). The method was originally developed to investigate reward mechanisms associated with addiction and during withdrawal from drugs of abuse (Phillips et al. 1983; Schaefer and Michael 1983). The procedure involves the implantation of an electrode into the medial forebrain bundle and the animal is trained to associated a lever press response with direct stimulation of the associated dopaminergic pathway (for review see Liebman 1983). To quantify the hedonic response, the threshold for stimulation is determined for each animal with a higher intensity of stimulation needed to maintain responding in animals exhibiting anhedonia. An alternative approach developed in the context of depression research is the SPT test or sucrose consumption test (Willner et al. 1987; Vogel et al. 1986). These assays depend on the animals' ability to experience reward associated with a weak sucrose solution (usually 1 %). Either total consumption or preference for the 1 % sucrose versus water can provide a measure of anhedonia in rodents (Willner et al. 1987; Vogel et al. 1986).

In terms of depression, there is good evidence for a stress-induced anhedonia in rodents following exposure to chronic mild stress (Willner et al. 1987) or chronic social defeat stress (Rygula et al. 2005). Studies have also shown that the stress-induced anhedonia is sensitive to chronic but not acute antidepressant drug treatment, mirroring clinical observations of the time course of therapeutic benefit (Willner et al. 1987; Vogel et al. 1986; Zacharko and Anisman 1991). Interestingly, treatment with the NMDA antagonist, ketamine, has been associated with a rapid reversal of SIB in patients (Diaz-Granados et al. 2010) although studies in animals using the SPT found effects with ketamine only after chronic administration (Garcia et al. 2009). Anhedonic changes similar to those seen in depression appear to be relatively well replicated in animals although as yet, only limited information is available for drug-induced anhedonia in the context of SIB (see Table 18.2). Studies using either ICSS or the SPT have investigated several different pro-depressant manipulations with the details of their findings summarised in Table 18.2. It is clear that consistency across drugs from different classes and tests of anhedonia has not been achieved although the number of studies reported in the literature is still very limited. Rimonabant has been shown to induce anhedonia following chronic but not acute administration when tested using the SPT (Rademacher and Hillard 2007) but effects measured using ICSS were inconsistent with some reports of an anhedonic effect following acute treatment whilst others report a lack of effect following either acute or chronic treatment (Deroche-Gamonet et al. 2001). Similar to the results for the FST, varenicline appeared to exhibit an antidepressant-like profile and in the ICSS paradigm it reduced the threshold for stimulation (Igari et al. 2014). Other drugs tested in models of anhedonia include retinoic acid, interferon-alpha and the anti-epileptics although their effects are also inconsistent (see Table 18.2). Thus, whilst the translational validity of animal models of anhedonia is high, the results to date do not provide evidence of good predictive validity for SIB.

18.3.3 Cognitive Neuropsychological Models of Depression

In 2003, studies using the antidepressant, reboxetine, found that acute treatments in healthy volunteers led to a positive shift in the processing of emotional information (Harmer et al. 2003). These changes were observed using neuropsychological tests of emotional behaviour and revealed that drug-induced changes in these cognitive processes were present in the absence of any subjective effects on mood (Harmer et al. 2003, see also reviews Harmer et al. 2009b Pringle et al. 2011; Harmer 2013). Cognitive processes in depression have been discussed for many decades with the first proposal of a cognitive theory of depression described in 1967 (Beck 1967, 1976). The more recent developments in computer-based neuropsychological tests have allowed for much more sensitive, objective measures of emotional behaviour to be made in human participants and renewed interest (For discussion see Robinson and Sahakian 2008; Clark et al. 2009; Harmer et al. 2009a; Elliott et al. 2011; Roiser et al. 2012; Roiser and Sahakain 2013). Studies in depressed patients have shown consistent deficits in emotion-related cognition including changes in emotional interpretation, learning and memory, with a shift towards a negative emotional interpretation (see Mathews and MacLeod 2005; Clark et al. 2009; Gotlib and Joormann 2010 for reviews). It is not yet known whether these *negative cognitive affective biases* (CAB) are a cause or consequence of the disease however, they appear to represent a possible biomarker for depression. This theory is supported by evidence that individuals with a vulnerability to MDD also exhibit similar negative biases without overt disease symptoms (Hayward et al. 2005; Joormann et al. 2007; Chan et al. 2007; Dearing and Gotlib 2009). Perhaps, the most important development from this work has been in the pharmacology of CABs and studies in healthy volunteers which suggest this type of biomarker may also provide an early indicator of both antidepressant efficacy and pro-depressant risk (see review by Pringle et al. 2011).

The majority of studies to date have focussed on whether early changes in CABs predict long-term antidepressant efficacy in patients (see review by Pringle et al. 2011). Using a range of antidepressant drugs from different classes and treatment regimes of single dose or 7 day of treatments, a positive bias in emotional processing, opposite to those seen in depression, has been reported (see review by Pringle et al. 2011). Although not all treatments act in an identical manner, all drugs which are effective antidepressants in humans induce a positive bias in one of more of the emotional processing tests carried out (for review see Pringle et al. 2011). Using a similar battery of neuropsychological tests, acute or short-term administration of the pro-depressant drug, rimonabant was shown to induce negative CABs (Horder et al. 2009, 2012). Interestingly, the partial agonist at the $\alpha_4\beta_2$ subtype of nicotinic acetylcholine receptor, varenicline, did not have any effects following short term treatment (Mocking et al. 2013). As well as the potential to use this type of neuropsychological approach to study pro-depressant risk in humans, methods assaying objective measures of emotional processing also provide the basis for the development of new, translational methods for use in animals.

Although studies in humans use language-based approaches or emotional facial expressions which cannot be directly translated to non-human tasks, the principles which underpin these tests can be translated (Paul et al. 2005). The first study to achieve this was reported by Harding et al. (2004) and described an assay to detect CABs in rodents. The study provided the first evidence that a translational method for studying emotional behaviour in a non-human species was achievable. The first rodent CAB task required animals to learn to associate two distinct auditory cues with different emotionally valenced outcomes: obtaining reward or avoidance of punishment. Once the animals had learnt the associations, CAB was investigated by presenting the animals with intermediate ambiguous tone cues and observing their responses. The 'optimistic' rat was predicted to make more responses in anticipation of reward whilst the 'pessimistic' rat would make more responses indicating anticipation of punishment. Using a chronic mild stress manipulation, this original study showed that rats in a putative negative affective state were more likely to anticipate negative events similar to what is seen in depressed patients (Wright and Bower 1992). A number of different laboratories have now replicated this work (Enkel et al. 2010; Anderson et al. 2012) and have refined the task design to reduce potential confounds associated with motivational state. There have also been task designs which use spatial cues in place of auditory cues to predict outcomes (for review see Hales et al. 2014). In both the original tone-based operant task and these spatial judgment tasks, a go/no-go task design is used. The potential problem with this design is that any change in motivation for the reward could impact on the ambiguous cue interpretation or the latency to approach the goal pot. In order to see a true *judgement bias*, go/go presentation of the tone-based operant task using active lever press responses to either obtain reward or avoid punishment has been developed (Enkel et al. 2010; Anderson et al. 2012; Rygula et al. 2012, 2013; Papciak et al. 2013). To date, the numbers of studies using this approach are limited and training protocols indicate that animals require long training periods of up to 3 months to reach a stable level of performance before drug testing can be carried out (for review see Hales et al. 2014). Pharmacological validation of these ambiguous cue interpretation or judgement bias methods is also limited (Anderson et al. 2013; Enkel et al. 2010) and studies investigating pro-depressant drugs have not yet been reported. Studies using the antidepressant fluoxetine have shown a tendency to reduce negative judgement biases following chronic but not acute administration (Anderson et al. 2013). In contrast, the antidepressant reboxetine either alone (Anderson et al. 2013) or in combination with corticosterone (Enkel et al. 2010) induced a negative bias and reduced anticipation of reward. Although the translational potential of this approach appears high, to date, the predictive validity is limited and further studies are needed before the value of this approach for SIB and depression-related studies can be fully evaluated.

An alternative method to study CAB in rodents has also recently been reported (Stuart et al. 2013). This assay uses a similar strategy of 'reverse translation' but is based on the memory biases observed in depressed patients as apposed to emotional interpretation biases (see Mathews and MacLeod 2005; Clark et al. 2009; Gotlib and Joormann 2010 for reviews). The rodent affective bias test (ABT) is similar conceptually to the conditioned place preference paradigm (CPP). The basis of the task is the hypothesis that memory for a specific experience is biased by affective state at the time the experience is learnt, which subsequently influences the memory of the relative value of that experience (Stuart et al. 2013). Studies using antidepressant drug treatments from different pharmacological classes suggest that a good correlation between their known clinical efficacy in patients and the drug's ability to induce a positive bias in the ABT. As well as pharmacological validation, experiments using psychosocial manipulations of affective state also resulted in biases in this assay consistent with their predicted effects on affective state. Exposure to social and environmental enrichment resulted in a positive bias whilst psychosocial stress induced a negative bias (Stuart et al. 2013). Together, these data support the translational and predictive validity of the ABT for depression-related research. In terms of SIB, studies using the ABT have also investigated a number of treatments known to induce depression and/or SIB. The CB_1-antagonist, rimonabant and the active ingredient of the anti-acne medication roaccutane, 13-cis-retinoic acid, induced a negative bias in this assay (Stuart et al. 2013, Fig. 18.1). Interestingly, the SSRI antidepressants tend to exhibit a bell-shaped dose response curve in the ABT (Stuart et al. 2013). This observation has not been further investigated but may be relevant to their proposed risks of inducing SIB in vulnerable individuals or at certain doses.

Considering all the different depression-related assays which have been used to investigate drugs with known neuropsychiatric risk, pharmacological data for the ABT test shows the greatest level of predictive validity when compared to data obtained from healthy human volunteers and/or patients. The assay has yet to be replicated in other laboratories and further validation data are needed. In particular studies using other drugs with a black box warning for SIB such as the anti-epileptics are needed. The current version of the task is also very labour intensive and would have greater value if it could be modified to an automated version.

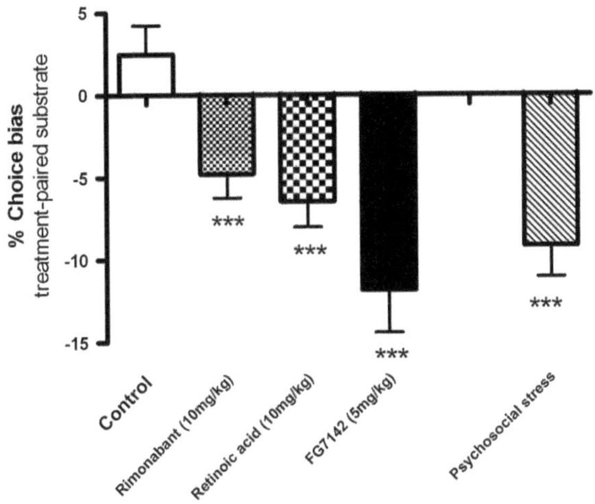

Fig. 18.1 Pharmacological evaluation of the ABT for predicting pro-depressant risk. In the ABT, the percentage choice bias is measured using a preference test where the animal bias towards or away from an experience encountered during antidepressant treatment is quantified. Results are shown the maximal effective dose and a positive control of psychosocial stress. Full dose-response data are given in Stuart et al. 2013. These studies show that three pharmacologically distinct pro-depressant treatments induce similar negative affective biases in the rat ABT. The magnitude of effect is similar to that seen following a stress manipulation (restraint stress and 24 h social isolation). Results are shown for mean ± sem for 16 animals tested using a within-subject affective bias test. $^{*}p < 0.05$, $^{**}p < 0.01$, $^{***}p < 0.001$ post-hoc one sample t-test versus no bias

18.4 Animal Models of Suicide-Related Behavioural Traits

Although animal models of depression are thought to be a good predictor of SIB and several of the drugs associated with these side effects also induce depression, other behavioural traits associated with suicide are also of potential interest. Suicide arises as a result of multiple behavioural traits, some or all of which may be present. Of specific relevance to SIB are the behavioural traits of hopelessness, impulsivity and aggression (for review see Brezo et al. 2006). Animal models to investigate these behaviours have all been described previously although usually in studies unrelated to SIB. The potential applications for animal models of these suicide-related behavioural traits have been reviewed previously (Malkesman et al. 2009; Preti 2011) and therefore only a brief synopsis is given here. As opposed to a detailed description of the specific methodologies, which are described in detail in Malkesman et al. (2009), particular attention has been made here to the pharmacological and translational validity of these approaches and any studies using drugs associated with SIB (Table 18.3).

Table 18.3 Effects of drugs associated with SIB in animal models of trait behaviours

Suicide-related trait behaviour	Animal model/assay	Summary of findings relevant to SIB	References
Hopelessness	Exposure to repeated inescapable stress e.g. footshock	No data	
Impulsivity	5-choice serial reaction time task (impulsive action) Stop-signal reaction time task (stopping an already initiated response) Delayed reward (impulsive choice)	↓Rimonabant, lithium ↔Carbamazapine, valproate No data ↔Rimonabant, valproate ↓Lithium	Wiskerke et al. (2011), Ohmura et al. (2011) Wiskerke et al. (2011), Halcomb et al. (2013)
Aggression	Resident intruder model	↓Rimonabant ↓Retinoic acid ↓Lithium, valproate	Griebel et al. (2005) Trent et al. (2009) Flaisher-Grinberg and Einat (2007)

18.4.1 Hopelessness

The most often used model for assessing hopelessness in animals is the learned helplessness paradigm (Maier and Seligman 1976), which has been conducted successfully in several species including rats and mice. In this paradigm, a presumed state of depression is induced in animals by exposing them to repeated inescapable, aversive stimuli (e.g. foot shock). The procedure results in long-lasting deficits in the animals' motivation and ability to escape in subsequent trials where escape is possible, as well as behavioural alterations such as vocalisations and passivity (Anisman et al 1979; Sherman and Petty 1982). The learned helplessness paradigm is used in pre-clinical pharmacological studies to assess the antidepressant effect of new compounds and it has been demonstrated that TCAs, MAOIs and SSRIs all prevent and/or reverse learned helplessness in animals (Martin et al 1990; Sherman and Petty 1982; Takamori et al 2001). Some studies also use the FST and TST to assess hopelessness although these assays are more commonly referred to as assays of behavioural despair which results from a relatively short-term exposure to an inescapable stress. Studies using the learned helplessness paradigm to investigate drug-induced SIB have not been reported.

18.4.2 Aggression

Laboratory research has produced detailed descriptions of aggression and defence patterns in rodents showing strong similarities across species (Blanchard and Blanchard 2003). Furthermore, research indicates that there are several similarities between offensive aggression in laboratory rodents and human aggression (Blanchard and Blanchard 2003). Various behavioural paradigms attempt to model aggression in animals (reviewed by Miczek et al, (2001)), but the resident intruder is the most frequently used. A naïve weight- and age-matched rodent ('intruder') is placed into the home cage of an experimental rodent and the aggressive behaviours of the resident rodent (e.g. attack bites, tail rattling and wrestling) are measured (Pellis and McKenna 1992). Notably, the ability to reduce aggressive behaviour in this paradigm is shared by acute treatment with all the pharmacologically disparate antidepressant compounds tested, including SSRIs, selective noradrenaline reuptake inhibitors (SNRIs), MAOIs, and TCAs (Mitchell 2005). Studies investigating drugs associated with SIB have so far been very consistent in their observations in terms of aggression with rimonabant, retinoic acid and the antiepileptic, valproate, all reducing aggression in the resident intruder paradigm (Table 18.3). These findings do not therefore support a predictive value for aggression and SIB.

18.4.3 Impulsivity

Impulsivity is not a unitary construct and subtypes, based on response inhibition versus impulsive choice, have been proposed in the context of animals and humans (Evenden 1999; Dalley et al. 2008). In rodents different aspects of impulsivity can be measured using operant behaviour paradigms (Fernando and Robbins 2011; Eagle and Baunez 2010; Winstanley et al. 2006). To measure impulsive actions in rodents, the 5-choice serial reaction time task (5-CSRTT) and modified forced choice version have both been used to study impulsivity associated with impaired response inhibition (Robbins 2002). The ability to stop an already initiated motor response can be quantified in both humans and rodents using the stop signal reaction time task (SSRT) (Eagle and Baunez 2010) and intolerance to delay of reward or impulse choice, is quantified using the delay discounting task (Cardinal et al. 2004). The delay discounting paradigm is based on the principle that the selection of a small but immediate reinforcer represents an 'impulsive' choice, whereas the opposite bias is an index of 'self control'. An extensive literature on the neural and neurochemical modulation of different types of impulse control exists and some insight into the possible link between key neurotransmitter systems and SIB may be feasible (Robbins 2002; Cardinal et al. 2004; Dalley et al. 2008). For example, the serotonin system has been shown to play an important modulatory role in impulse control in animals and evidence from post-mortem tissues have linked serotonin levels in the brain to suicide (for review see Bortolato et al. 2013). However, few studies have specifically investigated the relationship between SIB and impulsivity using these tasks. A couple of studies have investigate the effects of lithium and other antiepileptics and found they either reduce impulsivity or have no-effect depending on the task used (see Table 18.3). Studies using antidepressant drugs find either no effect or reduced impulsivity (Bizot et al 1999; Humpston et al. 2013).

18.5 Conclusions

Studies designed specifically to investigate the effects of novel drugs to induce SIB in animals as an approach to predict their effects in humans are still limited but the growing need for pre-clinical methods has seen an increase in publications in this area. The majority of researchers have sought to use animal models of depression to try to determine their predictive value for SIB. Conventional methods such as the behavioural despair assays or models of anhedonia have failed to provide consistent data and drugs from different pharmacological classes tend to have different effects suggesting these models may be limited to detecting drugs acting through specific mechanisms, such as the monoamine targets. Assaying trait behaviours such as aggression, hopelessness and impulsivity is potentially valuable within a full behavioural screen, however, the data for these methods also shows a lack of consistency in effects and evidence demonstrating their predictive validity for SIB is severely limited. Overall, the CAB studies have demonstrated the greatest potential for translational validity. They demonstrate the benefits which can be achieved by utilising developments in objective measures of mood-related symptoms in humans and related animal assays. Moving forward, more work into the potential of CABs as biomarkers for mood-related neurobiology in humans will also benefit animal studies. With a greater number of drugs tested across different pharmacological classes in humans, the translational validity of animal models can be better evaluated.

An important aim for future research is to try to not only develop methods which can predict risk but also try to find methods to help explain why certain drugs cause SIB and whether specific risk factors exist in a subpopulation of patients. The incidence of adverse neuropsychiatric side effects associated with treatments such as retinoic acid (Marqueling and Zane 2007) or rimonabant (Christensen et al. 2007) are not well defined and symptoms are seen in only a minority of patients. It is not yet possible to predict which patients will experience these side-effects meaning that all patients must be treated with the same degree of caution, therefore limiting the potential clinical use of the compound. If an animal model or series of behavioural tests can, together, provide a test battery from which vulnerability across different populations can be predicted, this can improve the safety of compounds as well as potentially offering an early screen to detect those most at risk.

References

Adamczyk P, Gołda A, McCreary AC, Filip M, Przegaliński E (2008) Activation of endocannabinoid transmission induces antidepressant-like effects in rats. J Physiol Pharmacol 59:217–228

Ahmed AI, Ali AN, Kramers C, Härmark LV, Burger DM, Verhoeven WM (2013) Neuropsychiatric adverse events of varenicline: a systematic review of published reports. J Clin Psychopharmacol 33(1):55–62

Anderson MH, Munafò M, Robinson EJ (2013) Investigating the psychopharmacology of cognitive affective bias in rats using an affective tone discrimination task. Psychopharmacology 226:601–613

Anderson MH, Hardcastle C, Munafò MR, Robinson ES (2012) Evaluation of a novel translational task for assessing emotional biases in different species. Cogn Affect Behav Neurosci 12:373–381

Anisman H, Matheson K (2005) Stress, depression, and anhedonia: caveats concerning animal models. Neurosci Biobehav Rev 29(4–5):525–546

Anisman H, Remington G, Sklar LS (1979) Effect of inescapable shock on subsequent escape performance: catecholaminergic and cholinergic mediation of response initiation and maintenance. Psychopharmacology (Berl) 61:107–124

Askew BM (1963) A simple screening procedure for imipramine-like antidepressant agents. Life Sci 2:725–730

Beautrais AL, Joyce PR, Mulder RT, Fergusson DM, Deavoll BJ, Nightingale SK (1996) Prevalence and comorbidity of mental disorders in persons making serious suicide attempts: a case-control study. Am J Psychiatry 153:1009–1014

Beck AT (1967) Depression: clinical, experimental, and theoretical aspects. Harper and Row, New York

Beck AT (1976) Cognitive therapy and the emotional disorders. New American Library, New York

Berton O, Hahn CG, Thase ME (2012) Are we getting closer to valid translational models for major depression? Science 338:75–79

Berton O, Nestler EJ (2006) New approaches to antidepressant drug discovery: beyond monoamines. Nat Rev Neurosci 7:137–151

Beyer CE, Dwyer JM, Piesla MJ, Platt BJ, Shen R et al (2010) Depression-like phenotype following chronic CB1 receptor antagonism. Neurobiol Dis 39:148–155

Bizot J, Le Bihan C, Puech AJ, Hamon M, Thiebot M (1999) Serotonin and tolerance to delay of reward in rats. Psychopharmacology (Berl) 146:400–412

Blanchard DC, Blanchard RJ (2003) What can animal aggression research tell us about human aggression? Horm Behav 44:171–177

Bortolato M, Pivac N, Muck Seler D, Nikolac Perkovic M, Pessia M, Di Giovanni G (2013) The role of the serotonergic system at the interface of aggression and suicide. Neuroscience 16 (236):160–185

Bremner JD, McCaffery P (2008) The neurobiology of retinoic acid in affective disorders. Prog Neuropsychopharmacol Biol Psychiatry 32(2):315–331

Brezo J, Paris J, Tremblay R, Vitaro F, Zoccolillo M, Hébert M, Turecki G (2006) Personality traits as correlates of suicide attempts and suicidal ideation in young adults. Psychol Med 36:191–202

Cai L, Yan XB, Chen XN, Meng QY, Zhou JN (2010) Chronic all-trans retinoic acid administration induced hyperactivity of HPA axis and behavioral changes in young rats. Eur Neuropsychopharmacol 20:839–847

Caldarone BJ, Wang D, Paterson NE, Manzano M, Fedolak A et al (2011) Dissociation between duration of action in the forced swim test in mice and nicotinic acetylcholine receptor occupancy with sazetidine, varenicline, and 5-I-A85380. Psychopharmacology (Berl) 217:199–210

Cardinal RN, Winstanley WA, Robbins TW, Everitt BJ (2004) Limbic corticostriatal systems and delayed reinforcement. Ann NY Acad Sci 1021:33–50

Chan SW, Goodwin GM, Harmer CJ (2007) Highly neurotic never-depressed students have negative biases in information processing. Psychol Med 37:1281–1291

Christensen R, Kristensen PK, Bartels EM, Bliddal H, Astrup A (2007) Efficacy and safety of the weight-loss drug rimonabant: a meta-analysis of randomised trials. Lancet. 370 (9600):1706–1713

Clark L, Chamberlain SR, Sahakian BJ (2009) Neurocognitive mechanisms in depression: implications for treatment. Ann Rev Neurosci 32:57–74

Cryan JF, Holmes A (2005) The ascent of mouse: advances in modelling human depression and anxiety. Nat Rev Drug Discov 4:775–790
Cryan JF, Mombereau C, Vassout A (2005a) The tail suspension test as a model for assessing antidepressant activity: review of pharmacological and genetic studies in mice. Neurosci Biobehav Rev 29:571–625
Cryan JF, Slattery DA (2007) Animal models of mood disorders: Recent developments. Curr Opin Psychiatry 20:1–7
Cryan JF, Valentino RJ, Lucki I (2005b) Assessing substrates underlying the behavioral effects of antidepressants using the modified ratforced swimming test. Neurosci Biobehav Rev 29 (4–5):547–569
Dalley JW, Mar AC, Economidou D, Robbins TW (2008) Neurobehavioral mechanisms of impulsivity: fronto-striatal systems and functional neurochemistry. Pharmacol Biochem Behav 90(2):250–260
Dearing K, Gotlib I (2009) Interpretation of ambiguous information in girls at risk for depression. J Abnorm Child Psychol 37:79–91
Deroche-Gamonet V, Le Moal M, Piazza PV, Soubrié P (2001) SR141716, a CB1 receptor antagonist, decreases the sensitivity to the reinforcing effects of electrical brain stimulation in rats. Psychopharmacology (Berl). 157(3):254–259
Detke MJ, Rickels M, Lucki I (1995) Active behaviors in the rat forced swimming test differentially produced by serotonergic and noradrenergic antidepressants. Psychopharmacology 121:66–72
DiazGranados N, Ibrahim LA, Brutsche NE, Ameli R, Henter ID, Luckenbaugh DA, Machado-Vieira R, Zarate CA Jr (2010) Rapid resolution of suicidal ideation after a single infusion of an N-methyl-D-aspartate antagonist in patients with treatment-resistant major depressive disorder. J Clin Psychiatry 71(12):1605–1611
DSM-V. American Psychiatric Association (2013) Diagnostic and statistical manual of mental disorders, 5th edn. American Psychiatric Publishing, Arlington
Eagle DM, Baunez C (2010) Is there an inhibitory-response-control system in the rat? Evidence from anatomical and pharmacological studies of behavioral inhibition. Neurosci Biobehav Rev 34(1):50–72
Elliott R, Zahn R, Deakin JF, Anderson IM (2011) Affective cognition and its disruption in mood disorders. Neuropsychopharmacology 36:153–182
Enkel T, Gholizadeh D, von Bohlen Und Halbach O, Sanchis-Segura C, Hurlemann R, Spanagel R et al (2010) Ambiguous-cue interpretation is biased under stress- and depression-like states in rats. Neuropsychopharmacology 35:1008–1015
Evenden JL (1999) Varieties of impulsivity. Psychopharmacology (Berl) 146:348–361
FDA draft guidance, Prospective assessment of occurrence in clinical trials, Revision 1, August 2012 http://www.fda.gov/downloads/Drugs/Guidances/UCM225130.pdf
Ferguson SA, Cisneros FJ, Gough B, Hanig JP, Berry KJ (2005) Chronic oral treatment with 13-cis-retinoic acid (isotretinoin) or all-trans-retinoic acid does not alter depression-like behaviors in rats. Toxicol Sci 87:451–459
Fernando AB, Robbins TW (2011) Animal models of neuropsychiatric disorders. Annu Rev Clin Psychol 7:39–61
Flaisher-Grinberg S, Einat H (2007) Strain-specific battery of tests for domains of mania: effects of valproate, lithium and imipramine. Front Psychiatry 1:10
Gamble-George JC, Conger JR, Hartley ND, Gupta P, Sumislawski JJ, Patel S (2013) Dissociable effects of CB1 receptor blockade on anxiety-like and consummatory behaviors in the novelty-induced hypophagia test in mice. Psychopharmacology (Berl) 228:401–409
Garcia LS, Comim CM, Valvassori SS, Réus GZ, Stertz L, Kapczinski F, Gavioli EC, Quevedo J (2009) Ketamine treatment reverses behavioral and physiological alterations induced by chronic mild stress in rats. Prog Neuropsychopharmacol Biol Psychiatry 33(3):450–455
Gartlehner G, Hansen RA, Morgan LC, Thaler K, Lux L, Van Noord M, Mager U, Thieda P, Gaynes BN, Wilkins T, Strobelberger M, Lloyd S, Reichenpfader U, Lohr KN (2011)

Comparative benefits and harms of second-generation antidepressants for treating major depressive disorder: an updated meta-analysis. Ann Intern Med 155(11):772–785
Geyer M, Markou A (1995) Animal Models of psychiatric disorders. In: Bloom F, Kupfer D (eds) Psychopharmacology: the fourth generation of progress. Raven Press, New York, pp 787–798
Gotlib IH, Joormann J (2010) Cognition and depression: current status and future directions. Annu Rev Clin Psychol 6:285–312
Griebel G, Stemmelin J, Scatton B (2005) Effects of the cannabinoid CB1 receptor antagonist rimonabant in models of emotional reactivity in rodents. Biol Psychiatry 57:261–267
Halcomb ME, Gould TD, Grahame NJ (2013) Lithium, but not valproate, reduces impulsive choice in the delay-discounting task in mice. Neuropsychopharmacology 38:1937–1944
Hales CA, Stuart SA, Anderson MH, Robinson ESJ (2014) Modelling cognitive affective biases in major depressive disorder using rodents. Br J Pharmacol. doi: 10.1111/bph.12603
Harding EJ, Paul ES, Mendl M (2004) Animal behaviour: cognitive bias and affective state. Nature 427:312
Harmer CJ, Hill SA, Taylor MJ, Cowen PJ, Goodwin GM (2003) Toward a neuropsychological theory of antidepressant drug action: increase in positive emotional bias after potentiation of norepinephrine activity. Am J Psychiatry 160(5):990–992
Harmer CJ, Goodwin GM, Cowen PJ (2009a) Why do antidepressants take so long to work? A cognitive neuropsychological model of antidepressant drug action. Br J Psychiatry 195:102–108
Harmer CJ, O'Sullivan U, Favaron E, Massey-Chase R, Ayres R, Reinecke A et al (2009b) Effect of acute antidepressant administration on negative affective bias in depressed patients. Am J Psychiatry 166:1178–1184
Harmer CJ (2013) Emotional processing and antidepressant action. Curr Top Behav Neurosci 14:209–222
Hayward G, Goodwin GM, Cowen PJ, Harmer CJ (2005) Low-dose tryptophan depletion in recovered depressed patients induces changes in cognitive processing without depressive symptoms. Biol Psychiatry 57:517–524
Hendrie C, Pickles A, Stanford SC, Robinson E (2013) The failure of the antidepressant drug discovery process is systemic. J Psychopharmacol 27:407–416
Horder J, Browning M, Di Simplicio M, Cowen PJ, Harmer CJ (2012) Effects of 7 days of treatment with the cannabinoid type 1 receptor antagonist, rimonabant, on emotional processing. J Psychopharmacol 26(1):125–132
Horder J, Cowen PJ, Di Simplicio M, Browning M, Harmer CJ (2009) Acute administration of the cannabinoid CB1 antagonist rimonabant impairs positive affective memory in healthy volunteers. Psychopharmacology (Berl) 205(1):85–91
Humpston CS, Wood CM, Robinson ES (2013) Investigating the roles of different monoamine transmitters and impulse control using the 5-choice serial reaction time task. J Psychopharmacol 27(2):213–221
Igari M, Alexander JC, Ji Y, Qi X, Papke RL, Bruijnzeel AW (2014) Varenicline and cytisine diminish the dysphoric-like state associated with spontaneous nicotine withdrawal in rats. Neuropsychopharmacology 39(2):455–465
Joormann J, Talbot L, Gotlib IH (2007) Biased processing of emotional information in girls at risk for depression. J Abnorm Psychol 116:135–143
Kelly JP, Wrynn AS, Leonard BE (1997) The olfactory bulbectomized rat as a model of depression: an update. Pharmacol Ther 74:299–316
Kentner AC, James JS, Miguelez M, Bielajew C (2007) Investigating the hedonic effects of interferon-alpha on female rats using brain-stimulation reward. Behav Brain Res 177:90–99
Kudryavtseva NN, Bakshtanovskaya IV, Koryakina LA (1991) Social model of depression in mice of C57BL/6J strain. Pharmacol Biochem Behav 38:315–320
Leonard BE (1984) The olfactory bulbectomized rat as a model of depression. Pol J Pharmacol Pharm 36:561–569
Liebman JM (1983) Discriminating between reward and performance: a critical review of intracranial self-stimulation methodology. Neurosci Biobehav Rev 17(1):45–72

Magin P, Pond D, Smith W (2005) Isotretinoin, depression and suicide: a review of the evidence. Br J Gen Pract 55(511):134–138
Maier SF, Seligman MEP (1976) Learned helplessness: theory and evidence. J Exp Psychol Gen 105:3–46
Makino M, Kitano Y, Komiyama C, Hirohashi M, Takasuna K (2000) Involvement of central opioid systems in human interferon-alpha induced immobility in the mouse forced swimming test. Br J Pharmacol 130:1269–1274
Malkesman O, Pine DS, Tragon T, Austin DR, Henter ID, Chen G, Manji HK (2009) Animal models of suicide-trait-related behaviors. Trends Pharmacol Sci 30(4):165–173
Marqueling AL, Zane LT (2007) Depression and suicidal behavior in acne patients treated with isotretinoin: a systematic review. Semin Cutan Med Surg. 26(4):210–220
Martin P, Soubrie P, Puech AJ (1990) Reversal of helpless behavior by serotonin uptake blockers in rats. Psychopharmacology (Berl) 101:403–407
Mathews A, MacLeod C (2005) Cognitive vulnerability to emotional disorders. Annu Rev Clin Psychol 1:167–195
Mathews A, Ridgeway V, Williamson DA (1996) Evidence for attention to threatening stimuli in depression. Behav Res Ther 34:695–705
McArthur and Borsini (2006) Animal models of depression in drug discovery: a historical perspective. Pharmacol Biochem Behav 84(3):436–452
McKinney WT (2001) Overview of the past contributions in animal models and their changing place in psychiatry. Semin Clin Psychiatry 6:68–78
Miczek KA, Maxson SC, Fish EW, Faccidomo S (2001) Aggressive behavioral phenotypes in mice. Behav Brain Res 125:167–181
Mitchell PJ (2005) Antidepressant treatment and rodent aggressive behaviour. Eur J Pharmacol 526:147–162
Mocking RJ, Patrick Pflanz C, Pringle A, Parsons E, McTavish SF, Cowen PJ, Harmer CJ (2013) Effects of short-term varenicline administration on emotional and cognitive processing in healthy, non-smoking adults: a randomized, double-blind, study. Neuropsychopharmacology 38(3):476–484
Moreau JL, Jenck F, Martin JR, Mortas P, Haefely WE (1992) Antidepressant treatment prevents chronic unpredictable mild stress-induced anhedonia as assessed by ventral tegmentum self-stimulation behavior in rats. Eur Neuropsychopharmacol 2:43–49
Mula M, Kanner AM, Schmitz B, Schachter S (2013) Antiepileptic drugs and suicidality: an expert consensus statement from the Task Force on Therapeutic Strategies of the ILAE Commission on Neuropsychobiology. Epilepsia 54(1):199–203
Nathan PJ, O'Neill BV, Napolitano A, Bullmore ET (2011) Neuropsychiatric adverse effects of centrally acting antiobesity drugs. CNS Neurosci Ther 17(5):490–505
Nestler EJ, Gould E, Manji H, Buncan M, Duman RS, Greshenfeld HK et al (2002) Preclinical models: status of basic research in depression. Biol Psychiatry 52:503–528
Nestler EJ, Hyman SE (2010) Animal models of neuropsychiatric disorders. Nat Neurosci 13:1161–1169
O'Reilly KC, Shumake J, Gonzalez-Lima F, Lane MA, Bailey SJ (2006) Chronic administration of 13-cis-retinoic acid increases depression-related behavior in mice. Neuropsychopharmacology 31:1919–1927
Ohmura Y, Tsutsui-Kimura I, Kumamoto H, Minami M, Izumi T, Yamaguchi T, Yoshida T, Yoshioka M (2011) Lithium, but not valproic acid or carbamazepine, suppresses impulsive-like action in rats. Psychopharmacology (Berl) 219:421–432
Osman A, Bagge CL, Gutierrez PM, Konick LC, Kopper BA, Barrios FX (2001) The Suicidal Behaviors Questionnaire-Revised (SBQ-R): validation with clinical and nonclinical samples. Assessment 8(4):443–454
Papciak J, Popik P, Fuchs E, Rygula R (2013) Chronic psychosocial stress makes rats more 'pessimistic' in the ambiguous-cue interpretation paradigm. Behav Brain Res 256:305–310
Paul ES, Harding EJ, Mendl M (2005) Measuring emotional processes in animals: the utility of a cognitive approach. Neurosci Biobehav Rev 29:469–491

Pellis SM, McKenna MM (1992) Intrinsic and extrinsic influences on play fighting in rats: effects of dominance, partner's playfulness, temperament and neonatal exposure to testosterone propionate. Behav Brain Res 50:135–145

Phillips AG, Broekkamp CL, Fibiger HC (1983) Strategies for studying the neurochemical substrates of drug reinforcement in rodents. Prog Neuropsychopharmacol Biol Psychiatry 7 (4–6):585–590

Platt JE, Stone EA (1982) Chronic restraint stress elicits a positive antidepressant response on the forced swim test. Eur J Pharmacol 82:179–181

Pollak DD, Rey CE, Monje FJ (2010) Rodent models in depression research: classical strategies and new directions. Ann Med 42:252–264

Porsolt RD, Le Pichon M, Jalfre M (1977) Depression: a new animal model sensitive to antidepressant treatments. Nature 266:730–732

Posner K, Brown GK, Stanley B et al (2011) The Columbia-Suicide Severity Rating Scale (C-SSRS): internal validity and internal consistency findings from three multi-site studies with adolescents and adults. Am J Psychiatry 168:1266–1277

Posner K, Oquendo MA, Gould M, Stanley B, Davies M (2007) Columbia Classification Algorithm of Suicide Assessment (C-CASA): classification of suicidal events in the FDA's pediatric suicidal risk analysis of antidepressants. Am J Psychiatry 164:1035–1043

Preti A (2011) Animal model and neurobiology of suicide. Prog Neuropsychopharmacol Biol Psychiatry 35(4):818–830

Pringle A, Browning M, Cowen PJ, Harmer CJ (2011) A cognitive neuropsychological model of antidepressant drug action. Prog Neuropsychopharmacol Biol Psychiatry 35:1586–1592

Pumariega, A, U Millsaps, K Posner et al (2011) C-SSRS: Evidence-based method for hospital-based suicide screening. Presented at Eastern nursing research society 23rd annual scientific sessions, Philadelphia, PA

Rademacher DJ, Hillard CJ (2007) Interactions between endocannabinoids and stress-induced decreased sensitivity to natural reward. Prog Neuropsychopharmacol Biol Psychiatry 31 (3):633–641

Reith DM, Edmonds L (2007) Assessing the role of drugs in suicidal ideation and suicidality. CNS Drugs 21(6):463–472

Robbins TW (2002) The 5-choice serial reaction time task: behavioural pharmacology and functional neurochemistry. Psychopharmacology (Berl) 163(3–4):362–380

Robinson OJ, Sahakian BJ (2008) Recurrence in major depressive disorder: a neurocognitive perspective. Psychol Med 38:315–318

Roiser JP, Elliott R, Sahakian BJ (2012) Cognitive mechanisms of treatment in depression. Neuropsychopharmacology 37:117–136

Roiser JP, Sahakian BJ (2013) Hot and cold cognition in depression. CNS Spectr 18:139–149

Rollema H, Guanowsky V, Mineur YS, Shrikhande A, Coe JW et al (2009) Varenicline has antidepressant-like activity in the forced swim test and augments sertraline's effect. Eur J Pharmacol 605:114–116

Rygula R, Abumaria N, Flugge G, Fuchs E, Ruther E, Havemann-Reinecke U (2005) Anhedonia and motivational deficits in rats: impact of chronic social stress. Behav Brain Res 162:127–134

Rygula R, Papciak J, Popik P (2013) Trait pessimism predicts vulnerability to stress-induced anhedonia in rats. Neuropsychopharmacology 38:2188–2196

Rygula R, Pluta H, Popik P (2012) Laughing rats are optimistic. PLoS One 7:e51959

Sammut S, Bethus I, Goodall G, Muscat R (2002) Antidepressant reversal of interferon-alpha-induced anhedonia. Physiol Behav 75:765–772

Sammut S, Goodall G, Muscat R (2001) Acute interferon-alpha administration modulates sucrose consumption in the rat. Psychoneuroendocrinology 26:261–272

Schaefer GJ, Michael RP (1983) Morphine withdrawal produces differential effects on the rate of lever-pressing for brain self-stimulation in the hypothalamus and midbrain in rats. Pharmacol Biochem Behav 18(4):571–577

Schmidt MV, Wang XD, Meijer OC (2011) Early life stress paradigms in rodents: potential animal models of depression? Psychopharmacology (Berl) 214:131–140

Semba J, Kuroda Y, Takahashi R (1989) Potential antidepressant properties of subchronic GABA transaminase inhibitors in the forced swimming test in mice. Neuropsychobiology 21:152–156
Sherman AD, Petty F (1982) Additivity of neurochemical changes in learned helplessness and imipramine. Behav Neural Biol 35:344–353
Slattery DA, Cryan JF (2012) Using the rat forced swim test to assess antidepressant-like activity in rodents. Nat Protoc 7:1009–1014
Sockalingam S, Links PS, Abbey SE (2011) Suicide risk in hepatitis C and during interferon-alpha therapy: a review and clinical update. J Viral Hepat 18(3):153–160
Steru L, Chermat R, Thierry B, Simo P (1985) The tail suspension test: a new method for screening antidepressants in mice. Psychopharmacology (Berl) 85:367–370
Stone M, Laughren T, Jones ML, Levenson M, Holland PC, Hughes A, Hammad TA, Temple R, Rochester G (2009) Risk of suicidality in clinical trials of antidepressants in adults: analysis of proprietary data submitted to US Food and Drug Administration. BMJ 339:b2880
Stuart SA, Butler P, Munafò MR, Nutt DJ, Robinson ESJ (2013) A translational rodent assay of affective biases in depression and antidepressant therapy. Neuropsychopharmacology 38:1625–1635
Takamori K, Yoshida S, Okuyama S (2001) Repeated treatment with imipramine, fluvoxamine and tranylcypromine decreases the number of escape failures by activating dopaminergic systems in a rat learned helplessness test. Life Sci 69:1919–1926
Tomasiewicz HC, Mague SD, Cohen BM, Carlezon WA Jr (2006) Behavioral effects of short-term administration of lithium and valproic acid in rats. Brain Res 1093:83–94
Topol EJ, Bousser MG, Fox KA, Creager MA, Despres JP, Easton JD et al (2010) Rimonabant for prevention of cardiovascular events (CRESCENDO): a randomised, multicentre, placebo-controlled trial. Lancet 376:517–523
Trent S, Drew CJ, Mitchell PJ, Bailey SJ (2009) Chronic treatment with 13-cis-retinoic acid changes aggressive behaviours in the resident-intruder paradigm in rats. Eur Neuropsychopharmacol 19:876–886
Turner JR, Castellano LM, Blendy JA (2010) Nicotinic partial agonists varenicline and sazetidine-A have differential effects on affective behavior. J Pharmacol Exp Ther 334:665–672
Vogel GW, Minter K, Woolwine B (1986) Effects of chronically administered antidepressant drugs on animal behavior. Physiol Behav 36:659–666
Willner P, Muscat R, Papp M (1992) Chronic mild stress-induced anhedonia: a realistic animal model of depression. Neurosci Biobehav Rev 16:525–534
Willner P, Towell A, Sampson D, Sophokleous S, Muscat R (1987) Reduction of sucrose preference by chronic unpredictable mild stress, and its restoration by a tricyclic antidepressant. Psychopharmacology (Berl) 93:358–364
Willner P (1984) The validity of animal models of depression. Psychopharmacology (Berl) 83:1–16
Willner P (1997) Validity, reliability and utility of the chronic mild stress model of depression: a 10-year review and evaluation. Psychopharmacology (Berl) 134:319–329
Willner P (2005) Chronic mild stress (CMS) revisited: consistency and behavioural-neurobiological concordance in the effects of CMS. Neuropsychobiology 52:90–110
Winstanley CA, Eagle DM, Robbins TW (2006) Behavioral models of impulsivity in relation to ADHD: translation between clinical and preclinical studies. Clin Psychol Rev 26:379–395
Wiskerke J, Stoop N, Schetters D, Schoffelmeer AN, Pattij T (2011) Cannabinoid CB1 receptor activation mediates the opposing effects of amphetamine on impulsive action and impulsive choice. PLoS One 6:e25856
Wright WF, Bower GH (1992) Mood effects on subjective probability assessment. Organ Behav Hum Decis Process 52:276–291
Zacharko RM, Anisman H (1991) Stressor-induced anhedonia in the mesocorticolimbic system. Neurosci Biobehav Rev 15:391–405

MIX
Papier aus verantwortungsvollen Quellen
Paper from responsible sources
FSC® C105338

If you have any concerns about our products,
you can contact us on
ProductSafety@springernature.com

In case Publisher is established outside the EU,
the EU authorized representative is:
Springer Nature Customer Service Center GmbH
Europaplatz 3, 69115 Heidelberg, Germany

Printed by Libri Plureos GmbH
in Hamburg, Germany